Nanotechnology Based Advanced Medical Textiles and Biotextiles for Healthcare

This book provides systematic coverage of research into medical and biotextiles based on nanomaterials as applicable in healthcare. Divided into three sections, it explains manufacturing, properties, types, and recent developments in nanotechnology based medical textiles backed by case studies. It includes a wide range of different clinical applications of biotextiles for healthcare including nanotextile scaffolds, nano-based artificial organs, surgical sutures, enzymatic assisted enhanced biotextiles, tissue engineering or drug delivery system via nanofibers, and so forth.

Features:

- Provides strong and broad overview of medical applications in the field of nano and biotextiles.
- Highlights different approaches, recent research, and emerging innovations.
- Covers designing or developing nanomaterials based antiviral surface disinfectants with self-cleaning property.
- Reviews different applications of nano based medical textiles such as deodorizing or pH control clothing for hygiene maintenance.
- Includes the real-life applications based descriptive case studies that offer a diverse range of perspectives.

This book is aimed at researchers and graduate students in textile technology and engineering, and medical textiles.

Nanotechnology Based Advanced Medical Textiles and Biotextiles for Healthcare

Edited by Prashansa Sharma,
Devsuni Singh, Suman Pant, and Vivek Dave

CRC Press
Taylor & Francis Group
Boca Raton London New York

CRC Press is an imprint of the
Taylor & Francis Group, an **informa** business

First edition published 2024
by CRC Press
2385 NW Executive Center Drive, Suite 320, Boca Raton FL 33431

and by CRC Press
4 Park Square, Milton Park, Abingdon, Oxon, OX14 4RN

CRC Press is an imprint of Taylor & Francis Group, LLC

© 2024 selection and editorial matter, Prashansa Sharma, Devsuni Singh, Suman Pant and Vivek Dave; individual chapters, the contributors

ISBN: 978-1-032-36375-2 (hbk)
ISBN: 978-1-032-36376-9 (pbk)
ISBN: 978-1-003-33161-2 (ebk)

DOI: 10.1201/9781003331612

Typeset in Times
by Apex CoVantage, LLC

Contents

PART 1   *Production Techniques*

Chapter 1   Description of the Processing Techniques Used in Biotextiles
for Medical Application 3

*Devsuni Singh, Prashansa Sharma, Suman Pant,
and Vivek Dave*

Vibeizonuo Rupreo and Jhimli Bhattacharyya

Pallerla Naveen Reddy, Vivek Dave, and Prashansa Sharma

PART 2   Applications of Medical Textiles for Non-Implants

Shovan Ghosh, Vivek Dave,
Prashansa Sharma, and Pranay Wal

PART 3   Applications of Biotextiles for Medical Implants

Preface

The association of the medicinal and textile fields is gaining enormous attention across the globe because of its ability to uplift human wellness. Over the last decade, the utilization of technical textiles in medical applications has emerged as a growing field within the textile industry. It has witnessed a substantial surge in research interest and has evolved into one of the rapidly expanding sectors in the worldwide technical textiles market. Its development has been greatly aided by the establishment of nanotechnology in the field of technical medical textiles and is taking an interesting and promising direction. This book explores the potential of nanotechnology-based medical textile enhancement by incorporating nanoparticles into fiber-forming polymers, producing electrospun nanofibers, and creating nano-enhanced antimicrobial textiles that work as barrier garments for healthcare workers, sutures, and implantable materials.

This book aims to offer an overview of how nanotechnology enhanced the medical textile sectors by representing various emerging non-implantable and implantable applications as well as novel innovative techniques related to producing and sterilizing nano-medical biotextiles that allow researchers and scientists to design or develop new advanced nanomaterials for healthcare purposes. Their comprehensive and in-depth coverage in this book makes it an indispensable resource for every reader.

The book *Nanotechnology Based Advanced Medical Textiles and Biotextiles for Healthcare* comprises three parts, and these parts are further divided into several chapters. The initial part of the book begins with manufacturing and bioprocessing techniques used for developing medical textiles. It also addresses the huge potential of nanotechnology to enhance various production or surface modification techniques for biotextiles. The second part highlights the various applications of medical textiles for non-implant materials. It extensively explores how textile materials and products can be utilized for infection control and protective materials. Advanced compression bandages, stockings, and wound care biomaterials with nanotechnology are critically discussed. Along with this, it also emphasizes the unique nanotechnology approaches for producing odor-control materials and nano-enhanced superabsorbent feminine hygiene napkins. The last part of the book covers five chapters that focus on the various approaches of medical textiles used for creating implantable materials including drug-loaded textile materials, vascular grafts, nanofibrous textile scaffolds for tissue engineering, surgical sutures, etc. It also deals with the advances in enzyme biotechnology applied as pre-treatment for medical textiles.

- The structure and content of this book were designed to ensure its utility for readers at various levels of expertise.
- The book is designed as both reference material and textbook material; its simple, comprehensive explanation and its unique features become a valuable reference for readers.

- Most of the key study areas have been addressed in each chapter, making the book very helpful for business professionals who deal with the real-world applications of technology in the field.
- The authors represent the variety of medical textiles in this book by hailing from different universities, institutions, and research organizations, and are leading experts in their field, which provides a diverse nature of knowledge to all readers.

This book has been edited to be as consistent and coherent as feasible. We would like to express our gratitude to all the authors and co-authors for their hard work in creating their outstanding manuscripts and for sharing with us their talent that accurately reflects the state of the art in each of their respective fields. We also would like to convey our appreciation to the publisher, Taylor & Francis, for granting us the opportunity to evolve this book. Last but not least, I'd like to share my sincere hope that every reader will find the book to be an engaging and informative read.

—**Prashansa Sharma**
Devsuni Singh
Suman Pant
Vivek Dave

About the Editors

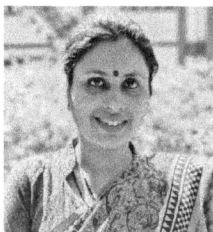

Prashansa Sharma is result-oriented, high energy, hands-on, and proficient with a successful record of achievements. Currently, she is Assistant Professor at the Department of Home Science, Mahila Maha Vidyalaya, Banaras Hindu University, Varanasi. She has completed her M.Sc and Ph. D from Banasthali Vidyapith Rajasthan India and received Gold Medal Award from Banasthali Vidyapith during her Post Graduation. She has almost 12 years of teaching experience in Banasthali Vidyapith Rajasthan along with research experience. She has drafted many research and review papers related to nanotechnology and nanotextile science in journals of national/international repute. She has been the recipient of several awards in various conferences, seminars, and conventions. Dr. Sharma is also acting as a regular reviewer of journals of national and international repute of different publishing houses. Her knowledge in this regard has promised to deliver the young and innovative minds a detailed informative description about novel and absolutely modern nanotechnology using Green synthesis and textile models.

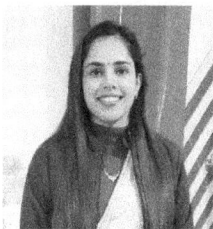

Devsuni Singh is in the Department of Clothing and Textile, Faculty of Home Science at Banasthali Vidhyapith, Rajasthan, India. She received her master's degree in clothing and textile with high grades from Banasthali Vidhyapith, Rajasthan, India. She has guided many M.Sc project students and actively engaged in research work. She served as an editor and author in edited books on nanotechnology and technical textiles. She is focused on her research work and is passionate about gaining deep knowledge of nanotextile science. Her research interests include the development of novel functionality nanotextiles, textile technology, nanotextile science, environmentally friendly 'green nanocomposites', healthcare textiles, textile designing, textile testing, and sustainable textiles. Her informative knowledge regarding nanotextiles and nanoparticles using green herbal synthesis in the textile material, helps to promote the emerging fields of nanotechnology and nanotextile science.

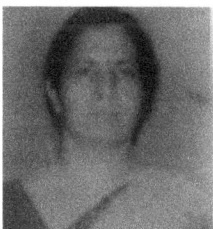

Suman Pant completed her M.Sc with specialization in clothing and textile from G. B. Pant University of Agricultural and Technology, Pantnagar, and Ph. D from Banasthali Vidhyapith, Rajasthan. Currently, she is working as Dean and Professor in clothing and textile at the Faculty of Home Science, Banasthali Vidhyapith. She has 34 years of diversified experience in teaching undergraduate and postgraduate students along with research experience. Dr. Suman has guided more than 100 PG students and research scholars on a wide range of topics related to clothing and textiles which include eco-friendly dyeing, printing, and finishing of textile; the blending of natural and manmade fibres, consumer studies, innovative techniques for designing and construction of garments for value, rejuvenation of traditional textiles, documentation of costumes and textiles, etc. She is also a member of the academic body of several universities and a life member of several professional organizations. She has presented many papers at several national and international conferences. She has around 150 papers on her credits in national and international journals of repute. She is also the author of a book.

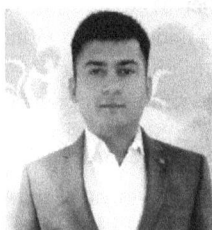

Vivek Dave, presently working in the capacity of Dean, School of Health Science and Head Department of Pharmacy at Central University South Bihar, Gaya, Bihar, has commendable experience skills coupled with sound theoretical background. His expertise on working with formulation and development of novel drug delivery systems like PEGylated liposome, ethosomes, nanoparticle, quantum dots, and nanotechnology has shaped this book into a modish platform that has promised to promote anticipated trends in the aspect of nanotechnology and nanotextile science. He has been working in the field of novel drug delivery system and nanotechnology and has already published several articles in journals of national/international repute. He has also recorded his expertise in the form of many chapters and books. He has been the recipient of several awards in various conference, seminars, and conventions. Dr. Dave is also acting as regular reviewer of journals of national and international repute of different publishing houses.

Contributors

Amisha Singh
Department of Home Science
Mahila Mahavidyalaya, Banaras Hindu
    University
Varanasi, India

Arijit Das
Department of Chemical Engineering
Visvesvaraya National Institute of
    Technology Nagpur
Maharashtra, India

Bharat H. Patel
Department of Textile Chemistry
Maharaja Sayajirao University of Baroda
Gujarat, India

Devsuni Singh
Department of Clothing and Textile
Banasthali Vidyapith, Banasthali
Rajasthan, India

Jhimli Bhattacharyya
National Institute of Technology, Nagaland
Nagaland, India

Khushboo Choudhary
Department of Pharmacology and
    Toxicology
National Institute of Pharmaceutical
    Education and Research
Hajipur, India

Kruthi Doriya
Institute of Chemical Technology
IOC Bhubaneswar, India
Hajipur, India

K S Rajmohan
Department of Chemical Engineering
National Institute of Technology
Warangal, India

Nitesh Kumar
Department of Pharmacology and
    Toxicology
National Institute of Pharmaceutical
    Education and Research
Hajipur, India

Om Prakash Ranjan
Department of Pharmaceutical
    Technology
National Institute of Pharmaceutical
    Education and Research
    (NIPER)
Guwahati, India

Pallerla Naveen Reddy
School of Health Sciences
Central University of South Bihar
Gaya, India

Pranay Wal
Department of Pharmacy
Pranveer Singh Institute of
    Technology
Kanpur, India

Prashansa Sharma
Department of Home Science
Mahila Mahavidyalaya,
    Banaras Hindu University
Varanasi, India

Radha Sachchidanand Wattamwar
Institute of Chemical Technology
    Mumbai
ICT-IOC, Bhubaneswar
Bhubaneswar, India

Rakesh Kumar
Department of Biotechnology
Central University of South Bihar
Gaya, India

Rashmi Bhushan
Department of Pharmacology and
  Toxicology
National Institute of Pharmaceutical
  Education and Research
Hajipur, India

Ruchi Pandey Sachindra Kumar
Department of Pharmacology and
  Toxicology
National Institute of Pharmaceutical
  Education and Research
Hajipur, India

Shilpi Shree Sahay
Department of Home Science
Mahila Mahavidyalaya, Banaras Hindu
  University
Varanasi, India

Shovan Ghosh
School of Health Sciences
Central University of South Bihar
Gaya, India

Srijita Sen
Department of Pharmaceutical
  Technology
National Institute of Pharmaceutical
  Education and Research (NIPER)
Guwahati, India

Suman Pant
Department of Clothing & Textile
Banasthali Vidyapith, Banasthali
Rajasthan, India

Sujot Sunil Borse
Institute of Chemical Technology
  Mumbai
ICT-IOC, Bhubaneswar
Bhubaneswar, India

Tasnim N. Shaikh
Department of Textile Engineering
The Maharaja Sayajirao University of
  Baroda
Vadodara, Gujarat

Vaibhav Verma
School of Health Sciences
Central University of South Bihar
Gaya, India

Vibeizonuo Rupreo
National Institute of Technology,
  Nagaland
Nagaland, India

Vivek Dave
School of Health Sciences
Central University of South Bihar
Gaya, India

Abbreviations

ACL	Anterior cruciate ligament
AFM	Atomic force microscopy
AgNPs	Silver nanoparticles
API	Active pharmaceutical ingredient
AUL	Absorbency under load
AuNPs	Gold nanoparticles
BC	Bacterial cellulose
BFE	Bacterial filtration efficiency
bFGF	Basic fibroblast growth factor
BHV	Bioprosthetic heart valves
BMCs	Bone Marrow Cells
BSA	Bovine serum albumin
BSA	Bovine serum albumin
CA	Cellulose acetate
CD	Circular dichroism
ClO$_2$	Chlorine dioxide
CLSD	CO$_2$ laser supersonic drawing
CMC	Carboxymethylcellulose
CNT	Carbon nanotubes
CTA	Cellulose triacetate
CTC	Circulating tumor cells
CVDs	Cardiovascular diseases
DDS	Drug delivery systems
DLS	Dynamic light scattering
DMAPS	3-dimethyl (methacryloyloxyethyl) ammonium propane sulphonate
ECG	Electrocardiogram
ECH	Epichlorohydrin
ECM	Extracellular matrix
ECMO	Extracorporeal Membrane Oxygenation
ECS	Extracellular space
EDTA	Ethylenediamine tetraacetic acid
EEG	Electroencephalogram
EP	European Pharmacopeia
ePTFE	Expanded polytetrafluoroethylene
ETFE	Ethylene-tetra fluoroethylene
EtO	Ethylene oxide
FCS	Fluorescence correlation spectroscopy
FDA	Food and Drug Administration
FGF	Fibroblast growth factor
GelMA	Gelatin methacrylate
GNPs	Gelatin-loaded nanoparticles

HDPE	High-density polyethylene
HEC	Hydroxyethyl cellulose
HEPA	High efficiency particulate matter
IPD	In-Patient Department
IR	Infrared spectroscopy
MHV	Mechanical heart valves
MS	Mass spectroscopy
NBR	Nitrile-butadiene rubber
NGC	Nerve Guidance Conduits
NICE	National Institute for Health and Care Excellence
OPD	Out Patient Department
OT	Operation Theatre
PAA	Polyacrylic acid
PANI	Polyaniline
PBS	Polybutylene succinate
PBT	Poly (butylene terephthalate)
PCL	Poly (ε-caprolactone)
PDGF	Platelet-derived growth factor
PDO	Poly (p-dioxanone)
PDS	polydioxanone
PEDOT	Poly (3, 4-ethylene dioxythiophene)
PEG	Polyethylene glycol
PEI	Poly (ether ketone)
PEN	Poly (ethylene napthalate)
PET	Poly (ethylene-terephthalate)
PETG	Polyethylene terephthalate copolymer
PGA	Polyglycolide acid
PLA	Polylactic acid
PLGA	Poly (lactide-co-glycolide)
PMP or TPX	Poly (methyl pentene)
PP	Polypropylene
PPCO	Poly (propylene co-polymer)
PPE	Personal protective equipment
PPO	Poly (phenyl oxides)
PPY	Polypyrrole
PS	Polystyrene
PTFE	Poly (tetrafluoroethylene)
PTT	Poy (trimethylene terepthalate)
PU	Polyurethanes
PVC	Polyvinyl chloride
PVD	Peripheral vascular illness
PVDF	Poly (vinylidene fluoride)
PVF	Polyvinylidene fluoride
RES	Reticuloendothelial system
RS	Raman scattering
SAL	Sterility assurance levels

SAPs	Superabsorbent polymers
SEM	Scanning electron microscopy
SHP	Sodium Hypophosphite
SMC	Smooth muscle cells
SPI	Soy protein isolate
TEHV	Tissue-engineering of heart valves
TEM	Transmission electron microscopy
TEVGs	Tissue-engineered vascular grafts
Tg	Glass transition temperature
TGF- β	Transforming growth factor
Tm	Melting temperature
TMMAAI	Trimethyl methacrylamidopropyl ammonium iodide
TSF	Tussah silk fibroin
UHMWPE	Ultra high molecular weight polyethylene
USP	United States Pharmacopeia
USPIO	Ultra-small superparamagnetic iron oxide nanoparticles
VEGF	Vascular endothelial growth factor
VEGF	Vascular endothelium growth factor
VFE	Viral filtration efficiency
ZnONPs	Zinc oxide nanoparticles
ZSM-5	Zeolite Socony Mobil-5

Part 1

Production Techniques

1 Description of the Processing Techniques Used in Biotextiles for Medical Application

*Devsuni Singh, Prashansa Sharma,
Suman Pant, and Vivek Dave*

1.1 INTRODUCTION

In recent times, biotextiles (or medical textiles) have gained lots of attention across the globe because of their capacity for treating and preventing infectious diseases in an individual. Biotextiles occupy around 9.5% of the market globally in 2022 and are expected to grow more until 2030 which justifies the popularity and efficacy of the products (Contrive Datum Insights Pvt Ltd, 2023). They could be developed from any synthetically or naturally derived fabrics that could be either biodegradable or non-biodegradable depending upon the need for research. Natural materials are obtained from plants, seeds, insects, and animals whereas synthetic materials are synthesized by altering the chemical or physical properties of natural materials. The fibres could be processed by some established methods such as electrospinning, melt spinning, wet spinning, and biocomponent or multicomponent spinning. The selection of a procedure to manufacture a fabric is decided on the basis of desired fibre needed that could be loaded with a drug and material of that fibre.

The usage of textiles is prevalent since ancient times. In Egypt, naturally derived fabrics such as cotton, silk, linen, and flax were used for ages to design bandages for wound healing. The selection of a fabric for loading a drug depends upon its close resemblance to the skin that slowly leaches out from the fabric and permeates the skin (Denton & Daniels, 2002). This could be fabricated to obtain a desired structure of the fibre which could deliver the sustained effect of a drug efficiently. For instance, knitted fabrics are porous in nature which serves better permeability of a drug along with the flexibility of the fabric. Contrarily, woven textiles are less porous compared to knits, but possess stable dimensions and result in a stronger fabric. The structure of nonwoven textiles could be altered by altering the dimensions of the fibre whereas braided fabrics possess high tensile strength resulting in instability of the fibre. Hence, the selection of a textile type is essential to obtain desired therapeutic efficacy of a drug (Qin, 2016).

DOI: 10.1201/9781003331612-2

The choice of manufacturing drug-eluting textiles is also an important step while designing a biotextile. There are a variety of approaches that could be employed to generate a drug-loaded fabric such as encapsulation, hollow fibres, nanoparticles, surface coating, and bioconjugation. Depending upon the rate of drug release, type of drug, and method of fibre development, a suitable method is elected to load the drug to the textile (Qin, 2016).

The chapter summarizes the role of biotextiles and the polymers required to prepare the fabric. The chapter also highlights different fibre manufacturing processes and various textile fabrication techniques along with a special emphasis on techniques to process drug-eluting textiles.

1.2 FIBRE-FORMING POLYMERS

1.2.1 Natural Polymers for Biotextile Construction

A number of natural polymeric composites have been widely used as films, fibres, and textiles for the production of medical products. Natural polymers are inexpensive, widely accessible, biodegradable, nontoxic, biocompatible, and readily available in many regions of the world. Natural polymers consist of cellulose materials; polysaccharides such as chitosan, chitin, alginate, or hyaluronic acid; and protein materials such as collagen, keratin, elastin, zein, and silk.

Cellulose is the most widely known carbohydrate polymer and is primarily derived from wood pulp, processed cotton, or bacterial sources. Cellulose and its derivatives are extensively utilized in the medical and biotextile applications, and they are classified into two categories: internal applications including dental applications, sutures, wound dressings, surgical applications, drug delivery, and tissue engineering, and external applications such as surgical covers (drapes, covers, etc.), beddings (blankets, pillow covers, sheets, and many more), absorbent pads, and surgical clothing (face masks, caps, robes, uniforms, etc.) (Khalaji & Lugoloobi, 2020). Due to its advantageous characteristics, such as appropriate gas permeability, high water absorption, and quick absorption of wound fluids including blood and plasma as well as other exudates in the wound area, cotton is remarkably employed as a wound dressing material as well as a most preferred option for drug delivery, due to its significant focus on slow or controlled drug administration system, high mechanical performance, large surface area, and ease of preparation.

Additionally, fibres derived from modified polysaccharides, such as reticulated cellulose and dextran from bacterial fermentation, chitosan from crustacean shells, alginates from algae, and hyaluronan from the extracellular matrix (ECM), are employed in medical and biotextile applications. Alginate is another natural biopolymer polysaccharide, which is extracted from brown seaweeds. They are made from two copolymers, α -L-guluronic acid and β -D-mannuronic acid, which provide strength and flexibility to alginates. Some of the alginates' appealing characteristics are biocompatibility, biodegradability, immunogenicity, antimicrobial properties, degradability, high porosity, and low toxicity. Alginate nanocomposites accelerate wound healing by generating a moist environment around the wound and eliminating wound exudate (Radoor et al., 2021). Alginate nanocomposites have a wide range of applications such as drug delivery excipients, nanocomposites for therapeutics delivery, surgical devices, and many more. Chitosan is a naturally occurring biopolymer polysaccharide generated from the deacetylation of chitin by the alkali of crustaceans and insects. Chitosan's molecular weight and degree of acetylation are its primary properties which determine its functional characteristics, including solubility, capacity to produce materials, biodegradability, and a variety of bioactive qualities. Chitosan possesses excellent properties like having bioadhesive, biodegradable, biocompatible, nontoxic, bacteriostatic, and fungicidal properties. These inherent properties increase the chitosan potential as an excellent choice for many medical and biotextile applications, in particular hemostatic wound care devices, antibacterial activity (Beulah et al., 2019), skin tissue engineering, surgical sutures, and scaffold material. Hyaluronic acid (also known as hyaluronan) is an anionic, linear polysaccharide that is composed of two consecutive disaccharide monomers $\beta(1{\rightarrow}4)$ D-glucuronic acid and $\beta(1{\rightarrow}3)$ N-acetyl-D-glucosamine. Hyaluronan is an ideal and secure biomaterial for a variety of medicinal applications because of its great biocompatibility, biodegradability, and lack of toxicity. HA is a new medical fibre and can be used in various applications of the medical and healthcare sector like nonwoven wound healing composites (Kubíčková et al., 2021), engineering of new tissue, postoperative adhesions, or hydration, antimicrobial dressings, and scaffolds materials, and osteochondral defects can be repaired with carbon nonwoven textiles (Rajzer et al., 2013).

1.2.2 Synthetic Polymers for Biotextile Construction

Synthetic polymers are derived from chemicals or petrochemicals based materials. They are split into two categories: thermoplastic polymers become soft when heated and can be melted temporarily, and thermoset polymers go through chemical reactions to produce insoluble materials. Synthetic polymers have drawn a lot of interest due to their high water resistance, good mechanical properties, biocompatibility, thermal stability, flexibility, good strength, controllable degradation rate, resistivity, easy manufacturing of scaffolds, and affordable nature. Some high degree of crystallinity polymers has greater influence in their mechanical qualities that can lead to advancement in medical textile applications including silk, poly(vinylidene fluoride) (PVDF), poly(tetrafluoroethylene) (PTFE), polyethylene, and polydioxanone. Permanent synthetic polymers, such as poly(ethylene-terephthalate) (PET), were initially developed for non-medical purposes, such as textile fibres for clothing. A variety of common nanofibrous polymers made of both natural and synthetic polymers are generated via the electrospinning process including polyglycolide (PGA), poly(ε-caprolactone) (PCL), poly(p-dioxanone) (PDO), and poly(lactide-co-glycolide) (PLGA).

Non-degradable polymers are frequently utilized in biomaterial as scaffolds for tissue engineering, fillings, vascular grafts, orthopedic implants, dentistry, heart valves, and bone cement (Subramaniam, 2014). Poly(ethylene terephthalate) (PET) is a non-biodegradable thermoplastic polyester, commercialized as

Dacron®, and has various medical applications such as vascular grafts, surgical sutures, anterior ligament prostheses, protective surgical, and arterial stent-grafts. Polytetrafluoroethylene (PTFE), also known as Teflon, is composed of a core of carbon atoms enclosed in a protective shell of fluorine atoms. However, the polymer is typically used in its expanded form, known as ePTFE, in medical textile applications such as surgical sutures, vascular grafts, heart valves, and AC ligaments. Poly(propylene) is a biostable polymer, trade name ACTISITE®. It has excellent stiffness and superior mechanical performance that can be used in orthopedic implants (Liu & Wang, 2007), surgical sutures, and ventral incisional hernia (San Pio et al., 2003).

A number of biodegradable aliphatic polyesters, such as polylactic acid (PLA), polydioxanone, polyglycolic acid (PGA), polyethylene glycol (PEG), polycaprolactone (PCL), and polyglactin, have been developed for use in medical biomaterials as biodegradable scaffold materials for tissue engineering, drug delivery, 3D scaffolds, or bone substitute material (Kundu et al., 2013). Table 1.1 shows the fibrous materials used for medical and healthcare applications.

TABLE 1.1
Fibrous materials used for medical and healthcare applications

Fibre	Morphology	Construction	Applications
Cotton	Hydrophilic; Crystallinity up to 65-70%; DP: 9,000-15,000; 99% cellulose	Spun by genus Gossypium seeds in the mallow family Malvaceae	Sutures, dressings, absorbent pads, and bandages
Viscose Rayon	1st regenerated cellulosic fibre, produced in 1892, also known as Artificial Silk, Hydrophilic; Crystallinity up to 35-40%; DP: 250-450	Wet spun from the wood pulp of alkali sodium hydroxide cellulose xanthate solution (NaOH) into continuous multifilaments	Wound dressing; disposable absorbent materials
Silk	Hydrophilic; Crystallinity 70%; natural bicomponent fibre made of two protein components: fibroin protein and sericin protein	Spun by Bombyx mori silkworm, coated with natural gum (sericin); sericin is removed in the finishing process	Sutures (Perma-Hand™; Sofsilk™)
Chitosan	Off-white powder; particle size: 80 μm; viscosity 150-200 mPa.s; degree of deacetylation: >90.0%	An amino polysaccharide, created by the deacetylation of chitin found in crustaceans and insects	Hemostat wound care products (Axiostat™; MaxioCel™)
Alginate	Hydrophilic; white to yellowish brown, edible polysaccharide; density: 1.601 g/cm³	Polysaccharides found in brown algae; consist of two repeating saccharides: L-glucuronic acid and D-mannuronic acid	Wound care devices (Algisite™; Repara®; Aiwryyi)

TABLE 1.1 (Continued)
Fibrous materials used for medical and healthcare applications

Fibre	Morphology	Construction	Applications
Nylon 6	Thermoplastic; Hydrophobic; Crystallinity 50% as spun; DP: 200; Tg = 45°C; Tm = 220°C; molecular weight: 20,000	Melt spun from monomer Caprolactam into monofilaments and multifilament yarns	Sutures (Nurolon™; Trulon™; Ethilon™), dressing (HydraFoam), tubular bandages
Nylon 6,6	Thermoplastic; Hydrophobic; Crystallinity 50% as spun; Tg = 60°C; Tm = 265°C; Molecular weight: 12,000-20,000; Ignition temp: 530°C	Melt spun from two monomers: Hexamethylenediamine and adipic acid into monofilaments and multifilament yarns	Sutures (Monosof™; Surglion™; Dermalon™)
Poly (tetrafluoroe-thylene) (PTFE)	Thermoplastic; Colourless gas; Hydrophobic; Tm = 325°C; Density:1.52 g/cm³; Crystallinity up to 50–75%	Melt extrusion from monomer (tetrafluoroethylene) into films and typically thermo-mechanically expanded into ePTFE	Commercialized as TEFLON®, Sutures; vascular and endovascular grafts; embolic vena cava filter; heart valve sewing rings; ACL ligaments
Poly(ethylene terephthalate) (PET)	Thermoplastic; Hydrophobic; Tm = 265°C; Tg = 65–105°C; 100% amorphous as spun so need to be drawn and annealed to have crystallinity	Melt spinning of monofilaments and multifilament yarns in the form of weaving, braiding, and knitting	Commercialized as DACRON®, sutures (Mersilene™; Surgidac™; Ticron™); hernia repair meshes; ACL prostheses; heart valve sewing rings; vascular and endovascular grafts
Polyglycolide (PGA)	Thermoplastic; Tm = 225°C; Tg = 40–45°C; Crystallinity up to 45–55%; simplest linear aliphatic polyester; rigid mechanical properties	Melt spun into monofilament and multifilament yarns; can be electrospun into nanofibres; can be copolymerized with other resorbable polymers	Sutures (Dexon™); meshes (for defect repairs and periodontal inserts); used as scaffolds in tissue engineering
Polypropylene (PP)	Predominantly isotactic Thermoplastic; Hydrophobic Tm = 165–175°C; Crystallinity up to 40–46%; higher fracture toughness than HDPE; susceptible to degradation from heat and radiation	Melt spinning into monofilaments, hollow fibres, or melt blown and spun-bonded to form nonwoven textiles	Commercialized as ACTISITE®; sutures (Prolene™; Surgipro™); hernia repair meshes; blood filters (e.g., renal dialysis machines

1.3   FIBRE PRODUCTION METHOD

1.3.1   Melt Spinning

Melt spinning, or melt extrusion, is one of the most economical spinning techniques for producing synthetic polymeric fibres and is widely used in the textile industry. It is the most applicable method when polymer yarns are spun from thermoplastics like nylon, polyester, polyethylene, olefin, glass fibres, or poly(ethylene terephthalate) PET, poly(butylene terephthalate)PBT, poy(trimethylene terepthalate)PTT, poly(ethylene napthalate)PEN, etc. In this process, the raw polymer materials are heated above their melting point to form a viscous polymer melt that is pumped and extruded through the spinneret under pressure, the spinneret containing a number of holes with defined geometry. The extruded long molten strand of polymer (monofilament or multifilament) is quenched by the blast of cold air or gas blower, which rapidly cools and solidifies into a continuous filament. It is then immediately collected on a take-up wheel, which stretches, lubricates, or twists the fibre, and it is then winded onto a spool depicted in Figure 1.1 (A), or the yarn is prepared for further processes, such as texturing, crimping, weaving, knitting, or braiding. The drawing operation facilitates the production of yarns with finer diameters, making them more parallel and enhancing their mechanical qualities. To minimize yarn resistance and enhance yarn handling, or efficacy, spin finishes are used as a lubricant. Melt-spun fibres can have a variety of unique cross-sectional forms, comprising round, square, or trilobites, depending upon the shape, size, and length of the spinneret holes. Sutures are the most common medical use of melt-spun fibres. Melt-spun multifilament yarns are frequently utilized as vascular grafts.

1.3.2   Dry Spinning

In dry spinning fibre formation method, the polymer solvent is extruded through a spinneret and passes into the warm air chamber, where it solidifies the fibres by condensing the solvent in a stream of warm air gas. The extrusion process is followed by washing for removing extra solvent, stretching, lubricating, and either take-up on a package or cutting to short-staple fibres as shown in Figure 1.1 (B). Heat transmission, mass transfer, and filament stress are the three main factors in dry spinning. Acetate, triacetate, acrylic, mod-acrylic, spandex, or some aramids fibres are the most significant polymers for dry spun fibres.

1.3.3   Wet Spinning/Gel Spinning

Wet spinning is capable of spinning a large number of non-thermoplastic polymers simultaneously meanwhile various spinnerets can be submerged in a coagulation bath. This process is used to produce viscose rayon, rayon, acrylic, mod-acrylic, lyocell, or spandex fibres. In this procedure, the raw polymeric material is solubilized in a solution and then extruded into a non-solvent in a coagulation bath by submerging a spinneret. When the fibres are pulled out from the bath, they precipitate and solidify. Then the filaments are washed and lubricated before they are dried on

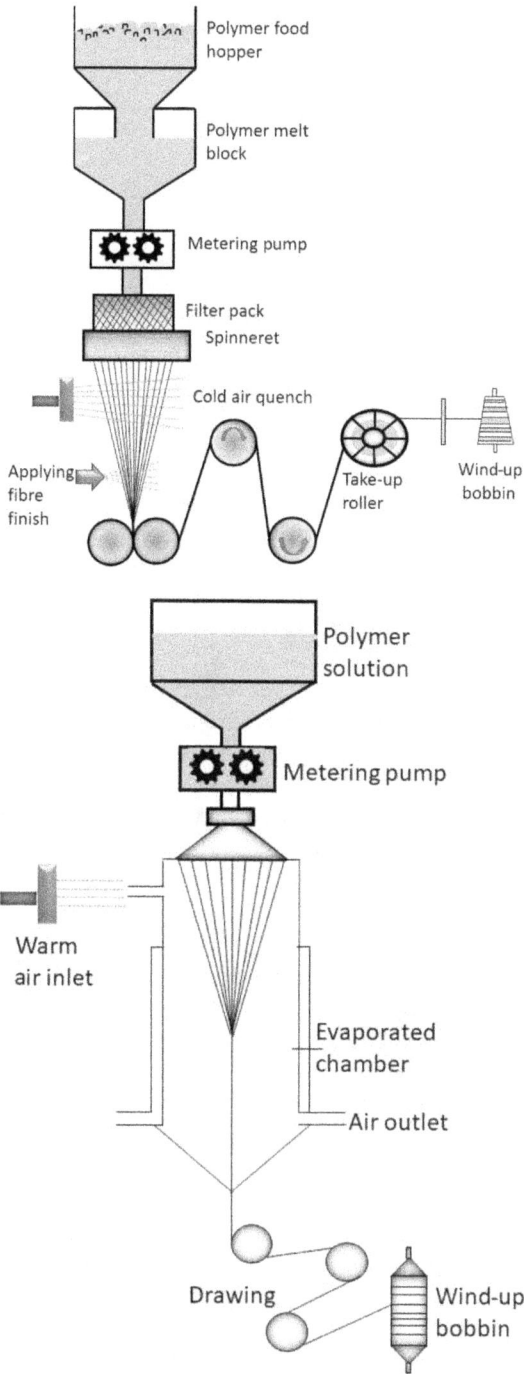

FIGURE 1.1   A. Schematic illustration of melt spinning process; B. Schematic of dry spinning process

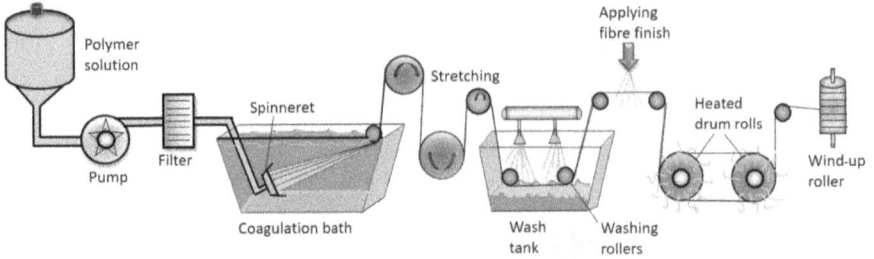

FIGURE 1.2   Schematic illustration of the wet spinning process

large heated drum rolls, and at the end winded up onto a bobbin for long continuous filament fibre or for short-staple fibre, and sent to the cutter as illustrated schematically in Figure 1.2. Wet spinning is a simple and older technique, although there is potential to generate microfibres (PLLA, PLGA) that could be used to produce scaffolds with both drug delivery system and tissue engineering. Lavin et al. (2012) presented more evidence that drug encapsulation through wet spinning enhances the mechanical characteristics of microfibrous scaffolds.

Gel spinning, often referred to as semi-melt spinning, is a technique that creates high-strength and high-elastic modular fibre in the gel condition. The polymeric solution or plasticized gel is extruded from the spinnerets, next cooled in a solvent or body of water, and then stretched into gel fibre by an extreme high extension (Kuo & Lan, 2014). Numerous synthetic and biological polymers, such as PLGA, PCL, chitosan, cellulose, collagen, fibrin, alginate, and cyclodextrin, can be spun using the wet/gel fibre method (Razal et al., 2009).

1.3.4   Electrospinning

The electrospinning technique to fabricate microfibres and nanofibres was first patented in 1934 by Formhals, when he reported his research on artificial threads produced with an electrostatic approach. With this technique, nonwoven fibrous materials can be fabricated with fibre diameters from tens of nanometers to microns. The extremely elevated surface-to-volume ratio, flexible porosity, controlled the matrix composition and malleability of electrospun nanofibre arrays, allowing them to be formed into a wide range of sizes and forms. The electrospinning process occurs when a strong electrostatic force is generated on polymer solvent or melt is exposed to an electric field through a syringe pump that regulates the flow rate of solvent and supplies a high static voltage to a liquid droplet, at a critical point liquid eruption from the surface called the Taylor cone. Thus, fibre can be fabricated to a collector electrode or collected on a grounded stationary or rotating metal screen shown in Figure 1.3. The ability to easily create fibres with a variety of morphologies and dimensions, the capacity to incorporate beneficial compounds into the polymer solution, the flexibility to orient the fibres either arbitrarily or in a well-arranged way are all benefits of using electrospinning

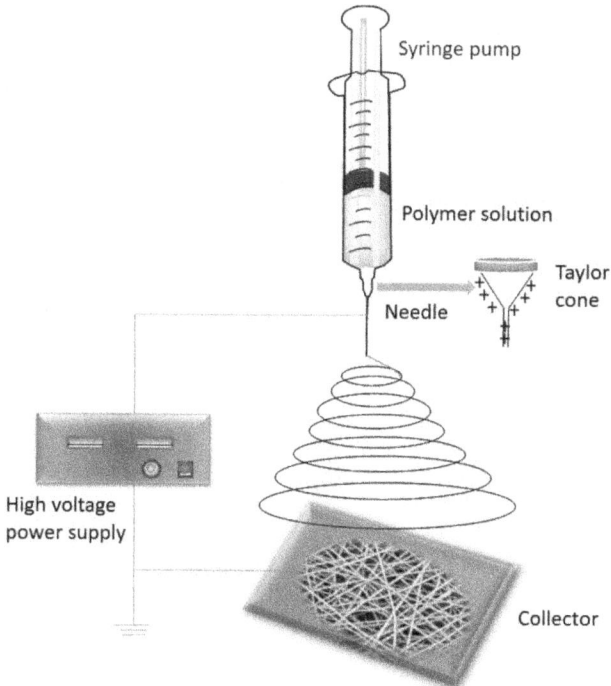

FIGURE 1.3 Schematic illustration of electrospinning

to create macro and nanofibres in drug delivery systems for tissue engineering related applications (Sill & Von Recum, 2008). The use of electrospun fibre structure in drug delivery systems has been extensively researched in the area of wound healing, but single material might not be strong enough mechanically or have less optimum drug loading capability into wounds. Bai et al. (2013) were able to successfully address both problems by using an electrospinning technique to create a chitosan/polycaprolactone (CS/PCL) nonwoven mat. The study by Chen et al. (2010) explores the utilization of the electrospinning method to fabricate composite PAN/PVP nanofibres, serving as a filament-forming matrix for drug delivery applications with controlled release.

1.3.5 BICOMPONENT SPINNING/MULTICOMPONENT SPINNING

Biocomponent spinning or multicomponent spinning is a technique that combines two or more different polymers to meet each other at the spinneret hole and form cross-sections in each spun filament (Durany et al., 2009). In 1960, Dupont created the first bicomponent fibres: a side by side fibre consisting of two varieties of polyamide fibres with varying retraction. Bicomponent spinning (Figure 1.4) can be used to generate nanofibres by using two vital techniques with desired configurations, which involves spinning two polymers via the spinning die 1)

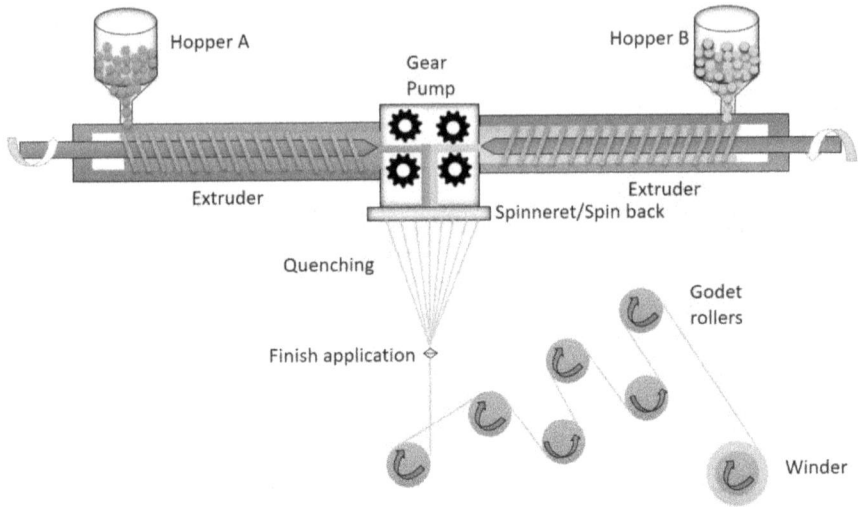

FIGURE 1.4   Schematic illustration of bicomponent spinning

islands-in-the-sea (I/S), 2) core/shell or core/sheath, 3) side by side or segmented pie fibers and removing one polymer. In the textile or medical industry, bicomponent fibres with shell/core structure are frequently used for the thermal bonding of nonwoven fabrics (Yeom & Pourdeyhimi, 2011) by depending on the variance in the melting temperatures of the polymers, where a lower melting temperature is utilized in the sheath structure, while a higher melting temperature is employed in the core structure (Durany et al., 2009; Yeom & Pourdeyhimi, 2011). Bicomponent fibres can be created by electrospinning, melt spinning, or wet spinning. Additionally, bicomponent fibres can be used to create ultrafine fibres by removing polymer matrix of some fibres' components through thermal treatment or dissolutions (Durany et al., 2009; Gong & Nikoukhesal, 2009). The benefit of employing this fibre arrangement in vascular applications lies in the sheath's ability to expedite an inflammatory or foreign body response and enhance the overall healing process. Simultaneously, the core component ensures the mechanical integrity of the device (King et al., 1999).

1.4   TEXTILE FABRICATION TECHNIQUES

When fibres or yarns are extruded through spinning they are then obtained by fabricating into a textile structure in order to obtain the necessary mechanical or biological properties. In the textile industry wovens, nonwovens, knitted, and braided textile structures are traditional methods used for manufacturing fabrics and can be applied for biotextile applications. Additionally, there are unconventional methods used for fabric construction such as bonding fibres via mechanical, chemical, thermal, or solvent.

1.4.1 KNITTED BIOTEXTILES

Knitted textiles are constructed by the continuous interlooping series of loop stitches made from one or more yarns. In a knitted structure, interlocking the loops along the lengthwise direction is called *wales* or warp knitted fabric and loops run across the widthwise direction called *courses* or weft knitted fabric. Knitted fabrics can be produced either in flat or tubular form, by intermeshing the stitches with the subsequent and preceding rows. As compared to woven, knitted structures are commonly more flexible, elastic, and inherently open porous structures with total porosity values exceeding 65%. Therefore, it is commonly used in sutures (Chang et al., 2020), tissue ingrowth (King & Chung, 2013), adhesive tapes, and medicated bandages (Spencer, 2001). Warp knits exhibit greater dimensional stability, reduced stretch, and less unraveling when cut in comparison to weft knits. Warp knits, exemplified by fabrics like velour or pile knits, tend to be more adaptable, allowing for further modification through the incorporation of additional yarn into the structure. This addition enhances thickness, bulk, and surface texture. The knitted loops in both the course and wales directions impart significant extensibility to knit fabrics, providing them with greater elasticity compared to woven fabrics. This characteristic makes knit fabrics a common choice for medicated bandages, adhesive tapes, or covering materials as shown in Table 1.2.

1.4.2 WOVEN BIOTEXTILES

Woven fabrics are created by using two or more sets of yarn interwoven at right angles to one another called warp and weft. Warp yarns are retained in the loom direction, whereas the weft or filling yarns are carried by shuttle in the cross-direction. For biotextile devices, woven constructions are frequently used, such as plain, twill, satin, and leno weaves or combinations of these woven designs. Contrary to twill and satin weaves, the plain weave may be produced very thinly, making it the preferred material for many endovascular graft designs. For long-lasting healing of vascular prostheses, it is preferable to use textured multifilament yarns in twill or satin weave as they offer additional open, porous, and bulkier construction that allows

TABLE 1.2

Commercial knitted biotextile products and their medical application

Application	Structure	Product	Company
Bandages	Warp knit (cotton, viscose)	Tensopress	Smith & Nephew Ltd.
Cardiac support device	Knit (Polyester (PET))	CorCap™	Acorn Cardiovascular
Skin graft	Knitted (PLGA)	Dermagraft®	Organogenesis
	Knitted (Nylon)	Biobrane®	Smith & Nephew Ltd.
	Knitted (Nylon/Collagen)	TransCyte®	Organogenesis
Wound dressing	Knitted (Jersey)	tg®	Lohmann & Rauscher
	Knitted/Nonwoven composite	Acticoat™	Smith & Nephew Ltd.

TABLE 1.3

Commercial woven biotextile products and their medical application

Application	Structure	Product	Company
Gauze dressings	Leno weave (cotton/ viscose rayon)	JELONET	Smith & Nephew
	Leno weave (100% cotton open weave)	Euronet Paraffin	Eurofarm S.P.A.
	Leno weave (cotton)	UniTulle	ZENTA
	Leno weave (cotton)	Sofratulle	Hoechst Marion Roussel Ltd
Wound dressing	Woven (cotton)	Kendall Curity	Kendall Healthcare Prod Inc.
	Woven (nylon)	3M™ Tegaderm™	3M
	Leno weave (nylon)	Tegapore	3M Healthcare Ltd.
Bandages	Woven	Tubifast tubigrip, tubipad	MOLNLYCKE
	Woven (nylon, cotton)	Setopress	Seton Healthcare Group Plc
	Woven	Granuflex®	ConvaTec
Vascular prostheses	Woven, weft knit, velour knit, warp knit, (PET)	DeBakey woven Dacron vascular prothesis	Bard
	Woven	Gelweave™	Valsalva

for more tissue penetration. Woven are used for several medical applications including drug delivery systems, wound dressing, compressing bandages, medical gauze, a variety of artificial skin grafts, vascular prostheses, and 3D woven scaffolds for tissue engineering, shown in Table 1.3. Gadkari et al. (2020) investigated the self-assembled coating on woven cotton fabrics using the layer-by-layer (L-B-L) process to obtain antibacterial characteristics. Bioactive woven cotton gauze can be used to make antimicrobial wound dressings. One type of medical gauze was treated with acacia gum and silver nanoparticles. Staphylococcus aureus and Pseudomonas aeruginosa, two contagious bacterial species, were found to be resistant to the woven fabric (El-Naggar et al., 2019). Through citric acid as a biodegradable cross-linker and spacers for anchoring Ag-NPs and TiO2-NPs to the processed fabric surface, NaH_2PO_2 (SHP), a catalyst, and the pad-dry-cure method were used by Ibrahim et al. (2013) to multi-functionalize cotton/spandex woven fabrics.

1.4.3 Nonwoven Biotextiles

Nonwoven fabrics are referred as sheet or porous uniform web structures bonded together by directly entangling the fibres or filaments without the intervening stage of yarn manufacturing, and interlocked together mechanically, thermally, chemically, or by using any adhesive or solvent means. Nonwovens are frequently used in medical application due to their short manufacturing cycles, great flexibility, dimensional stability, high porosity, and cost effective production. The current advancement in nonwoven materials is the formation of 2D and 3D nanofibre mats for implantable use as tissue scaffolds (Rostamitabar et al., 2021), the intestinal prosthesis (Liu et al., 2019),

TABLE 1.4

Commercial nonwoven biotextile products and their medical application

Application	Structure	Product	Company
Wound dressing	Nonwoven composite (PET Viscose rayon)	Mepore	Molnlycke
	Nonwoven (Carboxymethyl cellulose)	Aquacel	Convatec
	Nonwoven (Calcium alginate)	Kaltostat	Convatec
Vascular prosthesis	ePTFE membrane	Gore-Tex, Flixene	W. L. Gore & Associates, Getinge
Gauze	Nonwoven	Sterilux gauze	Hartmann USA Inc.
		Sterile gauze	McKesson

tendon grafts (Sensini & Cristofolini, 2018), drug-eluting devices, and blood filtration. For usage in drug administration applications, Balogh et al. (2015) researched the fabrication of a melt-blown nanofibre system based on a hydrophilic vinylpyrrolidonevinyl acetate copolymer and PEO plasticizer. Additionally, nonwoven fabrics can be produced directly from polymers using four processes: melt blowing, spun bonding, electrospinning, and the expansion of PTFE polymer. Melt blowing produces synthetic polymer-shaped products (polyethylene, polypropylene, or polyester) with micro denier-sized fibres that are generally utilized for fluid and gas filtration. Spun-bonding fabrics produce thin, porous, and robust fabrics that are typically created from the same polymers used for making melt-blowing fabrics. These fabrics are utilized in various medical devices but are most frequently used for absorbent feminine hygiene napkins, disposable baby care products, or wound care dressings, and nonwoven electrospun nanofibre webs are currently used as scaffolds for tissue engineering. The only nonwoven material utilized directly as implants (sutures, arterial grafts) is based on the expanded polytetrafluoroethylene (ePTFE) polymer that produces fine pores structure (Gupta, 2013). Table 1.4 displays the medical applications of commercial nonwoven biotextile products.

1.4.4 BRAIDED BIOTEXTILES

Braiding is the diagonal interlacing of three or more strands that overlap one another at different angles and frequencies and form a narrow strip of flat or circular fabric. The braided construction is defined by the horizontal repeat distance named as line and (denoted as l), the vertical repeat distance named as stitch (denoted as s), (w) is the width of the yarn, and the (θ) braid angle between the yarn and machine directions. The three primary varieties of braided constructions are regular, diamond, and hercules. Braiding technologies encompass machines designed for crafting delicate surgical sutures, as well as braiding machines for the manufacturing of stents and catheters. Notably, a specialized horizontal extra-fine-wire braiding technique has been developed, particularly suited for producing small-lumen stents and catheters

TABLE 1.5
Commercial braided biotextile products and their medical application

Application	Structure	Product	Company
Esophageal stent	Polyester (PET)	Polyflex®	Boston Scientific
Sutures	Nylon 6	Nurolon™	Johnson & Johnson
	Polyester (PET)	Mersilene™, Ethibond™, Ticron™	Johnson & Johnson, Medtronic
Resorbable sutures	Polyglycolide (PGA)	Stoelting™ Visob	Fisher Scientific
	PLGA	Vicryl™, Polysorb™	Johnson & Johnson, Medtronic
Prosthesis	UHMWPE	Richards handle prosthesis	Smithsonian
Ligaments	Polyester (PET)	Leeds-Keio	Leeds Orthotics®

using Nitinol wire (Aibibu et al., 2016). One notable application of braided hollow tubes is in vascular stents. The low bending rigidity and radial expandability of the braid make it an ideal structure for maintaining open arteries and preventing clots. Additionally, braided fabrics find common use in anterior cruciate ligament (ACL) prostheses (Chang et al., 2020) and their commercial biotextile products shown in Table 1.5. Three-dimensional (3D) braiding innovations have made it possible to create more intricate structures like "I" beams, hollow channels, and solid tubes. Additional innovative approaches include fabricating the braided structure from a single wire used for repairing the thoracic aortic aneurysm and for oesophageal stents (Polyflex) (Murgo et al., 1998).

1.4.5 Nanofibre Nonwoven Structure

Nanofibre-based highly porous nonwovens are produced through electrospinning. Electrospinning is a relatively easy and versatile method for creating continuous fibres with sizes varying from 10 nm to numerous micrometers. Nonwoven fabrics made with nanoscale fibres exhibit interconnected smaller pores or channels, high porosity, and a high specific surface area throughout the fabric, which shows that the surface of the fibre or channel becomes more exposed to functional molecules. A number of natural and synthetic polymers have all been effectively electrospun into fibrous scaffolds for various purposes including fibrinogen, elastin, collagen, gelatin, polylactic acid, polycaprolactone, polyg-lycolic acid, polylactide-co-glycolide, and polylactide-co-caprolactone (Gupta, 2013). Leading applications of nonwovens include highly efficient and selective filters for liquids, gases, or aerosols; carriers for heterogeneous or homogeneous catalysts; and inlets or surface membranes for textiles that introduce potent wind protection, self-cleaning effects, or even antibacterial properties. Additionally, very porous scaffolds for tissue engineering that can promote cell proliferation, and differentiation, or directing cell development in a certain direction are used (Hussain et al., 2010).

1.4.6   EXPANDED PTFE PROCESS AND STRUCTURE

The microporous structure of expanded polytetrafluoroethylene is achieved by the rapid stretching of the extruded tube at high temperature. Polytetrafluoroethylene (PTFE), a thermoplastic polymer, is the base for manufacturing ePTFE membranes and other goods. The structure is made by circumferentially arranged nodes, around 5–10 μm wide interconnected by longitudinal fibrils that are less than 0.5 μm in diameter. Expanded polytetrafluoroethylene membrane films are hydrophobic and oleophobic, making benefits for medical applications. The production of expanded polytetrafluoroethylene (ePTFE) membrane is a multistep procedure, briefly summarized in these steps: sieving PTFE resins of fine powder are blended with a propellant (usually, naphtha), now placing the mixture for the maturation process for 24 hours (curing time and temperature is earlier fixed) then carrying out for shaping (either rectangular, circular, tube, or even irregular form) by extrusion. Extrusion is carried out at a steady rate of the process that will ensure the material is stretched without breaking. In order to get the naphtha out of the material, drying is required. After drying, carrying out for calendaring process (by passing the material between the rollers) for stretching at a specific gravity of around 0.55 to 0.75, usually at the longitudinal direction, and then heated for composite shaping temperature is controlled at 300°C ~380 °C for reshaping or trimming the finally produced expanded polytetrafluoroethylene (ePTFE) membrane shown in Figure 1.5. Huang et al. (2007) and Ardakani et al. (2013) discovered that effectively raising the extrusion pressure may improve the accumulation of nearby powders, and increasing the degree of fibrillation in the extrudate can help to enable the formation of a stretched membrane with larger porosity and smaller mean pore diameters.

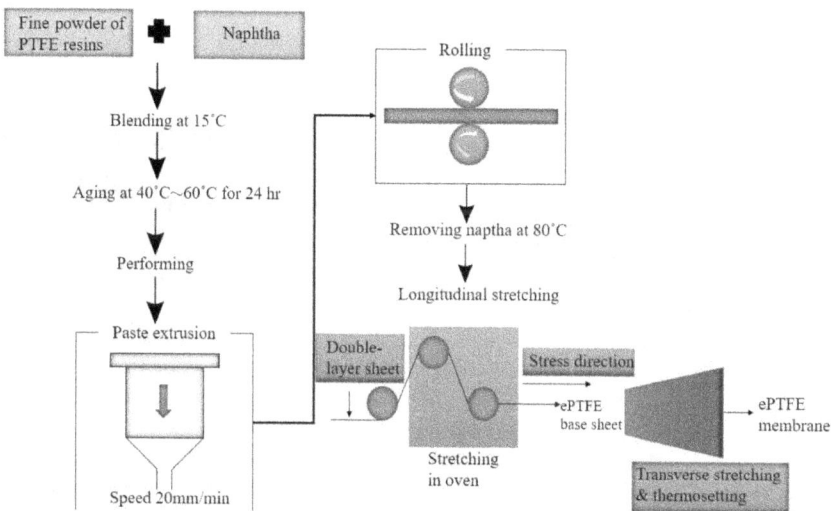

FIGURE 1.5   Schematic illustration of ePTFE porous membrane

1.5   DRUG RELEASING TREATMENT OF TEXTILE MATERIAL

The preparation of drug-releasing textiles is often considered a precise way for sustaining the release of an active compound. The technique is welcomed for the manufacturing of several drugs such as proteins, DNA, genes, antibiotics, vaccines, anti-inflammatory, and anticancer agents. Manufacturing of drug-eluted textiles is decided on the basis of the required duration of drug elution, preparation of fibre, and drug type. Several methods have been recognized for the development of these types of textiles, such as encapsulation, nanoparticles, coating, supercritical impregnation, hollow fibres, and bioconjugation (Tiwari et al., 2012; Banik & Brown, 2014). These techniques are discussed briefly in this section.

1.5.1   ENCAPSULATION

The technique is suitable for the textile that can be soaked in drug-filled liquid and swells the fibre after the drug diffuses through it. Drug solubility and diffusion play a crucial role in terms of manufacturing a medical textile product (Natu et al., 2011). Drug-polymer suspensions could be an ideal option to design the medical textile if the drug's solubility is low. This is prepared by converting the particles into a fine powder that is further subjected to agitation, followed by exposure to UV waves (Perelshtein et al., 2008). The fibre could also be prepared by the process of wet spinning (requires a particular antisolvent that could solidify the fabric and results in partial dissolution of the active compound) and electrospinning (Yan et al., 2009; Yu et al., 2009). The encapsulation can also be done at the initial stage of fibre development. This could be done by mixing the polymer and drug homogeneously. The encapsulation method serves efficient release of the drug and permeation of air, and provides a specific surface area to the fibre as the fibre gets entrapped with solvent and non-solvent molecules and pores formed resulting in sustained release of drug (Qin, 2016).

1.5.2   NANOPARTICLES

Textile materials have the potential to undergo nanoparticle treatment, incorporating bioactive agents. These nanoparticles can be permanently affixed to the fabric through chemical bonds, achieved either by the direct reaction of the particle's side groups with the textile material or through the utilization of a linker molecule. The nanoparticles could be either degradable or non-degradable particles and are selected on the basis of priorities set by a researcher. Microbial infections caused by unhygienic clothes and bedding could be treated with medical textiles prepared by nano-encapsulation. The nanoparticles are prepared by adding the drug to a polymeric shell and encapsulated by the process of precipitation, microemulsion, and interfacial polymerization (Rajendran et al., 2011). Nanoparticles are incorporated in either synthetic (such as cellulosic fibres) or natural (wool and other animal fibres) fibres. In the nanoparticle-prepared solution, suspension, or emulsion the fibre is either soaked, sprayed, padded, or dipped in it under a specific temperature and pressure for some minutes to a few days (Qin, 2016).

1.5.3 Surface Coating

This technique is performed by immersing the fabric into the drug solution or fabricating the fibre using a nanoparticle-filled drug. Coating techniques are selected on the basis of the desired pH, the thickness of the coating, and the solid content that needs to be coated. The coating should not vanish after one to two cycles of washing as it may devaluate its medicinal use (Ma et al., 2009). After evaluating these parameters, methods such as dispersion, ultrasound, electrochemical deposition, ion beam, curtain coating, irradiation, or immersion could be selected (Wang et al., 2018; Yao et al., 2014; Klueh et al., 2000; Shah & Halacheva, 2016). The coatings enhance the sustained effect of a drug if coated precisely.

1.5.4 Supercritical Impregnation

The technique has gained lots of attention across the globe because of its certain prominent advantages which include low surface tension, high diffusion tendency, and easy-to-remove solvent after completing the impregnation. The process utilizes supercritical fluid that must possess temperature and pressure above critical values at the same time. The most precise temperature and pressure for drug loading range from 35–55°C and 90–200 bar, respectively. The technique is employed in various fields of textiles ranging from dyeing, extraction, cleaning, fractionation, and impregnation. Impregnation refers to the infusion of a drug into a polymeric matrix that alters the physical and chemical characteristics of the fibre. The method possesses several benefits such as pure fibre free from residual solvent containing a high amount of drug.

The process comprises three steps, i.e. dissolution of the drug into $scCO_2$ followed by exposure of the polymer to it resulting in diffusion of the drug to the polymer. Later, carbon dioxide and left-over drugs that could not bind to the fibre are removed by the process of depressurization and develop a medicated fibre (Abate et al., 2019).

1.5.5 Bioconjugation

This method aims to achieve sustained release of a compound by binding it to the fibre after applying either physical or chemical modifications to the fabric. It is essential that certain functional groups such as amines, sulfonic, and carboxyl groups must present on the surface of the fibre or it can be generated with the help of some known methods such as wet chemical method, graft copolymerization, plasma treatment, and co-spinning (Yoo et al., 2009).

(i) **Wet chemical method:** The technique increases the ester linkages in the water insoluble polymer that generates carboxylic and hydroxyl groups on the surface of polymer resulting in increase in conjugation sites. Biodegradable polyesters showed increased number of conjugation sites developed after chemically cleaving the ester linkage (partial surface hydrolysis) in an either acidic or basic environment (Yoo et al., 2009).

(ii) **Graft copolymerization:** The method develops conjugates either by chemical modification or through radiation. For instance, antibacterial fabrics could be processed by adding sulfonic groups in a polyethylene fibre with the help of the radiation of methacrylate (Yoo et al., 2009).

(iii) **Cospinning:** The functional group can be located on a fabric by mixing all the polymers possessing different functional groups to fabricate a conjugated textile product. For instance, an antibacterial fabric was prepared by incorporating repeated units of serine, glutamate, and glutamate three times (Sun et al., 2007).

(iv) **Plasma treatment:** A biocompatible surface can be produced by chemically modifying the fabric containing several types of functional groups (such as amine and carboxyl). The conjugation sites are generated on the basis of gas used to prepare the plasma. Protein-based components such as collagen, fibronectin, gelatin, and laminin enhance cell proliferation and adhesion (Baek et al., 2008).

1.5.6 HOLLOW FIBRES

Hollow fibres recently have been explored commercially because of their capacity to mould themselves into any shape without any need for a complex installation procedure. The hollow fibres are generally available in the shape of a small tube that carries a certain amount of drug which permeates sustainably. The fibre is flexible which makes it an ideal choice for manufacturers to load the desired quantity of compound. In the preparation process, drugs are initially blended with a polymer material to create a core granulate loaded with the drug. Subsequently, this mixture undergoes coextrusion to shape the core of the hollow fibre. Another polymer is coated on the fibre to prepare its outer shell to toughen the fibre (Dukhov et al., 2021).

1.6 CONCLUSION

The expansion of the biotextiles market is expected to grow in the near future as it is an efficient preventive measure for infectious diseases. Biodegradable materials such as cellulose and its derivatives are used for external as well as internal medical applications because of their gas permeability and absorption ability. The alginates and chitosan extracted from brown seaweeds and crustaceans, respectively are also being employed as biotextiles. Additionally, the non-biodegradable fabric is utilized as biomaterials. Different processing methods such as melt, dry, wet/gel, and electrospinning are some of the widely exercised methods to produce biomaterials. Commonly, traditional structures used in the textile industry are wovens, nonwovens, knitted, and braided textile structures; usually they are also used for biotextile production. The preparation of drug-releasing textiles is often considered a precise way for sustaining the release of an active compound. Techniques such as encapsulation, nanoparticles, coating, supercritical impregnation, hollow fibres, and bioconjugation are used to prepare drug-releasing textiles.

REFERENCES

Abate, M.T., Ferri, A., Guan, J., Chen, G., Nierstrasz, V. (2019). Impregnation of materials in supercritical CO2 to impart various functionalities. In I. Pioro (Ed.), *Advanced Supercritical Fluids Technologies* (pp. 1–3). London, NY: IntechOpen. doi:10.5772/intechopen.89223.

Aibibu, D., Hild, M., Cherif, C. (2016). An overview of braiding structure in medical textile. In Y. Kyosev (Ed.), *Advances in Braiding Technology* (pp. 171–190). Amsterdam, NY: Elsevier.

Ardakani, H.A., Mitsoulis, E., Hatzikiriakos, S.G. (2013). Polytetrafluoroethylene paste extrusion: A fibrillation model and its relation to mechanical properties. *Int. Polym. Process*, 28, 306–313.

Baek, H.S., Park, Y.H., Ki, C.S., Park, J.C., Rah, D.K. (2008). Enhanced chondrogenic responses of articular chondrocytes onto porous silk fibroin scaffolds treated with microwave-induced argon plasma. *Surface and Coatings Technology*, 202(22–23), 5794–5797.

Bai, M.Y, Chou, T.C, Tsai, J.C, Yang, H.C. (2013). Active ingredient-containing chitosan/polycaprolactone nonwoven mats: Characterizations and their functional assays. *Materials Science and Engineering: C.*, 33, 224–233.

Balogh, A., Farkas, B., Faragó, K., Farkas, A., Wagner, I., Van, Assche I., Verreck, G., Nagy, Z.K., Marosi, G. (2015). Melt-blown and electrospun drug-loaded polymer fibre mats for dissolution enhancement: A comparative study. *J. Pharm. Sci.*, 104(5), 1767–1776.

Banik, B.L., Brown, J.L. (2014). Polymeric biomaterials in nanomedicine. In A.C. Laurencin, B. M. Deng, C.S. Kumbar (Eds.), *Natural and Synthetic Biomedical Polymers* (pp. 387–395). Amsterdam, NY: Elsevier.

Beulah, P., Jinu, U., Ghorbanpour, M., Venkatachalam, P. (2019). Green engineered chitosan nanoparticles and its biomedical applications—An overview. In M. Ghorbanpour, S.H. Wani (Eds.), *Advances in Phytonanotechnology* (pp. 329–341). London: Academic Press Inc.

Chang, C., Ginn, B., Livingston, N.K., Yao, Z., Slavin, B., King, M.W., Chung, S., Mao, H-Q 2020. Medical fibres and biotextiles. *Biomaterials Science (Fourth Edition)*, 575–600.

Chen, H.M., Yang, M., Wei, B., Ren, Z., Yu, D.G. (2010). Property improvement of electrospun drug-loaded nanofibres using composite PAN/PVP as filament-forming matrix. In *4th International Conference on Bioinformatics and Biomedical Engineering* (pp. 1–4). IEEE, China.

Contrive Datum Insights Pvt Ltd. [cited 11.01.2023], Biotextiles market to rise at a CAGR of 9.5% during forecast period, data by Contrive Datum Insights. *GlobeNewswire News Room*, Available from https://www.globenewswire.com/news-release/2023/01/11/2587292/0/en/Biotextiles-Market-to-Rise-at-a-CAGR-of-9-5-during-Forecast-Period-Data-by-Contrive-Datum-Insights.html.

Denton, M., Daniels, P. (2002). *Textile Terms and Definitions*, Textile Institute, 11th Ed. UK, NY: Manchester.

Dukhov, A., Pelzer, M., Markova, S., Syrtsova, D., Shalygin, M., Gries, T., Teplyakov, V. (2021). Preparation of hollow fibre membranes based on poly(4-methyl-1-pentene) for gas separation. *Fibres*, 10(1), 1.

Durany, A., Anantharamaiah, N., Pourdeyhimi, B. (2009). High surface area nonwovens via fibrillating spunbonded nonwovens comprising Islands-in-the-Sea bicomponent filaments: Structure—Process—Property relationships. *Journal of Materials Science*, 44, 5926–5934.

El-Naggar, M.E., Abdelgawad, A.M., Elsherbiny, D.A., El-shazly, W.A., Ghazanfari, S., Abdel-Aziz, M.S., Abd-Elmoneam, Y.K. (2019). Bioactive wound dressing gauze loaded with silver nanoparticles mediated by acacia gum. *J. Cluster Sci.*, 31, 1349.

Gadkari, R.R., Ali, S.W., Joshi, M., Rajendran, S., Das, A., Alagirusamy, R. (2020). Leveraging antibacterial efficacy of silver loaded chitosan nanoparticles on layer-by-layer self-assembled coated cotton fabric. *Int. J. Biol. Macromol.*, 162, 548–560.

Gong, R.H., Nikoukhesal, A. (2009). Hydro-entangled bi-component microfiber nonwovens. *Polym. Engg. Sci.*, 49(9), 1703–1707.

Gupta, B.S. (2013). Manufacture, types and properties of biotextiles for medical applications. In M.W. King, B.S. Gupta, R. Guidoin (Eds.), *Biotextiles as Medical Implants* (pp. 3–47). London, NY: Woodhead Publishing.

Huang., R., Hsu., P-S., Kuo., C-Y., Chung, S., Lai, J-Y., Lee, L.J. (2007). Paste extrusion control and its influence on pore size properties of PTFE membrane. *Adv. Polym. Technol.*, 26(3), 163–172.

Hussain, D., Loyal, F., Greiner, A., Wendorff, J.H. (2010). Structure property correlations for electrospun nanofibre nonwovens. *Polymer*, 51(17), 3989–3997.

Ibrahim, N.A., Amr, A., Eid, B.M., Almetwally, A.A., Mourad, M.M. (2013). Functional finishes of stretch cotton fabrics. *Carbohydr. Polym.*, 98(2), 1603–1609.

Khalaji, M.S., Lugoloobi, I. (2020). Biomedical application of cotton and its derivatives. In A.H. Wang, B.H. Memon (Eds.), *Cotton Science and Processing Technology* (pp. 393–416). New York, NY: Springer.

King, M.W., Chung, S. (2013). Medical fibres and biotextiles. *Biomaterials Science*, 301–320.

King, M.W., Ornberg, R., Marois, Y., Marinov, G., Cadi, R. (1999). Healing responses of partially bioresorbable bicomponent fibers: A subcutaneous rat study. *25th Annual Meeting Society for Biomaterials*, 22, 60.

Klueh, U., Wagner, V., Kelly, S., Johnson, A., Bryers, J.D. (2000). Efficacy of silver-coated fabric to prevent bacterial colonization and subsequent device-based biofilm formation. *Journal of Biomedical Materials Research Part B: Applied Biomaterials*, 53, 621–631.

Kubíčková, J., Medek, T., Husby, J., Matonohová, J., Vágnerová, H., Marholdová, L., Velebný, V., Chmelař, J. (2021). Nonwoven textiles from hyaluronan for wound healing applications. *Biomolecules*, 12(1), 16.

Kundu, J., Pati, F., Jeong, Y.H., Cho, D-W. (2013). Biomaterials for biofabrication of 3D tissue scaffolds. *Biofabrication*, 23–46.

Kuo, C.J., Lan, W.L. (2014). Gel spinning of synthetic polymer fibres. In D. Zong (Ed.), *Advances in Filament Yarn Spinning of Textiles and Polymers* (pp. 100–112). Cambridge, NY: Woodhead Publishing.

Lavin, D.M., Stefani, R.M., Zhang, L., Furtado, S., Hopkins, R.A., Mathiowitz, E. (2012). Multifunctional polymeric microfibres with prolonged drug delivery and structural support capabilities. *Acta Biomater.*, 8, 1891–1900.

Liu, Y., Wang, M. (2007). Fabrication and characteristics of hydroxyapatite reinforced polypropylene as a bone analogue biomaterial. *J. Appl. Polym. Sci.*, 106(4), 2780–2790.

Liu, Y., et al. (2019). Comparison of polyglycolic acid, Polycaprolactone, and collagen as scaffolds for the production of tissue engineered intestine. *J. Biomed. Mater. Res. B Appl. Biomater.*, 107(3), 750–760.

Ma, Z.H., Yu, D.G., Branford-White, C.J., Nie, H.L., Fan, Z.X., Zhu, L.M. (2009). Microencapsulation of tamoxifen: Application to cotton fabric. *Colloids and Surfaces B: Biointerfaces*, 69(1), 85–90.

Murgo, S., Dussaussois, L., Golzarian, J., Cavenaile, J., Abada, H., et al. (1998). Penetrating atherosclerotic ulcer of the descending thoracic aorta: Treatment by endovascular stent-graft. *CardioVascular and Interventional Radiology*, 21, 454–458.

Natu, M.V., De Sousa, H.C., Gil, M.H. (2011). Electrospun drug-eluting fibres for biomedical applications. In M. Zilberman (Ed.), *Active Implants and Scaffolds for Tissue Regeneration* (pp. 57–85). Berlin, NY: Springer.

Perelshtein, I., Applerot, G., Perkas, N., Guibert, G., Mikhailov, S., Gedanken, A. (2008). Sonochemical coating of silver nanoparticles on textile fabrics (nylon, polyester and cotton) and their antibacterial activity. *Nanotechnology*, 19(24), 245705.

Qin, Y. (2016). Medical textile materials with drug-releasing properties. In *Medical Textile Materials* (pp. 175–189). London, NY: Woodhead Publishing.

Radoor, S., Karayil, J., Jayakumar, A., Radhakrishnan, E.K., Parameswaranpillai, J.K., Siengchin. S. (2021). Alginate-based bionanocomposites in wound dressings. In A.S. Ahmed, B. Annu (Eds.), *Bionanocomposites in Tissue Engineering and Regenerative Medicine* (pp. 351–375). Cambridge, NY: Woodhead Publishing.

Rajendran, R., Radhai, R., Maithili, N., Balakumar, C. (2011). Production of herbal-based nanoparticles for medical textiles. *International Journal of Nanoscience*, 10, 209–212.

Rajzer, I., Menaszek, E., Bacakova, L., Orzelski, M., Błażewicz, M. (2013). Hyaluronic acid-coated carbon nonwoven fabrics as potential material for repair of osteochondral defects. *Fibres Text. East. Eur.*, 99, 102–107.

Razal, J.M., Kita, M., Quigley, A.F., Kennedy, E., Moulton, S.E., Kapsa, R.M., Clark, G.M., Wallace, G.G. (2009). Wet-spun biodegradable fibers on conducting platforms: Novel architectures for muscle regeneration. *Advanced Functional Materials*, 19(21), 3381–3388.

Rostamitabar, M, Abdelgawad, A.M., Jockenhoevel, S., Ghazanfari, S. (2021). Drug-eluting medical textiles: From fibre production and textile fabrication to drug loading and delivery. *Macromol Biosci.*, 21(7), 2100021.

San Pio, J.R., Damsgaard, T.E., Momsen, O., Villadsen, I., Larsen, J. (2003). Repair of giant incisional hernias with polypropylene mesh: A retrospective study. *Scand. J. Plast. Reconstr. Surg. Hand Surg.*, 37(2), 102–106.

Sensini, A., Cristofolini, L. (2018). Biofabrication of electrospun scaffolds for the regeneration of tendons and ligaments. *Materials*, 11(10), 1963.

Shah, T., Halacheva, S. (2016). Drug-releasing textiles. In L. van Langenhove (Ed.), *Advances in Smart Medical Textiles: Treatment and Health Monitoring* (p. 119). London, NY: Woodhead Publishing.

Sill, T.J., Von Recum, H.A. (2008). Electrospinning: Applications in drug delivery and tissue engineering. *Biomaterials*, 29, 1989–2006.

Spencer, D.J. (2001). *Knitting Technology: A Comprehensive Handbook and Practical Guide*. Cambridge, NY: Woodhead Publishing.

Subramaniam, A. (2014). Biomedical applications of nondegradable polymers. In S.G. Kumbar, C.T. Laurencin, M. Deng (Eds.), *Natural and Synthetic Biomedical Polymers* (pp. 301–308). Amsterdam, NY: Elsevier Science.

Sun, X.Y., Shankar, R., Börner, H., Ghosh, T., Spontak, R. (2007). Field-driven biofunctionalization of polymer fibre surfaces during electrospinning. *Adv. Mater.*, 19(1), 87–91.

Tiwari, G., Tiwari, R., Sriwastawa, B., Bhati, L., Pandey, S., Pandey, P., Bannerjee, S. K. (2012). Drug delivery systems: An updated review. *International Journal of Pharmaceutical Investigation*, 2(1), 2–11.

Wang, Y., Gao, Y., Xu, G., Liu, H., Xiang, Y., Cui, W. (2018). Accelerated fabrication of antibacterial and osteoinductive electrospun fibrous scaffolds via electrochemical deposition. *RSC Adv.*, 8(17), 9546–9554.

Yan, S., Xiaoqiang, L., Lianjiang, T., Chen, H., Xiumei, M. (2009). Poly (1-lactide-co-ε-caprolactone) electrospun nanofibres for encapsulating and sustained releasing proteins. *Polymer*, 50(17), 4212–4219.

Yao, Y., Wang, J., Cui, Y., Xu, R., Wang, Z., Zhang, J., Kong, D. (2014). Effect of sustained heparin release from PCL/chitosan hybrid small-diameter vascular grafts on anti-thrombogenic property and endothelialization. *Acta Biomaterialia*, 10(6), 2739–2749.

Yeom, B., Pourdeyhimi, B. (2011). Web fabrication and characterization of unique winged shaped, area-enhanced fibers via a bicomponent spunbond process. *J. Mater. Sci.*, 46, 3252–3257.

Yoo, H.S., Kim, T.G., Park, T.G. (2009). Surface-functionalized electrospun nanofibres for tissue engineering and drug delivery. *Advanced Drug Delivery Reviews*, 61(12), 1033–1042.

Yu, D., Shen, X., Zhang, X., Zhu, L., Branford-White, C., White, K. (2009). Symposium on Photonics and Optoelectronics (pp. 1–4). Wuhan, China.

2 Nanofiber Production Techniques for Medical Biotextiles

Radha Sachchidanand Wattamwar,
Sujot Sunil Borse, Kruthi Doriya, and K S Rajmohan

2.1 INTRODUCTION

Nanofibers are conventionally considered as having a nanoscale diameter and a length-to-diameter ratio greater than 100. Nanofibers have significantly better physiochemical properties as opposed to fibers of greater diameter. Due to their distinctive properties, such as a high surface area-to-volume ratio, strength, porosity, and flexibility, medical and healthcare industries evinced interest late in the nanofibers (Shuakat & Lin, 2014). Table 2.1 illustrates numerous applications of nanofibers and fabrication strategy.

Linen textile has been used since ancient times as a bandage to treat injuries. Over the last few years, nanofibers have been extensively used as a medical biotextile. Moreover, nanofibers-based scaffolds have been widely adopted in tissue engineering and implants for refining surgical interventions. In developing tissue engineering-based scaffolds, the scaffold must resemble the structure and biological function of the corresponding extracellular matrix (ECM). Polymeric nanofiber matrix has greater potential in contrast to nonwoven nanofibrous ECM protein because nanofiber matrix has a comparable physical structure to fibrous protein in native ECM. In addition, fabricated nanofibers can accelerate the wound healing process by regulating skin cell responses like proliferation, differentiation, and extracellular matrix deposition (Chen et al., 2017). An effective wound dressing or healing patch must exhibit properties such as antibacterial, rapid hemostasis, and cell proliferation. Owing to these properties, nanofiber mats have greater potential for wound healing and hemostatic properties (Liu et al., 2017). Another potential use of nanofibers is in the drug delivery, as the use of nanofibers as drug carriers will help in sustained release of the drug. Nanofibers are distinguished based on drug release approach in the drug delivery field. For instance, immediate drug release requires a simple structure of nanofibers, whereas prolonged, biphasic, and stimulus-activated drug release requires nanofibers with swellable and degradable polymer characteristics. Hence, it is essential to design a scaffold with nano-sized fibers with various intrinsic features such as fine pores and interconnected network for easy commercialization in the medical field (Kajdič et al., 2019). Figure 2.1

TABLE 2.1

Applications of nanofibers and fabrication strategy

Source	Nanofiber application	Nanofiber preparation method	Major outcomes	Reference
Natural	Wound dressing for diabetic foot ulcer	Cellulose acetate/gelatin electrospun nanofibers were fabricated in association with berberine as a wound dressing	Fabricated cellulose acetate/gelatin/beri dressing was appropriate to enhance the healing process of diabetic foot ulcers with enhanced antibacterial properties	(Samadian et al., 2020)
Synthetic	Tissue regeneration (tendon graft)	Polycaprolactone nanofibers were fabricated using a novel electrospinning method. Modification such as a rotating metal disc as well as a neutral hollow metal rod placed oppositely to collect nanofibers was made	The novel nanofibers formed had strong tensile strength and suture-retention strengths as well as a larger pore size	(Wu et al., 2017)
Synthetic	Implantable nanosensors for blood glucose monitoring	Fabricated nanofibers were plasticized with polycaprolactone and then loaded with alizarin and boronic acid. Glucose levels were detected through fluorescence	These nanosensors were sub-dermally implanted and showed greater residence time than the spherical nanosensors which have early diffusion	(Balaconis et al., 2015)
Synthetic/ natural	Biomarker detection	Mesoporous zinc oxide nanofibers are fabricated via electrospinning	The biomarker detector showed good reproducibility, selectivity, and femtomolar sensitivity	(Ali et al., 2015)
Synthetic	Cancer detection	Microchip embedded electrospun PGLA nanofibers for capturing circulating tumor cells in metastatic breast cancer	Fabricated nanofibers not only promote in situ culture of captured CTC but also allow subsequent visualization through the optical microscope	(Xu et al., 2017)
Synthetic	Biomimetic actuator	Bundle biohybrid artificial muscle with the integration of human skeletal muscle and hydrophilic polyeurethane/ carbon nanofibers via the electrospinning method	Improved mechanical strength to achieve a strong and flexible scaffold	(Jang et al., 2021)

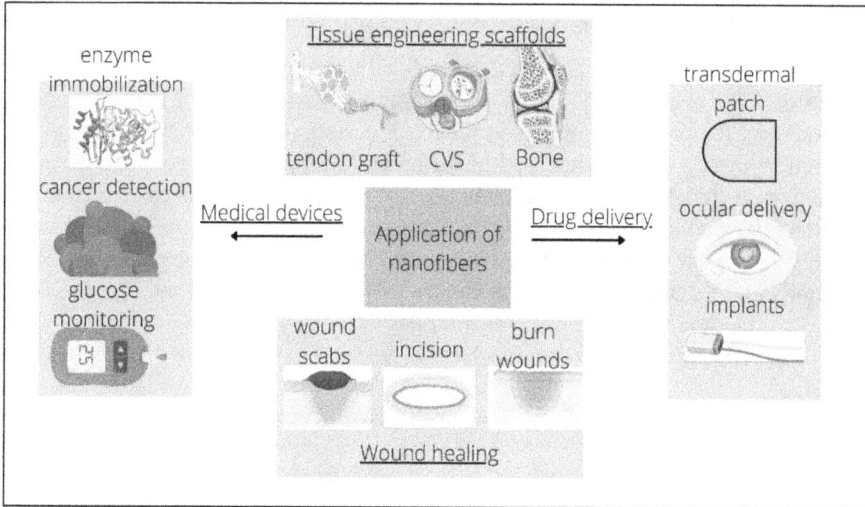

FIGURE 2.1 Applications of nanofibers in various medical fields

represents an application of nanofibers in various medical procedures such as controlled drug release, wound epithelialization, tissue engineering, diagnosis, and regenerative medicine.

Various techniques were tested out in the recent past to produce nanofibers with much-needed characteristics. Since the 1930s the electrospinning technique was the most preferred way to synthesize synthetic and natural polymers. Nanofiber manufacturing is done through electrospinning and non-electrospinning methods. Electrospinning techniques use electrostatic forces to create nanofibers. Electrospinning, template synthesis, extrusion, drawing, phase separation, self-assembly, laser, sonochemical, and plasma-induced synthesis are utilized to produce nanofibers. The simplest and the most proven method to produce nanofibers is through electrospinning, as it helps control the fiber diameter, various production materials, inclination, and layers. Nanofibers are made from a variety of materials (metals, ceramics, metal oxides, polymers, proteins, polysaccharides, and lipids) using electrospinning and non-electrospinning techniques. Various natural polymers such as, viz., collagen, gelatin, elastin, fibrinogen, chitosan, hyaluronic acid, cellulose acetate, and chitin are used in the formation of tissue engineering scaffolds. And synthetic polymers such as polyglycolide (PGA), poly (glycolic acid) (PGA), poly (ε-caprolactone) (PCL), polyurethane (PU), and poly (lactic acid) (PLA) are commonly used in medical applications as biodegradable polyesters (Zahmatkeshan et al., 2019).

The numerous techniques for synthesizing nanofibers are highlighted in the current chapter. This chapter also describes how different parameters affect the final qualities of the nanofibers. Finally, diverse applications of nanofibers in healthcare will be examined, alongside their potential applications in the future.

2.2   SYNTHESIS OF NANOFIBERS VIA DIFFERENT METHODS

In general, different composites have been constituted into nanofibers with or without needles for nanofiber synthesis. Electrospinning is considered the most adaptable method for producing thin nanofibers. Synthesis of the nanofiber procedure in electrospinning can be executed in different ways, including co-axial electrospinning, multi-jet electrospinning, blend, centrifugal, and emulsion electrospinning. Additionally, methods like drawing techniques, sonochemical synthesis, solution blowing or air jet spinning, phase separation/inversion, template synthesis, self-assembly, and plasma-induced synthesis have been introduced. Table 2.2 provides a list of all the non-electrospinning techniques used in synthesizing nanofibers with their properties, advantages, and disadvantages.

TABLE 2.2

List of all the non-electrospinning techniques used in the synthesis of nanofibers with their properties, advantages, and disadvantages

Technique	Advantage	Disadvantage	Properties of the nanofiber	Reference
Phase separation	Phase separation offers more control over the scaffold's porosity and thickness	Drawbacks include the labor-intensive method, manufacture on a small scale, structural instability, difficulty in maintaining porosity, and polymer specificity	Fabricated nanofibers are 50–500 nm in diameter, porous structure with a network of endless filaments	(Alghoraibi & Alomari, 2018)
Drawing method	Provide more flexibility while drawing continuous fibers in any arrangement	Fibers with diameters larger than 100 nm can be generated	Fabricated nanofibers are formed with strong deformations	(Alghoraibi & Alomari, 2018)
Template synthesis	Using this method, aligned polymer micro-/nanotubes and wires with controllable lengths and diameters can be synthesized	This method cannot produce nanofibers with long fiber lengths	Fabricated nanofibers which are synthesized are porous in nature	(Ma et al., 2005)
Self-assembly	Amphiphilic peptides have been specially created and self-assembled into nanofibers	The fundamental drawback of the approach is its length, complexity, and level of elaborateness, which results in low production and a lack of precise control over the fiber dimensions	The morphology of nanofibers was strongly influenced by the substrate, solvent, and preparation technique	(Ma et al., 2005)

TABLE 2.2 (Continued)

List of all the non-electrospinning techniques used in the synthesis of nanofibers with their properties, advantages, and disadvantages

Technique	Advantage	Disadvantage	Properties of the nanofiber	Reference
CO_2 supersonic laser technique	This process does not involve the use of any solvent or any other process which makes it more feasible to use	In some cases, the polymers can have two degrees of polymerization so can have two different melting points, so the final evaluation of behavior of polymers becomes difficult	Fabricated nanofibers were first prepared as monofilaments and then subjected to laser irradiation	(Suzuki & Aoki, 2008)
Solution blow spinning	SBS can deposit fibers onto any target; SBS is a more cost-effective and rapid technique for generating nanofibers	Low production rate, requiring the application of high voltages, and the use of solutions	The fabricated nanofibers have unique mechanical properties and bundled morphology	(Daristotle et al., 2016)
Interfacial polymerization	Interfacial polymerization results in controllable fabrication of films or fibers	Formation of liquid-liquid interface results in usage of large amounts of solvents	Fabricated nanofibers which are formed show homogenous nucleated growth	(Zhang et al., 2004)
Sonochemical synthesis	Ease in alteration of the operational parameters, such as ultrasonic power, current density, and deposition potential	The method is restricted to metals and its alloys	The fabricated nanofibers use physical and chemical effects of high intensity ultrasound for its shape and morphology	(Jing et al., 2007)
Plasma induced synthesis	No reducing agents are required	Ionic liquid decomposition by plasma can contaminate nanomaterials	Plasma modifications can result in high quality of electrospun nanofibers	(Kaushik et al., 2019)
Microfluidic spinning	Final controllability of fibers is an important advantage	Requires special equipment for regulating state of each phase of the microenvironment	Well-defined micro/nanoscale fibers have novel physical/chemical properties, controlled compositions, and intricate structures	(Du et al., 2019)

2.2.1 ELECTROSPINNING AND MODIFICATION OF ELECTROSPINNING METHODS

Electrospinning is one of the earliest and most straightforward technologies for producing highly porous nanofiber structures. There are more than 49,000 publications available to date on electrospinning, when the query string 'electrospinning' was used in the SCOPUS database. A syringe made of glass with a tiny needle, a vital voltage source, and a metal plate for collection are common elements of an electrospinning procedure. This method involves forcing a polymer solution via an electrically charged needle. Following solution charging, a droplet forms at the syringe's tip that started to expand due to the applied voltage, eventually producing a Taylor-cone shape. Once the electrostatic attraction is overcome, the repulsive force between the similar charges in an electrically conductive liquid can be countered by producing desired electric field. Once the pressure is countered, the polymer jet is discharged (Merritt et al., 2012). Electrospun nanofiber structures can be meticulously managed by operating parameters such as electric field, polymer solution properties, and environmental factors. The needle's diameter, flow rate, the gap between the tip of the needle and metal plate collector, and provided electric energy are some electrospinning parameters. The solution criteria are solvent, viscosity, polymer concentration, and solution conductivity. Temperature and humidity are the environmental factors. Figure 2.2 shows various electrospinning techniques and their respective methodology (Alghoraibi & Alomari, 2018).

2.2.1.1 Multi-Jet Electrospinning

Despite several advantages, the industrial application of electrospinning is limited. Numerous multi-jet electrospinning techniques have been created and tested to address this issue. The multi-jet electrospinning method was introduced to increase

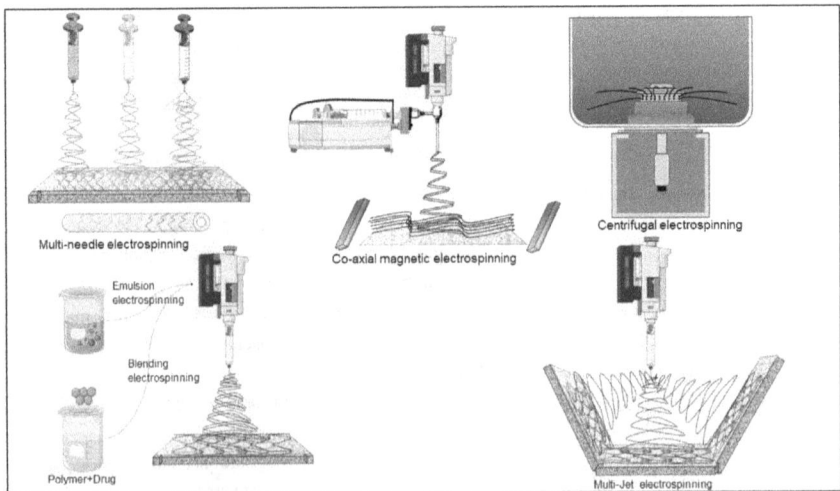

FIGURE 2.2 Schematic representation of various electrospinning techniques and their respective methodology, redrawn (Alghoraibi & Alomari, 2018)

productivity and enable mass production. Vaserano et al. designed a multi-jet electro-spinning system using polyethylene oxide, which included numerous nozzles ranging from 2–16, and obtained good quality nanofibers (Varesano et al., 2009). In another study, a 3D hybrid scaffold made of poly(ε-caprolactone), chitosan, and poly(vinyl alcohol) was created using the multi-jet electrospinning technique for application in regenerative medicine and tissue engineering. The findings from the study indicate how these nanofibrous scaffolds can successfully support the adhesion of rat mesen-chymal stem cells and osteogenic differentiation (Mohammadi et al., 2007).

2.2.1.2   Coaxial Electrospinning

Although significant effort was made to increase electrospinning productivity, most of the techniques only result in single structure-based nanofibers. Core-sheath bio-component nanofiber structures are created via co-axial electrospinning, also known as a two-fluid electrospinning technique. This method is shown to create multilay-ered hollow nanofibers. Multiple feed systems that can electrospin multiple polymer solutions to create coaxial capillaries have been added as modifications to the tra-ditional electrospinning technique (Qin, 2017). Because of their high encapsulation efficiency, huge surface area, multidrug loading capacity, solid mechanical qualities, and ability to control drug release kinetics, coaxial electrospun nanofibers have been used in the treatment of cancer (Li et al., 2022). In a separate study, two materials (hydrophilic polyvinylpyrrolidone and hydrophobic poly (3-hydroxybutyric acid-co-3-hydroxyvaleric acid)) were blended to form coaxial fibers for optimal release of poorly soluble medication. The features of two polymer materials were merged in this drug loading technique, which aids in constructing an improved fiber structure. A novel approach for drug delivery systems is offered by this fiber arrangement for drugs like curcumin, which has a low water solubility (Liu et al., 2022).

2.2.1.3   Emulsion Electrospinning

The emulsion electrospinning technique is used by pharma and food industries in the production of core/shell nanofibers that can hold enzymes, proteins, and drugs. This method is more stable than the ones produced by traditional electrospinning. To obtain the desired morphology, emulsion type, and composition, conductivity of a solution, the strength of the electric field, electrode configuration, surface tension, time required for the solution to cool, solution flow rate and dissolution temperature should be precisely controlled (Nikmaram et al., 2017). Using a single-step emulsion electrospinning method, Wang et al. developed a novel nanofibrous scaffold that simultaneously releases epidermal growth factor, useful in wound dressing applica-tions (Wang et al., 2016).

2.2.1.4   Blend Electrospinning

Blend electrospinning is an alternative for introducing functional components such as drugs. In this method, a polymer solution is mixed with a drug before the elec-trospinning process starts. Additionally, in blended polymer electrospinning, the desired polymer is initially mixed with a protein that adheres to cells, encasing the protein within the overall fibrous framework. This method enables the prolonged release of the encapsulated drug when appropriate favorable conditions such as dissolution-erosion or desorption-diffusion of the polymer network are governed (Buzgo et al., 2018). A more straightforward strategy was used by Li et al., who just combined a pH-responsive polymer (EL100–55) and a thermosensitive polymer (poly (N-isopropylacrylamide)). Blend electrospinning was employed for preparing poly(N-isopropyl acrylamide)/EL100–55 composite fibers. The cross fibers were then combined with the non-steroidal anti-inflammatory medicine ketoprofen to create a responsive system for drug delivery (Li et al., 2018).

2.2.1.5   Centrifugal Electrospinning

The centrifugal electrospinning method is effective in generating ultrathin nanofibers. In this technique, a rotating platform or spinneret is employed, from where the solution of polymer is jetted toward a metal plate collector by the action of centrifugal force. This process aids in creating thin fibers from various polymeric melts (Müller et al., 2020). Modifying centrifugal electrospinning technique to a multi-compartment centrifugal electrospinning technique is offered as an enhanced centrifugal electrospinning setup for specialized biometric applications (Wang et al., 2017).

2.2.2   Phase Separation

As the term suggests, phase separation is a frequently used method of nanofiber preparation that involves the separation of phases as polymer-rich and solvent-rich portions (Zumei Ma et al., 2005). This method involves four steps. Step 1 includes the dissolution of the polymer at room or higher temperature. Step 2 requires gelation, wherein the time duration determines the nanofiber morphology and structure. Also, parameters such as type of polymer, solvent type polymer concentration, solvent concentration, time-frequency of gelation, and temperature of gelation affect the final morphology of nanofibers (Garg et al., 2015). In step 3, solvent is extracted which is incorporated into the gel through water. Step 4 involves the formation of nanofiber through freezing, drying/lyophilization. Though electrospun nanofibers are widely used to synthesize Janus fiber (side-by-side structure formed by combining multifunctional materials) phase separation-based electrospinning technique is used. Recently, Janus-structured nanofibers were prepared from polyvinylpyrrolidone and polycaprolactone to create a versatile dressing for healing of wounds (Ji et al., 2021). The merit of utilizing this technique is that it does not require large scale commercial equipment. However, it cannot synthesize long fibers, and very limited polymer such as polylactic acid, polyglycolide, etc. are applied. Figure 2.3 shows various non-electrospinning techniques and their respective methodology (Alghoraibi & Alomari, 2018).

2.2.3   Drawing

In the drawing method, a polymer solution drop is applied to the surface, and then, using a microtip pipette, a polymer solution is applied on a pre-deposited substrate. In the next stage, a solidified solution is drawn out using hollow glass

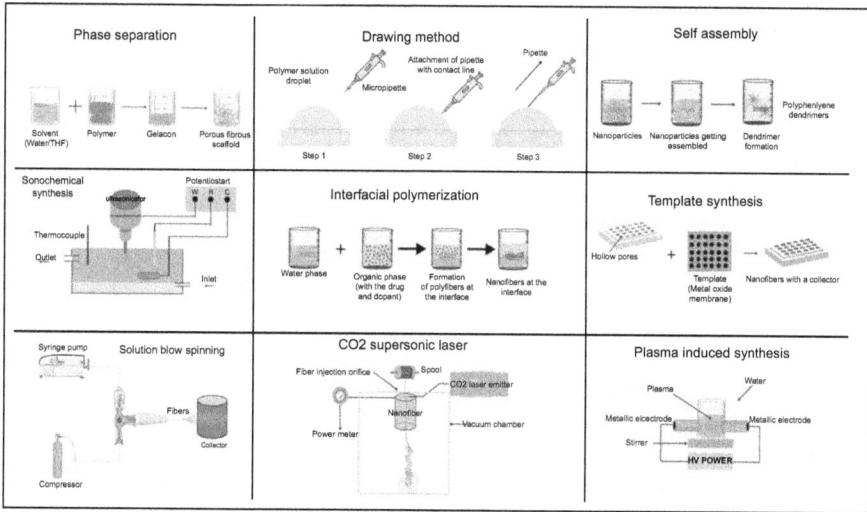

FIGURE 2.3 Schematic representation of various non-electrospinning techniques and their respective methodology, redrawn (Alghoraibi & Alomari, 2018)

micropipettes, and this locomotion fabricates nanofibers. The final dimensions and structure of nanofibers depend on solution drawing speed and viscosity (Garg et al., 2015). In the recent work by Wu et al., a novel nanofiber forming system was introduced, which integrates electrospun nano-yarn with a hot drawing method for developing efficient nanoyarn made of poly L-lactic acid. Synthesized poly L-lactic acid nano-yarn exhibited better orientation, crystallinity, and mechanical properties, and fabricated nano-yarn was able to promote the adhesion, proliferation, and survival of mesenchymal stem derived from human adipose cells (Wu et al., 2021).

2.2.4 TEMPLATE SYNTHESIS

In this technique for the nanofiber's fabrication, a template is required to synthesize a desired component or structure. In fabricating templates, nanofibers are created by allowing a polymer solution to extrude through holes with a diameter of only a few nanometers. Later on, association with the solidified solution yields nanofibers. One of the advantages of this method is that control of fiber dimensions would be possible by varying the template. The disadvantage is that this method cannot synthesize long nanofibers (Alghoraibi & Alomari, 2018). A 3D 58S bioglass scaffold made of very tiny nanofibers with a mean size of 30 nm was created by Luo et al. A sacrificial template approach was used to develop the nanofibrous 58S scaffold that would likely be used in regenerative medicine and bone tissue engineering. The template used was natural 3D bacterial cellulose (Luo et al., 2017).

2.2.5 SELF-ASSEMBLY

This method is a reversible spontaneous process in which random components form hierarchically arranged patterns or structures. It involves the formation of structures or patterns of molecules without human interference through hydrogen bonding, hydrophobic forces, and electrostatic interactions. Generally, peptides and proteins are used for rebuilding damaged cells that contains functional peptide regions and a carbon alkyl tail (Ma et al., 2005). The shape of macromolecular nanofibers can be altered by various solvents used during self-assembly on hydrophobic surfaces. Compared to other techniques, self-assembly is a complicated process, as it is lengthy (Alghoraibi & Alomari, 2018). Factors such as pH, amino acid sequence, and type of electrolyte medium affect the self-assembly of peptides, which in turn affects the nanofibers, which are rearranged to form the hydrogel. Self-assembling peptide hydrogels offer several advantages, such as biocompatibility and biodegradability that help in creating a natural habitat or microenvironment of cells in mammalian tissues (Koutsopoulos, 2016).

2.2.6 CO$_2$ LASER SUPERSONIC DRAWING

Suzuki et al. developed CO$_2$ laser supersonic drawing (CLSD) as a method that employs just CO$_2$ laser irradiation without any additional solvents or processes since electrospinning cannot be used for polymers that are not soluble in a variety of solvents, such as fluoropolymers and polyolefins (Suzuki & Aoki, 2008). Scattering of nanofibers is prevented, as this process is done in a closed system under a vacuum that utilizes CO$_2$ laser radiation. A supersonic jet was created when air was forced into a high vacuum through the inlet to inject the fiber into the chamber. The jet is cooled by the adiabatic process of air across the orifice. The fiber is instantaneously melted by the intense laser beam exposed to cold supersonic jet. Consequently, compared to melt-blowing or electrospinning, this approach is more reliant on environmental health and welfare. CLSD nanofibers may be created endlessly as long as the fiber is continually exposed to radiation with a laser beam and supplied consistently. Polylactic acid, polypropylene, as well as tetrafluoroethylene nanofibers were created in a solvent-less manner, or the second component is taken out when the monofilament forms (Suzuki et al., 2014). Due to the lack of solvents needed in the manufacturing process, nanofibers from CLSD can be employed as scaffolds in medicinal applications and tissue engineering (Suzuki & Ohta, 2018).

2.2.7 SOLUTION BLOW SPINNING

Solution blow spinning (SBS) combines electrospinning and melt-blowing process. The benefit of SBS is it can achieve an efficient spinning that is at least 10 times greater than that of electrospinning, requiring a low voltage and allowing easy device construction (Gao et al., 2021). Two adjacent concentric dynamic flows are required for SBS: a polymer dissolved in a volatile solvent and pressured gas circulating the polymer solution. The fiber generated in the process gets transferred towards the gas flow. SBS based nonwoven fibers are employed in scaffold regeneration, filtration, and electronics. Similar to electrospinning, polymer solution properties and flow rates affect the final fiber structure (Daristotle et al., 2016). Most recently, utilizing SBS technology, functionalized cellulose nanofibers were developed as a colorimetric sensor. This sensor was successfully used in the on-site determination of urea (El-newehy et al., 2021).

2.2.8 INTERFACIAL POLYMERIZATION

Monomer-anion aggregate, formed during interfacial polymerization, initiates a nucleation site for the formation of fibril. This process does not require a predetermined template. For instance, the chemical oxidative polymerization of aniline to polyaniline occurs at the boundary between two immiscible liquids. Polyaniline powder with alternate features can be synthesized when aniline is polymerized with dopants like camphorsulfonic acid. Single-phase mechanism initiates spontaneous polymer growth and results in changes to fibril morphology (Zhang et al., 2004). In contrast, interfacial polymerization uses two monomers in different phases. Hence nanofibers are made by nucleating homogeneous growth of polymers (Alghoraibi & Alomari, 2018).

2.2.9 SONOCHEMICAL SYNTHESIS

Sonochemical synthesis is another chemical fabrication technique for the production of nanofibers. In this procedure, ultrasonic radiation ranging from 20 KHz to 10 MHz is used to alter molecules chemically (Gugulothu et al., 2018). Jing et al. synthesized polyaniline nanofibers using an ultrasonicated system and found that in comparison to the magnetic stirred system, the ultrasonic synthesis approach represents a more simplistic and scalable form (Jing et al., 2007). Green sonochemical synthesis was used by Oorji et al. to create mesoporous Fe3O4@SiO2-hydroxyapatite nanocomposites for their application in sulfasalazine delivery. Results indicated that synthesized nanocomposites were effective carriers in drug delivery systems (Orooji et al., 2020).

2.2.10 PLASMA INDUCED SYNTHESIS

As the name suggests, this technique utilizes plasma in gas and water. Two electrodes are placed parallel to each other, and in the gap, high-energy free radicals are generated, which further form metal nanomaterials. This method does not require any chemical addition or a template. Nanomaterials, however, may become contaminated when ionic liquids decompose in plasma. For example, Hu et al. synthesized CuO nanoflowers using plasma-induced synthesis (Hu et al., 2014). Another work by Annuur et al. showed that the plasma-induced silver nanoparticles boosted the electrospun chitosan nanofibers' ability to inhibit bacteria (Annur et al., 2015).

2.3 APPLICATION OF NANO-BASED FABRICS

2.3.1 WOUND HEALING

Traditionally, plant fibers are used as wound healing materials to prevent infections. Any functional wound dressing material or bandage should have extraordinary properties such as healing time, and bioactive ingredients that exhibit antimicrobial and anti-inflammatory activity. Acute wounds and chronic wounds are the two main categories of wounds. During the healing process of any wound, based on the cell type, five different phases occur, such as inflammation, hemostasis, proliferation, migration, and remodeling (Zahedi et al., 2010). Nanotechnology has made it possible to heal wounds and scar formation effectively. As a result of their enhanced specific surface area and decreased diameter, nanofibers are widely employed in the recovery of wounds. In addition, extracellular matrix (ECM) nanofibril mimicking characteristics make it a reliable solution for biomedical applications. Due to their customizable morphology and surface function, electrospun nanofibers have drawn the most interest out of all micro/nanofibers. In order to improve the overall performance, variations in the structures such as a sheath, Janus, and triaxial structures were developed using side-by-side electrospinning, coaxial electrospinning, and triaxial electrospinning. Additionally, better absorption and permeability of nanofiber enables better healing habitat. The polymers used can be natural or synthetic, and some commonly used polymers are collagen, chitosan, hyaluronic acid, polyvinyl alcohol, polyacrylic acid, cellulose, and nylon-6,6 (Liu et al., 2021). For instance, using a one-step electrostatic spinning technique, Xia et al. developed perforated cellulose membranes with nanofibers coated with chitosan. Resultant nanofibers exhibited outstanding antibacterial activity. Additionally, histological analysis and in vivo tests showed that nanofibers with chitosan coating used to form cellulose membranes might be suitable for wound dressing (Xia et al., 2020). Similarly, Sylvester et al. performed a systematic review and demonstrated that polymorphic or composite nanofibers would improve wound healing by suppressing biofilm formation (Sylvester et al., 2019). Integrating electrospun materials and bioactive ingredients, such as drugs or cells, helps stimulate good mechanical properties for uses such as tissue engineering and wound dressing (Ghorbani et al., 2018). Hence, the final nanofiber fabrication method must emphasize green solvents, fabrication technique without any template, affordable costs, and successful clinical trials for accelerating the development of wound dressing materials and technologies.

2.3.2 DRUG DELIVERY

In general, the mode of drug administration and associated physical and microenvironment parameters play a crucial role in therapeutic efficiency. Due to excellent patient compliance, oral medication delivery is the most favored method of drug administration. However, repeated oral administration of drugs at frequent points is troublesome due to allied hypersensitive, and immunomodulatory effects caused by rapid drug release. Therefore, the sustained release of the drug and combination of bioactive ingredients with polymer fillers has attracted enormous attention. Applying different nano/microfibers in other drug delivery systems for various diseases has shown promising results. Triaxial electrospinning was used by Yu et al. to establish nanofibers with distinct functional compositions in each layer but with similar polymer matrix. The idea of creating nanofibers with the same polymer present in all three working fluids but varying drug contents has led to the development of functional nanofibers with advanced properties (Yu et al., 2015).

Moreover, the manipulation of fibers to achieve desired properties can be beneficial for drug loading and sustained release capabilities. In the case of transdermal drug delivery, they are in the form of a textile bandage, ion exchange fibers, and electrospun mats, etc. (Zhu & Yu, 2013). Canbolat et al. chose poly (ε-caprolactone) as the polymer matrix for Naproxen (drug with poor water solubility, and anti-inflammatory properties) drug delivery system. Beta-cyclodextrin and the drug were complexed to create an inclusion complex, which was subsequently electrospun. According to scanning electron microscopy analysis, the fibers had a diameter of around 300 nm. Moreover, the fabricated complex improved the drug's solubility, and the complexed drug was released better than the unaggregated drug from the fibers (Canbolat et al., 2014). A lot of research has been done to evaluate nanofiber mats as a drug delivery method. For instance, Cui et al. fabricated chitosan and polyvinyl alcohol nanocomposite through electrospinning for their intended use in transdermal drug delivery. This network structure was cross-linked and was successful in regulating the drug release rate. This was demonstrated by drug release assays (Cui et al., 2018). Nanofibers are used in gastro-retentive drug administration parallelly to transdermal drug delivery. This is done by delivering the drug directly to the target location while retaining the appropriate drug concentration. In such a situation, nanofiber systems can replace the current methods, making nanofiber an excellent choice for gastric retaining of the drug (Malik et al., 2015). Deepak et al. emphasized that electrospun nanofibers are applied in oral, buccal, sublingual, ocular, nasal, and vaginal drug delivery systems because of their distinguishing surface and functional characteristics such as porosity, high surface area, biodegradability, controlled release, and mucosal surface availability (Deepak et al., 2018). Recently, several modifications have been added to the electrospinning process to create nanofibers that can aid in preventing burst release and sustained release for a prolonged duration. Core-sheath nanofibers are reportedly known to be favored in the controlled release of incorporated active drugs (Pant et al., 2019).

2.3.3 Tissue Regeneration/Scaffolds

Nanofibrous scaffolds enable the development and regeneration of new tissues with specific cellular and anatomical makeups. A synergistic combination of various nanofiber production techniques and traditional textile forming methods has become an avenue for synthesizing nanofibrous biotextiles. In this manner, the electrospun nano-yarns were built and then processed into various nanofibrous textiles with desired properties. With these structures, it is possible to repair and regenerate different tissues, bones, tendons, and peripheral nerves (Wu et al., 2022). Creating scaffolds for tissue engineering with a three-dimensional (3D) habitat is particularly appreciated if the original structure is mimicked. Wang et al. prepared a 3D scaffold that can mimic native skeletal tissue. Additionally,

C2C12 myoblasts were implanted on the oriented nanofiber yarns, and culture process showed better compatibility to cellular elongation and alignment (Wang et al., 2015). In another investigation, Kitsara et al. combined electrospinning and plasma treatment methods to develop a new scaffold for bone tissue. Resultant polyvinylidene fluoride nanofibrous scaffolds exhibit durable hydrophilic characteristics that may activate osteoblasts cells without the use of an outside source of energy (Kitsara et al., 2019).

2.3.4 MEDICAL DIAGNOSIS

Early and effective diagnosis requires quick and easy points along the way in medical diagnostic instruments. Because nanofibers contain more binding areas, which are sensitive and have a lower detection limit, a variety of nanofibers have been produced as diagnostic instruments for the detection of a wide range of chemicals, infections, and metastatic tumors (Prabhu, 2019). By monitoring several data, such as pressure created by bodily movements, intelligent wearable technology needs to be used to determine health issues. These wearable sensors are available in different forms such as lens, clothes, and wristbands. Various micro/nanostructures such as particles, fibers, wires, and tubes are fabricated and utilized to prepare sensors. Of all the forms, fibrous structures are widely evaluated for fabricating highly wearable sensors (Ghosh et al., 2020). For enzyme-based glucose detection, Sapountzi et al. synthesized electrospun nanofibers with a layer of gold electrodes. Hence, adding metal nanoparticles to electrospun nanofibers enhances their mechanical, electrical, optical, and thermal capabilities. Fabricated nanosensors exhibited efficient glucose selectivity and operational stability (Sapountzi et al., 2017). Furthermore, during the recent outbreak of COVID-19, cotton swabs for biological assessment are requisite for accurate testing of the disease. McCarthy et al. recently developed a unique swab with cylindrical nanofiber tips made from electrospun membranes that expanded gas-foam along a fixed axis. Similarly, preparations based on nanofibers have enormous promise in the medical and forensic domains (McCarthy et al., 2021).

2.4 CONCLUSION AND FUTURE PERSPECTIVE

Nanofibers are high-performance nanostructures with a unique size, structure, and stability. Various fabrication strategies have been proposed for the past three decades, and remarkable advancements have been made to improve productivity and prepare novel composites for their possible application as medical or biotextile. Numerous methods based on electrospinning and non-electrospinning technologies have been investigated for the fabrication of nanofibers. Among all the techniques, electrospinning is extensively studied for its application in wound healing, drug delivery, biosensors in the health sector, and tissue engineering. Since electrospun nanofibers exhibit large surface area and tunable pore size in addition to other electrochemical and mechanical properties, modifications in electrospinning setup and process parameters would affect the final nanofiber structure and morphology, as centrifugal electrospinning can produce ultrathin nanofibers. Various non-electrospinning methods such as sonochemical synthesis, templated assisted, solution blow spinning, and self-assembly have been studied to date and reported in this chapter for their potential application in healthcare. In addition, the development of various structures such as core-sheath and Janus has provided more support in improving the overall performance of tissue engineering and therapeutic delivery. Regardless of the multiple studies listed, still there have not been broader implications of nanofibers as medical biotextile on a larger scale. From this chapter, it is clear that significant developments have transformed the conventional wound dressing into a nanofibrous cover that is biocompatible and biodegradable. Hence, for developing a biomimetic nanofiber matrix/scaffold material, *future research can be more inclined towards many aspects as listed next*:

- Further research focuses on blending various polymeric materials through multi-jet electrospinning would enhance the productivity of nanofibers. Combining multiple polymer materials, integrating electrospun materials and bioactive ingredients, and modification in the electrospinning construction would enable various fibrous structures like multi-layered and garland-shaped fibers (Srivastava, 2017). On the other hand, optimization of various electrospinning parameters, polymer concentration, and bioactive ingredient concentration would affect the thickness and morphology of nanofibers, which are significant in the preparation of 3D scaffolds and control of drug delivery.
- To commercialize any nanofiber-based wound dressing, it is essential to identify the aspects of the healing process for wounds. Furthermore, many clinical evaluations are necessary to understand the biosafety and stability of nanofiber-based wound dressings.
- The development of functionalized polymer nanofibers will offer a new competence in modern medicine. Preliminary in-depth studies on optimization of hybrid nanofiber morphology, chemical composition, and in vivo and in vitro compatibility studies enable a desired platform for synthesizing an efficient polymer matrix in case of drug delivery and improved nanofibrous scaffolds can be analogous to native ECM in the case of tissue engineering.

REFERENCES

Alghoraibi, I., Alomari, S. (2018). Different methods for nanofiber design and fabrication. In A. Barhoum, M. Bechelany, A. Makhlouf (Eds.), *Handbook of Nanofibers* (pp. 1–46). Cham, NY: Springer. doi:10.1007/978-3-319-42789-8_11-2.

Ali, M.A., Mondal, K., Singh, C., Dhar Malhotra, B., Sharma, A. (2015). Anti-epidermal growth factor receptor conjugated mesoporous zinc oxide nanofibers for breast cancer diagnostics. *Nanoscale*, 7, 7234–7245.

Annur, D., Wang, Z.K., Liao, J. der, Kuo, C. (2015). Plasma-synthesized silver nanoparticles on electrospun chitosan nanofiber surfaces for antibacterial applications. *Biomacromolecules*, 16, 3248–3255.

Balaconis, M.K., Luo, Y., Clark, H.A. (2015). Glucose-sensitive nanofiber scaffolds with an improved sensing design for physiological conditions. *Analyst*, 140, 716–723.

Buzgo, M., Mickova, A., Rampichova, M., Doupnik, M. (2018). Blend electrospinning, coaxial electrospinning, and emulsion electrospinning techniques. In A.M.L. Focarete, B.A. Tampieri (Eds.), *Core-Shell Nanostructures for Drug Delivery and Theranostics* (pp. 325–347). Amsterdam, NY: Elsevier. doi:10.1016/b978-0-08-102198-9.00011-9.

Canbolat, M.F., Celebioglu, A., Uyar, T. (2014). Drug delivery system based on cyclodextrin-naproxen inclusion complex incorporated in electrospun polycaprolactone nanofibers. *Colloids Surf. B Biointerfaces*, 115, 15–21.

Chen, S., et al. (2017). Recent advances in electrospun nanofibers for wound healing. *Nanomedicine*, 12, 1335–1352.

Cui, Z., et al. (2018). Electrospinning and crosslinking of polyvinyl alcohol/chitosan composite nanofiber for transdermal drug delivery. *Advances in Polymer Technology*, 37, 1917–1928.

Daristotle, J.L., Behrens, A.M., Sandler, A.D., Kofinas, P. (2016). A review of the fundamental principles and applications of solution blow spinning. *ACS Appl. Mater. Interfaces*, 8, 34951–34963.

Deepak, A., Goyal, A.K., Rath, G. (2018). Nanofiber in transmucosal drug delivery. *J. Drug Deliv. Sci. Technol.*, 43, 379–387.

Du, X.Y., Li, Q., Wu, G., Chen, S. (2019). Multifunctional micro/nanoscale fibers based on microfluidic spinning technology. *Advanced Materials*, 31, 1–38.

El-newehy, M.H., El-hamshary, H., Salem, W.M. (2021). Solution blowing spinning technology towards green development of urea sensor nanofibers immobilized with hydrazone probe. *Polymers (Basel)*, 13, 1–14.

Gao, Y., et al. (2021). Recent progress and challenges in solution blow spinning. *Mater. Horiz.*, 8, 426–446.

Garg, T., Rath, G., Goyal, A.K. (2015). Biomaterials-based nanofiber scaffold: Targeted and controlled carrier for cell and drug delivery. *J. Drug Target.*, 23, 202–221.

Ghorbani, S., et al. (2018). Combined effects of 3D bone marrow stem cell-seeded wet-electrospun poly lactic acid scaffolds on full-thickness skin wound healing. *International Journal of Polymeric Materials and Polymeric Biomaterials*, 67, 905–912.

Ghosh, R., et al. (2020). Micro/nanofiber-based noninvasive devices for health monitoring diagnosis and rehabilitation. *Appl. Phys. Rev.*, 7.

Gugulothu, D., Barhoum, A., Nerella, R., Ajmer, R., Bechlany, M. (2018). Fabrication of nanofibers: Electrospinning and non-electrospinning techniques. In A.A. Barhoum, B.M. Bechelany, C.A.S.H. Makhlouf (Eds.), *Handbook of Nanofibers* (pp. 45–77). New Yorl, NY: Springer. doi:10.1007/978-3-319-42789-8_6-2.

Hu, X., et al. (2014). Plasma-induced synthesis of CuO nanofibers and ZnO nanoflowers in water. *Plasma Chem. Plasma Process.*, 34, 1129–1139.

Jang, Y., et al. (2021). Biomimetic cell-actuated artificial muscle with nanofibrous bundles. *Microsyst. Nanoeng.*, 7.

Ji, X., et al. (2021). Phase separation-based electrospun Janus nanofibers loaded with Rana chensinensis skin peptides/silver nanoparticles for wound healing. *Mater. Des.*, 207, 109864.

Jing, X., Wang, Y., Wu, D., Qiang, J. (2007). Sonochemical synthesis of polyaniline nanofibers. *Ultrason. Sonochem.*, 14, 75–80.

Kajdič, S., Planinšek, O., Gašperlin, M., Kocbek, P. (2019). Electrospun nanofibers for customized drug-delivery systems. *J. Drug Deliv. Sci. Technol.*, 51, 672–681.

Kaushik, N.K., et al. (2019). Plasma and nanomaterials: Fabrication and biomedical applications. *Nanomaterials*, 9, 1–19.

Kitsara, M., et al. (2019). Permanently hydrophilic, piezoelectric PVDF nanofibrous scaffolds promoting unaided electromechanical stimulation on osteoblasts. *Nanoscale*, 11, 8906–8917.

Koutsopoulos, S. (2016). Self-assembling peptide nanofiber hydrogels in tissue engineering and regenerative medicine: Progress, design guidelines, and applications. *J. Biomed. Mater. Res. A*, 104, 1002–1016.

Li, H., et al. (2018). Dual-responsive drug delivery systems prepared by blend electrospinning. *Int. J. Pharm.*, 543, 1–7.

Li, J., Liu, Y., Abdelhakim, H.E. (2022). Drug delivery applications of coaxial electrospun nanofibres in cancer therapy. *Molecules*, 27.

Liu, M., Duan, X.P., Li, Y.M., Yang, D.P., Long, Y.Z. (2017). Electrospun nanofibers for wound healing. *Mater. Sci. Eng. C*, 76, 1413–1423.

Liu, X., Xu, H., Zhang, M., Yu, D.G. (2021). Electrospun medicated nanofibers for wound healing: Review. *Membranes (Basel)*, 11.

Liu, Y., Chen, X., Liu, Y., Gao, Y., Liu, P. (2022). Electrospun coaxial fibers to optimize the release of poorly water-soluble frug. *Polymers (Basel)*, 14, 1–13.

Luo, H., et al. (2017). Sacrificial template method for the synthesis of three-dimensional nanofibrous 58S bioglass scaffold and it's in vitro bioactivity and cell responses. *J. Biomater. Appl.*, 32, 265–275.

Ma, Z., Ph, D., Kotaki, M., Ph, D., Inai, R. (2005). Potential of nanofiber matrix as tissue-engineering scaffolds. *Tissue Eng.*, 11, 101–109.

Malik, R., Garg, T., Goyal, A.K., Rath, G. (2015). Polymeric nanofibers: Targeted gastro-retentive drug delivery systems. *J. Drug Target*, 23, 109–124.

McCarthy, A., et al. (2021). Ultra-absorptive nanofiber swabs for improved collection and test sensitivity of SARS-CoV-2 and other biological specimens. *Nano Lett.*, 21, 1508–1516.

Merritt, S.R., Exner, A.A., Lee, Z., von Recum, H.A. (2012). Electrospinning and imaging. *Adv. Eng. Mater.*, 14, 266–278.

Mohammadi, Y., et al. (2007). Nanofibrous poly (ε-caprolactone)/poly(vinyl (alcohol)/chitosan hybrid scaffolds for bone tissue engineering using mesenchymal stem cells. *International Journal of Artificial Organs*, 30, 204–211.

Müller, F., Jokisch, S., Bargel, H., Scheibel, T. (2020). Centrifugal electrospinning enables the production of meshes of ultrathin polymer fibers. *ACS Appl. Polym. Mater.*, 2, 4360–4367.

Nikmaram, N., Roohinejad, S., Hashemi, S. (2017). Emulsion-based systems for fabrication of electrospun nanofibers: Food, pharmaceutical and biomedical applications. *RSC Adv.*, 7, 28951–28964.

Orooji, Y., Mortazavi-Derazkola, S., Ghoreishi, S.M., Amiri, M., Salavati-Niasari, M. (2020). Mesopourous Fe3O4@SiO2-hydroxyapatite nanocomposite: Green sonochemical synthesis using strawberry fruit extract as a capping agent, characterization and their application in sulfasalazine delivery and cytotoxicity. *J. Hazard. Mater.*, 400, 123140.

Pant, B., Park, M., Park, S.J. (2019). Drug delivery applications of core-sheath nanofibers prepared by coaxial electrospinning: A review. *Pharmaceutics*, 11.

Prabhu, P. (2019). Nanofibers for medical diagnosis and therapy. In *Handbook of Nanofibers*. doi:10.1007/978-3-319-53655-2_48.

Qin, X. (2017). Coaxial electrospinning of nanofibers: Electrospun nanofibers. In *Electrospun Nanofibers* (pp. 41–71). Cambridge, NY: Woodhead Publishing. doi:10.1016/B978-0-08-100907-9.00003-9.

Samadian, H., et al. (2020). Electrospun cellulose acetate/gelatin nanofibrous wound dressing containing berberine for diabetic foot ulcer healing: In vitro and in vivo studies. *Sci. Rep.*, 10, 1–12.

Sapountzi, E., et al. (2017). Gold nanoparticles assembly on electrospun poly(vinyl alcohol)/poly(ethyleneimine)/glucose oxidase nanofibers for ultrasensitive electrochemical glucose biosensing. *Sens. Actuators B Chem.*, 238, 392–401.

Shuakat, M.N., Lin, T. (2014). Recent developments in electrospinning of nanofiber yarns. *J. Nanosci. Nanotechnol.*, 14, 1389–1408.

Srivastava, R.K. (2017). Electrospinning of patterned and 3D nanofibers. In M. Afsheri (Ed.), *Electrospun Nanofibers* (pp. 399–447). Amsterdam, NY: Elsevier. doi:10.1016/B978-0-08-100907-9.00016-7.

Suzuki, A., Aoki, K. (2008). Biodegradable poly(l-lactic acid) nanofiber prepared by a carbon dioxide laser supersonic drawing. *Eur. Polym. J.*, 44, 2499–2505.

Suzuki, A., Mikuni, T., Hasegawa, T. (2014). Nylon 66 nanofibers prepared by CO2 laser supersonic drawing. *J. Appl. Polym. Sci.*, 131, 1–11.

Suzuki, A., Ohta, K. (2018). Mechanical properties of poly(ethylene terephthalate) nanofiber three-dimensional structure prepared by CO2 laser supersonic drawing. *J. Appl. Polym. Sci.*, 135, 1–9.

Sylvester, M.A., Amini, F., Keat, T.C. (2019). Electrospun nanofibers in wound healing. *Mater. Today Proc.*, 29, 1–6.

Varesano, A., Carletto, R.A., Mazzuchetti, G. (2009). Experimental investigations on the multi-jet electrospinning process. *J. Mater. Process. Technol.*, 209, 5178–5185.

Wang, L., Ahmad, Z., Huang, J., Li, J.S., Chang, M.W. (2017). Multi-compartment centrifugal electrospinning based composite fibers. *Chem. Eng. J.*, 330, 541–549.

Wang, L., Wu, Y., Guo, B., Ma, P.X. (2015). Nanofiber yarn/hydrogel core-shell scaffolds mimicking native skeletal muscle tissue for guiding 3D myoblast alignment, elongation, and differentiation. *ACS Nano*, 9, 9167–9179.

Wang, Z., et al. (2016). Evaluation of emulsion electrospun polycaprolactone/hyaluronan/epidermal growth factor nanofibrous scaffolds for wound healing. *J. Biomater. Appl.*, 30, 686–698.

Wu, S., et al. (2021). Combining electrospinning with hot drawing process to fabricate high performance poly (L-lactic acid) nanofiber yarns for advanced nanostructured biotextiles. *Biofabrication*, 13.

Wu, S., et al. (2022). State-of-the-art review of advanced electrospun nanofiber yarn-based textiles for biomedical applications. *Appl. Mater. Today*, 27.

Wu, S., Wang, Y., Streubel, P.N., Duan, B. (2017). Living nanofiber yarn-based woven biotextiles for tendon tissue engineering using cell tri-culture and mechanical stimulation. *Acta Biomater.*, 62, 102–115.

Xia, J., Zhang, H., Yu, F., Pei, Y., Luo, X. (2020). Superclear, porous cellulose membranes with chitosan-coated nanofibers for visualized cutaneous wound healing dressing. *ACS Appl. Mater. Interfaces*, 12, 24370–24379.

Xu, G., et al. (2017). Hyaluronic acid-functionalized electrospun PLGA nanofibers embedded in a microfluidic chip for cancer cell capture and culture. *Biomater. Sci.*, 5, 752–761.

Yu, D. G., et al. (2015). Nanofibers fabricated using triaxial electrospinning as zero order drug delivery systems. *ACS Appl. Mater. Interfaces*, 7, 18891–18897.

Zahedi, P., Rezaeian, I., Ranaei-Siadat, S.O., Jafari, S. H., Supaphol, P. (2010). A review on wound dressings with an emphasis on electrospun nanofibrous polymeric bandages. *Polym. Adv. Technol.*, 21, 77–95.

Zahmatkeshan, M., et al. (2019). Polymer-based nanofibers: Preparation, fabrication, and applications. In A.A. Barhoum, B.M. Bechelany, C.A.S.H. Makhlouf (Eds.), *Handbook of Nanofibers* (pp. 1–47), New York, NY: Springer. doi:10.1007/978-3-319-53655-2_29.

Zhang, X., Chan-Yu-King, R., Jose, A., Manohar, S.K. (2004). Nanofibers of polyaniline synthesized by interfacial polymerization. *Synth. Met.*, 145, 23–29.

Zhu, L.M., Yu, D.G. (2013). Drug delivery systems using biotextiles. In A.M.W. King, B.B.S. Gupta, C.R. Guidoin (Eds.), *Biotextiles as Medical Implants* (pp. 213–231), Cambridge, NY: Woodhead Publishing. doi:10.1533/9780857095602.2.213.

3 Nanotechnology and Biomaterials for Hygiene and Healthcare Textiles

Shilpi Shree Sahay, Prashansa Sharma, and Vivek Dave

3.1 INTRODUCTION

In hospitals, health safety concerns have always been a great challenge as they endanger human well-being and reduce the quality of life. The maintenance of hygienic conditions and hygiene standards is an essential requisite for the control of infections and the spreading of germs. It should however be noted that the risks associated with the impact of hygiene are devastating and thus cannot be neglected. Hospital textile material is the major driving force for the spread of infection that jeopardizes healthcare. This crucial area needs to be addressed because the contagious matter, microbes, get tremendously transmitted via different routes. Presently, the medical sector is struggling to cope with poor or compromised hygienic practices, as millions of the population are vulnerable to fatal diseases. Challenges concerning the control and elimination of inevitable threats and biomedical hazards remain constant.

The recognition of the risk of contracting or spreading infectious diseases and facing future health threats has underscored the necessity for incorporating advanced technology in the medical field for new product development. The key strategy for better infection control focused on the recent breakthrough development of nanotechnology.

Nanotechnology served as an important impetus that caused the rapid advancement of medical science. Additionally, this technology has huge potential to serve diverse disciplines. Textile serves as a pervasive interface and a perfect material for integrating electronics, nanomaterials, and optical devices. Scientific research and technological development have led to the rapid expansion of textile auxiliaries to produce high-performance and functional products by fabricating functional properties. Medical application of textiles covers a wide spectrum of materials and products. The functional requirements and performance for medical textiles are complex. We can still note, however, that the usage of the material is defined by the type of material, structural configuration, and target area. Owing to modern technological development, nanotechnology has brought imperative enhancement in the various approaches to the healthcare aspect. The nano-assisted system with highly precise, fast, and accurate treatment brought much improvement in the quality of healthcare

DOI: 10.1201/9781003331612-4

systems. New optic materials are being evaluated for sensing, actuation, and monitoring of involuntary mechanical and biophysical parameters. Healthcare products containing nanostructures are commercially available. Likewise, nano-finishes on medical textile products enabled manipulation of the basic structural composition of fibre. Nano-coatings represent an important facet of this progress. They entail the application of nanoscale materials onto the surfaces of medical textiles, endowing them with enhanced properties. These coatings offer advantages like improved water repellency, antimicrobial activity, and stain resistance. The nanoscale nature of these coatings allows for precise control over the properties and interactions at the surface, resulting in improved performance and durability. They can be engineered to release antimicrobial agents, inhibiting the growth of bacteria and other pathogens on the textile surface which is particularly important for medical garments and dressings that come into direct contact with the patient's skin, helping to prevent infections. Additionally, they can impart hydrophobic qualities, making medical textiles resistant to fluids, stains, and bodily secretions, an essential attribute for maintaining hygiene. Furthermore, nano-coatings can also be designed to promote wound healing by providing an environment conducive to tissue regeneration, facilitating controlled moisture levels, preventing bacterial contamination, and even delivering therapeutic agents to the wound site. They can also enhance the durability of medical textiles by providing a protective barrier against wear, tear, and abrasion, crucial for garments used in demanding medical environments.

Nanoencapsulation is another remarkable advancement in the field. It involves the confinement of active substances within nanoscale carriers or capsules. In the context of medical textiles, nanoencapsulation can be used to incorporate various functional agents into the textile materials itself, including drugs, vitamins, fragrances, or other bioactive compounds. Nanoencapsulation allows for controlled and sustained release of drugs from the textile material, which can be especially useful for wound dressing that needs to deliver medication directly to the wound site over time. Beyond drug release, encapsulating fragrances, or odour-neutralizing agents, medical textiles can be designed to minimize unpleasant odours from the garments worn by patients and healthcare professionals. Furthermore, it enables the integration of protective layers, on the textile surface releasing beneficial substances like moisturizers or sunscreens catering to the individual needs of patients with sensitive or compromised skin. Nanoencapsulation transforms conventional textiles into "smart" textiles.

Focused efforts are made to eliminate hygiene-related issues and ensure sustained progress toward emerging health threats. To impart antimicrobial characteristics, several organic and inorganic agents have been systematically studied for their potential effectiveness. Despite the usage of disinfectant liquids and detergents, it is challenging to fully control the growth of microbes and pathogens. The notion of protective clothing is attractive to all. It ensures the safety of the medical professionals who come in direct contact with patients suffering from various types of diseases. In response to this type of issue, reinforcement of hygienic practices acts as the frontline warriors in resolving the health agenda but the uptake of positive hygienic practices alone is not sufficient. To address the issue, protective textiles assist healthcare professionals. The protective textile provides reasonable assurance against exposed biomedical infection and hazards. The ever-rising variant of microbes imposes strains on health. To enhance the surface characteristics of clothing, such as microbicidal, durability, and resistance to dirt, odour, stain, and wrinkle, and better thermal performance, nanoparticles are increasingly employed in combination with fibres or as a coating on textile substrates. To achieve an anti-bacterial, anti-fungal, and anti-microbial surface inhibiting the growth of microbes, a thin layer of chemicals is deposited on the base material which improves the functionality of the product. The textile materials are either treated with metallic nanoparticles or embedded with a surface coating to impart functionality to the textile material. As reported by the Business Research Company, the worldwide market for nanotechnology-integrated clothing witnessed significant growth, achieving a cumulative annual growth rate (CAGR) of 24.6%, escalating from \$4.61 billion in 2021 to \$5.75 billion in 2022. Projections indicate that the market for clothing infused with nanotechnology is poised to further expand, reaching an estimated value of \$13.83 billion by the year 2026, driven by a projected CAGR of 24.6%. A significant trend driving the market's expansion is the introduction of new products that incorporate wearable technology.

Currently, extensive research is underway to explore optimal methods for synthesizing various nanomaterials including polymers, micelles, dendrimers, liposomes, emulsions, nano-capsules, and nanoparticles (Sahu et al., 2021).

Biomaterials serve as a fundamental component in healthcare applications due to their unique properties that interact with biological systems. These materials are specifically designed to interface with living tissues, organs, or bodily fluids to enhance medical treatments and interventions. Their significance in healthcare lies in their ability to provide support, replace damaged tissues, or deliver therapeutic agents. Thus, biomaterials are non-drug substances appropriate for use in systems that support or take the place of physiological tissues or organ functions. The term biomaterials can be simply understood as a substance that can imitate or substitute biological function. These biomaterials are typically compatible with the human body. Natural biomaterials, derived from organic sources, have garnered attention for their biocompatibility and bioactive properties. Among these, collagen and chitin have emerged as notable contenders in the development of wound dressing and tissue engineering scaffolds. Synthetic biomaterials have paved the way for innovative solutions in implantable medical textiles. Polymers like polyethylene and polyurethane, engineered with specific properties, are gaining prominence in the development of implants and medical devices.

The tissue response to biomaterials can range from minimal inflammation to complete integration. Biocompatible biomaterials are designed to induce minimal or no adverse reactions when in contact with living tissues. They interact harmoniously with the body, promoting healing and tissue integration without eliciting an immune response or inflammation. These biomaterials are often used for temporary implants, drug delivery systems, and wound dressings. Bioinert biomaterials are characterized by their lack of reactivity with surrounding tissues. They are generally stable and do not provoke significant immune responses. These materials are used in applications where the main goal is structural support or protection. Bioinert biomaterials are commonly employed in orthopaedic implants, dental prosthetics, and other load-bearing applications. Bioactive biomaterials actively engage with the surrounding tissues, stimulating specific cellular responses that enhance tissue integration. These materials often contain components that can elicit controlled reactions, such as promoting bone growth or encouraging the formation of blood vessels. Bioactive biomaterials are commonly used in orthopaedics and dentistry to facilitate bone healing and regeneration. Biodegradable biomaterials have the unique property of breaking down over time and being absorbed by the body. As these materials degrade, they release by-products that are metabolized and eliminated. Biodegradable biomaterials are used in applications where temporary support is needed, such as sutures, drug delivery devices, and tissue engineering scaffolds. They eliminate the need for surgical removal of implants after they have fulfilled their purpose. Bioresorbable biomaterials closely resemble biodegradable materials but have a specific focus on tissue replacement. These materials degrade over time as the body's natural healing processes replace them with newly formed tissue. Bioresorbable materials are frequently used in tissue engineering to provide temporary support while new tissue regenerates. They are commonly utilized in cardiovascular stents and wound dressings. The Bioactive Resorbable Biomaterials category combines the features of both bioactive and resorbable biomaterials. These materials not only stimulate tissue growth and integration but also gradually break down and get replaced by the body's tissues. They are often used in applications where long-term tissue integration is required, such as in bone grafts and some tissue engineering constructs. The choice of biomaterial category depends on factors such as the intended use, duration of implantation, and desired tissue response.

3.2 FIBRES IN MEDICAL TEXTILES

Yarns are spun from fibres made of synthetic or natural polymers. Subsequently, these fibres are interlaced or intertwined through weaving or knitting processes to form fabrics tailored for specific products. Only a select few polymers may be processed into fibres for use in the production of medical fabrics because the appropriate polymer must satisfy specific criteria for an effective conversion into a fibrous product. For extrusion, polymers must be meltable or soluble, and they must have linear, long, flexible chain groups that can be orientated and crystallized. By utilizing various natural and synthetic fibre-forming polymers, a wide variety of fibres have been created over time (Morris & Murry, 2020).

According to their intended use, several fibre types, including specialized fibres, commodity fibres, biodegradable fibres, and non-biodegradable fibres, are used in medical textiles.

1) Natural/regenerated fibres and
2) Synthetic fibres.

Cotton, silk, and viscose are two naturally occurring examples of natural fibres that are used in hygiene products as well as non-implantable materials, but there are also regenerated cellulosic fibres (viscose rayon) that are widely utilized in non-implantable applications. In contrast, polyester, polyamide, polypropylene, glass fibre, carbon fibre, and polytetrafluoroethylene (PTFE) are examples of synthetic fibres.

The second categorization is based on the fibre's biodegradability.

1) Biodegradable fibres, and
2) Non-biodegradable fibres.

1) **Biodegradable fibres**: These fibres encompass a group of materials that hold the remarkable capability to undergo degradation over time through natural processes. These fibres are often composed of bio-absorbable materials that feature intricate interconnections of polymer chains. The breakdown process occurs as these polymer chains gradually disintegrate into smaller, water-soluble molecular compounds. This disintegration is facilitated by the hydrolysis of bonds like peptide, hemiacetal, ester, and phosphate and phosphate in the fibre's primary structure. One significant advantage of biodegradable fibre lies in its compatibility with the human body. After degradation, the resulting low molecular weight compounds are assimilated by fluids present in the immediate vicinity of the affected area. Examples of biodegradable fibres frequently employed in the medical sector include cotton, viscose rayon, polyamide, polyurethane, collagen, and alginate. One of the distinguishing characteristics of these fibres is their relatively swift absorption by the body. Within a span of two to three months following implantation, these materials naturally break down, minimizing the need for subsequent removal procedures. This feature is particularly advantageous for applications like wound dressing, surgical sutures, and temporary implants. Likewise, synthetic polymers found in hydrolyzable units such as anhydride, carbonate, ester, and orthoester can also be absorbed into bodily tissue.

2) **Nonbiodegradable fibres:** In contrast, non-biodegradable fibre encompasses materials that do not undergo natural degradation as rapidly as their biodegradable counterparts. These fibres retain their structural integrity over an extended period, offering durability and stability that can be advantageous for certain medical applications. However, their relatively slower rate of breakdown necessitates careful consideration when used within the human body. Materials falling within the category of this fibre include polyester (such as Dacron), polypropylene, polytetrafluoroethylene (PTFE), and carbon. These materials exhibit a more gradual absorption process when introduced into the body. Consequently, they require a longer time frame, generally exceeding six months, for a complete breakdown to occur. This fibre finds its utility in medical applications where prolonged structural support or stability is required. Orthopaedic implants, cardiovascular stents, and certain tissue engineering scaffolds are some examples where non-biodegradable fibres contribute to maintaining the structural integrity of the implant site while allowing for tissue regeneration and healing.

3.3   SPECIALTY FIBRES UTILIZED IN MEDICAL TEXTILES

Polymers offer a high degree of flexibility since their composition and structure can be altered and customized to fit a variety of criteria. Natural polymers encompass chitin, chitosan, alginate, catgut, gelatin, collagen, pectin, heparin, lignin, silk fibroin, and hyaluronan whereas polylactic acid (PLA), polyglycolic acid (PGA), polypropiolactone, and polycaprolactone (PCL) are synthetic polymers the most widely used for inhibiting bacterial activity and fungal growth. Owing to unique biochemical properties, these polymers have unique structural compositions, biocompatibility, biodegradability, and nontoxicity. It paves the way for lightweight implantable materials. But both natural and synthetic polymers also have certain drawbacks. Natural polymers have weak mechanical strength and they degrade fast while synthetic polymers proliferate less and exhibit lower cell adhesion properties. Compared to synthetic polymers, natural polymers exhibit less immunogenicity, and some of them even have innate antimicrobial properties. Synthetic polymers exhibit greater synthesis and modification flexibility, but they have lower cell affinities.

3.3.1 CHITIN NANOFIBRE

It is highly insoluble, inelastic, and the most abundant natural amino polysaccharide polymer. It is obtained from insects, invertebrates, fungi, and the exocuticle portion of crustacean (crab, shrimp, shellfish, and squid) shells. The most important characteristics of this include structural integrity, biodegradability, non-toxicity to cells, and excellent healing. This occurs as crystalline microfibrils and possesses a high percentage of nitrogen. It is employed as dressings for artificial skin. Artificial skin made of chitin nonwoven textiles adheres to the body, promoting the growth of new skin, which accelerates the recovery process and lowers pain. Through advanced processing techniques, chitin is broken down at nanoscale fibres often referred to as chitin nanofibres. Chitin nanofibres possess an impressive combination of mechanical strength, flexibility, and biocompatibility, making them versatile candidates for applications ranging from biomedicine to environmental engineering. The chitin nanofibres exhibit biodegradability and low immunogenicity, rendering them suitable for wound healing scaffolds, drug delivery carriers, and tissue engineering constructs. Their high surface area-to-volume ratio also enhances their interaction with biological systems, enabling efficient absorption of bioactive molecules and facilitating controlled release. Chitin can be transformed into its widely recognized derivative, chitosan, through an enzymatic or chemical deacetylation process (Rasouli et al., 2019).

3.3.2 CHITOSAN NANOFIBRE

Chitosan nanofibres, stemming from this transformation, inherit the same advantageous properties of the precursor, chitin, while also offering tailored personalities due to chitosan's unique chemical composition. These properties include antimicrobial activity, cellular adhesion promotion, and enhanced mechanical properties which collectively make chitosan nanofibres even more appealing for specialized applications. Chitosan is a biodegradable polymer that can be produced synthetically through a process called thermochemical chitin deacetylation in an alkaline environment. It exhibits intrinsic antibacterial properties and high porosity. Owing to unique biochemical properties, these biomaterials can be utilized for tissue engineering, wound dressing, antiaging cosmetics, stem cell technology, and drug and gene delivery. Thus, chitin- and chitosan-based adhesive formulations have

promising applications in medicine and surgery as bioproducts can be easily processed into a wide array of products like hydrogels, membranes, nanofibres, scaffolds, and sponges. Slow drug-release membranes made of chitosan are currently
being developed. Their inherent properties, combined with the ability to customize
their features through modification, underscore their role as a promising platform
for addressing diverse challenges across various disciplines (Kalantari et al., 2019).

3.3.3 ALGINATE NANOFIBRE

Alginate nanofibres, akin to chitin and chitosan, have emerged as a dynamic biomaterial with exceptional attributes and versatile applications. Alginate, a naturally occurring polysaccharide, derived from brown seaweed has gained substantial
attention due to its unique properties such as biocompatibility, biodegradability, and
ability to form hydrogels. Manufacturing Alginate nanofibres involves intricate electrospinning or self-assembly techniques resulting in the development of nanoscale
structures that mimic the extracellular matrix, providing an ideal environment for
cellular growth and tissue regeneration. In the medical field, alginate nanofibres are
harnessed as wound dressings that create a moist environment, enhancing wound
healing while preventing infections. The controlled release of bioactive agents, such
as growth factors or antimicrobial agents, through alginate nanofibres enhances
wound healing processes and reduces patient discomfort. Their high water retention
capacity also aids in maintaining proper moisture levels for optimal healing conditions. Alginate nanofibres are being explored as carriers for controlled drug delivery.
Their porous and interconnected network allows for the encapsulation and sustained
release of therapeutic agents. This control delivery mechanism not only improves
treatment efficacy but also reduces side effects by minimizing systematic exposure
to the drugs. In tissue engineering, alginate nanofibre serves as an essential scaffold
material for cultivating cells and promoting tissue growth. Their porous structure
facilitates nutrient exchange and cell attachment, crucial factors in tissue regeneration. The compatibility with different cell types allows for the creation of tailored
constructs for various applications, ranging from bone and cartilage regeneration to
neural tissue repair. Furthermore, these also hold promise in bio-fabrication and 3D
bioprinting. Their ability to form hydrogels upon contact with divalent ions, such
as calcium, enables the creation of complex three-dimensional structures with high
precision. This is particularly advantageous for engineering intricate tissue architectures for transplantation and regenerative medicine. Alginate nanofibre scaffolds
serve as a foundation for tissue engineering, enabling the regeneration of damaged
or lost tissue like bone, cartilage, and blood vessels. The integration of alginate
nanofibres with living cells generates bioengineered constructs that hold immense
promise in organ transplantation and regenerative medicine. As research in alginate
nanoparticles continues to evolve, ongoing efforts are directed toward optimizing
their mechanical properties, degradation rates, and biocompatibility for specific
applications. The high surface area-to-volume ratio enables efficient interaction with
biological systems. This opens up possibilities for tailored functionalities and applications across different domains. Alginate nanofibres have demonstrated impressive
potential as wound dressing. Their gel-forming ability allows for moisture retention,

essential for maintaining a favorable wound environment providing a conducive environment for tissue regeneration and wound healing. The integration of these innovative biomaterials into the healthcare landscape signifies a transformative step towards more effective and patient-centric approaches to healing, regeneration, and disease management.

3.3.4 CATGUT

Catgut, derived from the submucosa of sheep or goats, is a natural material historically employed as a suture material in medical procedures. This versatile substance owes its unique properties to its biodegradability, characterized by gradual absorption within the body over time, eliminating the need for suture removal. This inherent quality obviates the need for suture removal, thereby reducing the risk of wound complications and the need for additional medical interventions. This is particularly advantageous in challenging surgical sites or in settings where follow-up care might be limited. Beyond sutures, catgut's bio-compatibility and biodegradability have spurred interest in biomedical and pharmaceutical contexts. Catgut's compatibility with living tissue is another significant advantage. It elicits minimal inflammation and tissue reaction, contributing to better wound healing outcomes. Catgut is distinguished by its uniformly fine-grained tissue structure, excellent elasticity, and tensile strength. It has low knot security but is simple to handle. Although synthetic sutures are more commonly used today, catgut's natural origin and gradual absorption continue to find application in specialized surgeries.

3.3.5 COLLAGEN NANOFIBRE

Collagen, a major structural protein in the extracellular matrix of tissues, has gained significant attention in the field of nanotechnology due to its versatile properties and inherent biocompatibility. When processed into nanofibres, collagen exhibits unique features that make it an exciting material for various biomedical applications. Collagen nanofibres can be produced through various techniques including electrospinning, self-assembly, and phase separation. The nanoscale architecture resembles the native structure of tissues, facilitating cellular attachment and growth. This property is particularly advantageous in tissue engineering, where collagen nanofibres serve as scaffolds to support the regeneration of damaged or lost tissues. Their biodegradability aligns with the pace of tissue regeneration, ensuring the scaffold degrades as new tissue forms. Collagen's natural affinity for bioactive molecules allows for precise loading and release, enabling targeted therapies. Moreover, these nanofibres have been explored for wound-healing applications. Their porous structure promotes efficient moisture management and gas exchange, facilitating wound healing and minimizing scarring. Furthermore, collagen fibres have a unique triple helical structure that imparts exceptional mechanical strength and resilience, vital for maintaining structural integrity in biomedical constructs. Importantly, collagen's natural abundance and low immunogenicity enhance its appeal for medical applications. It also displays a distinct hyper-elastic characteristic identical to human tissue in its natural state. Collagen is bacteriostatically resistant which has the innate ability to fight infection and helps to keep the wound clean. When used as a burn dressing, collagen promotes the rapid growth of healthy granulation tissue and speeds up the healing process. It is commonly used in burn recovery, bone reconstruction, and in a variety of dental, orthopedic, cosmetic surgery, and surgical operations. To harness collagen's benefit even further, researchers have explored the integration of collagen fibres with polymeric materials to create composite structures. For making collagen composite fibre, typical polymers include Polylactic acid (PLA), polyurethane (PU), polycaprolactone (PCL), polydioxanone (PDO), hydroxyapatite (HAP), chitosan, poly(N-isopropyl) acrylamide, and others. Collagen is converted into gelatin by denaturing the triple-helix structure. The synergy between collagen fibres and polymeric materials presents a promising avenue for developing advanced biomaterials that cater to the specific needs of diverse biomedical applications (Lin et al., 2019).

3.3.6   GELATIN NANOFIBRE

Gelatin nanofibres are nanoscale fibres composed of gelatin which is obtained from the hydrolysis of collagen-rich animal tissues. They can be engineered to carry bioactive molecules, growth factors, or drugs, enabling controlled release and targeted therapies. Gelatin nanofibres can be fabricated using techniques such as electrospinning, enabling the creation of nanoscale fibrous structures with high surface area and controlled porosity. The mechanical properties of gelatin nanofibres can be tailored by adjusting parameters during the fabrication process. This customization ensures that nanofibres can match the mechanical demands of different tissues. The natural biopolymer is known for its biocompatibility, biodegradability, non-antigenicity, and low immunogenicity. The inherent biocompatibility ensures that gelatin nanofibres interact favorably with cells, promoting cell attachment, proliferation, and tissue regeneration. Gelatin nanofibre is gradually degraded in the body, aligning with the natural degradation processes. These nanofibres gradually break down over time, avoiding the need for scaffold removal in tissue engineering applications. The gelatin nanofibres' surface chemistry allows for easy modification with bioactive molecules, growth factors, and other functional groups. This property enables the precise control of cellular behaviour and tissue-specific responses. Gelatin nanofibres have been explored in regenerating various tissues including skin, bone, cartilage, and nerve. The porous structure and biodegradability make them suitable candidates for wound dressings. Gelatin nanofibres have shown promise in dental and orthopaedic applications, such as guided tissue regeneration, bone regeneration, and heart disease repair. Their ability to support cell adhesion and mimic native structures enhances effectiveness in these contexts.

3.3.7   HYALURONIC ACID (HA) NANOFIBRE

Hyaluronic acid (HA), a naturally occurring glycosaminoglycan, is a key component of the extracellular matrix in connective tissues. Hyaluronic acid nanofibres possess several characteristic properties that make them well-suited for biomedical applications. HA is known for its exceptional water-binding capacity, enabling it to maintain optimal hydration levels in tissues. This property is harnessed in wound healing and skin care applications, where HA nanofibre-based dressing or patches can help create a moist wound environment, facilitating tissue regeneration and reducing scarring. Additionally, HA has inherently immunogenic, biodegradable, and biocompatible properties. Although it occurs naturally in many tissues and fluids, articular cartilage and synovial fluid contain higher concentrations of hyaluronic acid (also known as hyaluronan or hyaluronate). HA is a naturally occurring, non-sulfated, non-protein glycosaminoglycan with unique physicochemical characteristics. It exhibits exceptional viscoelastic properties, characterized by its ability to combine both viscosity and elasticity. This unique combination contributes to its role as an effective lubricant and shock absorber in various biological systems. Furthermore, hyaluronic acid is renowned for its remarkable moisture retention capacity. Its molecular structure enables it to bind and retain water molecules ensuring optimal hydration levels in tissues. The distinct viscoelastic properties of HA give the skin its firmness and flexibility. As a result, HA is extensively utilized for cosmetics and skin care applications. In ophthalmology, HA's are explored for their potential to mimic the natural environment of the cornea. These nanofibres can serve as substrates for corneal cell growth and are investigated for applications such as corneal wound healing. Hyaluronic acid's hygroscopic characteristic is also noteworthy. It has an inherent affinity for water molecules making it effective in creating and maintaining hydrated environments. The inherent lubricating properties make it suitable for eye-related applications including artificial tears and contact lenses that enhance comfort. These nanofibres can be loaded with therapeutic agents enabling targeted delivery and sustained release particularly valuable in localized treatments for conditions like arthritis. Thus, it is used to treat ophthalmic, cutaneous, burns, wounds, and a variety of other medical problems.

3.4 BIORESORBABLE FIBRES UTILIZED IN MEDICAL TEXTILES

3.4.1 POLYLACTIC ACID (PLA)

Polylactic acid (PLA) is a biodegradable polymer with high mechanical strength and processability. Additionally, this aliphatic polymer is thermoplastic with high biocompatibility and high versatility. PLA nanofibres can be produced using various techniques, with electrospinning being one of the most widely employed methods. In this technique, a polymer solution is subjected to an electric field, leading to the formation of ultra-fine fibres with diameters in the nanometer range. This process offers precise control over fibre dimensions, porosity, and architecture (Singhvi et al., 2019). PLA has been used to make sutures and bio-absorbable medical implants. Lactic acid-based melt-spun fibres are biodegradable and have strength and heat resistance characteristics that are comparable to nylon. PLA has proven to be an effective bio-absorbable polymer for orthopaedic implants like resorbable pins, plates, and screws. Bio-absorbable implants don't need to be removed via a second surgery, which minimizes medical expenditures and permits the progressive restoration of tissue over time. The ability of PLA nanofibres to create a moist wound environment, promote gas exchange, and provide a barrier against external contaminants makes them suitable for wound dressing applications. The controlled drug release is particularly valuable in therapies requiring precise dosing over extended periods, such as cancer treatments, wound healing, and localized interventions. Thermoplastic PLA has a broad range of mechanical properties and is highly biocompatible and biodegradable. Resorbable implants also don't interfere with computed tomography scans once they've been resorbed, making it easier for subsequent medical imaging evaluations.

3.4.2 POLYDIOXANONE (PDO)

Polydioxanone (PDO) is a synthetic, biodegradable polymer that has gained prominence in the biomedical field, particularly in the form of nanofibres. A polymer with outstanding mechanical characteristics, shape memory, and minimal inflammatory response is frequently utilized as a commercially available suture. As PDO degrades, it is replaced by new tissue, making it suitable for wound healing and tissue regeneration. Despite its biodegradability, PDO maintains adequate mechanical strength during its functional life. This property is essential for maintaining support and integrity in applications such as tissue engineering scaffolds or surgical sutures. This is well tolerated by the body and exhibits minimal immune response or adverse reactions. These fibres are highly flexible, allowing them to conform to complex anatomical structures. PCL is a semi-crystalline, aliphatic polymer that exhibits adequate biocompatibility.

3.4.3 POLYGLYCOLIC ACID (PGA)

Polyglycolic acid is a highly crystalline, biodegradable, linear aliphatic polyester. It is a synthetic biodegradable polymer that has gained prominence in the medical field, particularly when processed into nanofibres. PGA nanofibre-based wound dressing can also be designed to incorporate bioactive agents, growth factors, or antimicrobial agents, thereby promoting accelerated healing and reducing the risk of infection. These fibres can be loaded with drugs and released in a controlled manner, offering targeted therapies and reducing the frequency of administration. The tunable degradation rate of PGA nanofibres enables the sustained release of drugs over a desired period, optimizing treatment outcomes. When processed into nanofibres, PGA sutures exhibit enhanced flexibility and reduced tissue damage during suturing. These PGA nanofibre sutures are commonly used in various surgical procedures, including gastrointestinal anastomosis, cardiovascular surgeries, and orthopaedic applications.

3.4.4 εPTFE

ePTFE is made up of fluorocarbon polymer in which an elastic, microporous central layer is surrounded by two layers of fibrous polymer producing a three-layered polymer. High strength-to-weight ratio, lower thrombogenicity, and high resistance to allergic reactions and inflammation have made ePTFE a suitable material for valve repair.

3.4.5 POLYETHYLENE TEREPHTHALATE (PET)

Polyethylene terephthalate (PET) is a widely used topical polymer known for its durability, strength, and versatility. In recent years, PET has been explored in nanofibre form for various applications. PET nanofibres exhibit excellent biocompatibility, making them suitable for applications that come into direct contact with their skin or bodily fluids. They have been tested for cytotoxicity and have shown minimal adverse effects on the cell. Additionally, PET nanofibres can undergo various sterilization methods, ensuring their suitability for medical textiles intended for clinical use. PET nanofibre-based dressing can provide a moist wound healing environment while preventing bacterial infiltration, which is essential for promoting rapid and infection-free healing. They have been explored for creating implantable devices such as hernia meshes or vascular grafts, due to their strength and ability to integrate with surrounding tissues. PET nanofibres can be engineered to create barrier fabrics with enhanced properties such as water repellency, breathability, and protection against airborne particles. These fabrics can find application in medical gowns, face masks, and other protective wear. Additionally, the surface modification of PET nanofibres with antimicrobial agents can lead to the development of textiles that inhibit the growth of bacteria, reducing the risk of healthcare-associated infections.

3.5   FIBRE PRODUCTION TECHNIQUES

These techniques involve processes that transform raw materials into fibres with specific properties, ensuring they meet the stringent requirements of medical applications. Fibre production techniques play a critical role in determining the properties, characteristics, and suitability of fibre used in medical textiles. Several common techniques are employed in the medical textile industry for producing fibres.

Spinning: Both synthetic and natural fibres are spun to achieve various properties. Synthetic fibres like polyester or polypropylene are produced through melt spinning where the polymer is melted and extruded through fine nozzles, solidifying as it cools. Natural fibres like silk or cotton are obtained through a process involving the separation of fibres from plant or animal sources, followed by twisting and combing to enhance their strength.

Extrusion: It is commonly used to produce synthetic fibres. It involves melting polymer granules and forcing the molten material through a small hole in a spinneret to create a continuous filament. These filaments are then cooled and solidified to form fibres. The versatility of extrusion allows for control over fibre diameter, shape, and other characteristics.

Electrospinning: This is an advanced technique that involves using an electrical field to draw a charged polymer solution or melt into fine fibres. This process results in fibre with a diameter in the nano-meter to micro-meter range (Chen et al., 2018). These nanofibres find application in wound dressing, drug delivery systems, and tissue engineering scaffolds due to their enhanced interaction with biological environments. Nanofibres featuring different surface morphology (porous, hollow, helicoidal, patterned, aligned, core-shell, and ribbon form) can be produced by carefully choosing the electrospinning technique (coaxial electrospinning, solution electrospinning, melt electrospinning, near field electrospinning, magnetically assisted electrospinning, rotating wire electrospinning), regulating the processing parameters (such as solvent type, its concentration, applied voltage, nozzle collector distance, fibre collector design, temperature, and the rate of ejecting polymer), and adjusting the physicochemical characteristics (Pamu et al., 2022). The process of electrospinning is quick and easy and also it allows for greater control over the morphology of nanofibres. This process entails applying a high voltage into a syringe containing polymeric solution. The self-assembly method produces nanofibres with a lower diameter but as compared to electrospinning, it is more complex to use (Dos Santos et al., 2020).

In spite of electrospinning's high degree of adaptability, the convenience of its use, and the low price of the processing system, there are still several obstacles preventing its widespread industrial implementation.

Wet spinning: This technique is utilized to produce fibre from polymers that are dissolved in a solvent. The polymer solution is extruded into a coagulating bath, where the solvent is removed, causing the fibres to solidify. This technique is commonly employed for producing fibres with specific properties such as high tensile strength or biocompatibility. Depending on the needs of the intended substance, they are made from a variety of monomers in variable amounts (Vaishya et al., 2018).

Melt blowing: It is used to produce nonwoven fibres by extruding a melted polymer through a fine nozzle onto a moving conveyor. The fibres solidify quickly forming a nonwoven mat. These fibres have their application in surgical masks, and wound dressing due to their filtration and absorption capabilities.

Layer-by-layer fabrication: It is an advanced additive manufacturing technique used for producing fibres with complex structures. This technique involves depositing layers of material on a substrate, building up the fibre's structure layer by layer. This is used for creating innovative medical textiles such as artificial tissues or implants with precisely controlled properties.

Electrostatic Spinning (Electro-spraying): Similar to electrospinning, it employs an electric field to generate fibres, droplets, or particles from a liquid solution. It is utilized for drug delivery systems, wound healing dressings (Chen et al., 2017), and controlled release applications (Mohandas et al., 2021).

Melt electrospinning: It is a specialized variant of the electrospinning technique. This is particularly useful for processing high melting point polymers that cannot dissolve in solvents. It is primarily used to make fibres from polymers, such as polypropylene (PP) and polyethylene (PE). It offers solvent-free fibre deposition that can be controlled precisely at a cheaper cost of production with improved safety and an enhanced method of manufacturing.

Self-assembly techniques: It involves a spontaneous arrangement of molecules in ordered structures driven by their inherent properties. These fibres can exhibit controlled drug release, enhanced mechanical properties, and improved biocompatibility. They are utilized in drug delivery systems and tissue engineering scaffolds.

3D printing/Additive manufacturing: Additive manufacturing is revolutionizing the production of fibres for medical textiles. It allows for the precise layer-by-layer deposition of materials, enabling the creation of complex and customized fibre structures. They are used to produce implants, prosthetics, tissue scaffolds, and even wearable medical devices. This technique offers unmatched versatility in tailoring fibres to meet specific patient needs.

Surface modification: This technique alters the surface properties of fibres to achieve specific functionalities. Techniques like plasma treatment, chemical grafting, and nanoparticle deposition can introduce antimicrobial properties, enhanced biocompatibility, or increased adhesion to biological tissues. Surface-modified fibres are valuable for wound dressings, implants, and surgical textiles.

Smart fibre technologies: Smart fibres incorporate sensors, actuators, or responsive materials to detect and respond to external stimuli. These fibres can monitor physiological parameters, deliver drugs in response to specific conditions, or adapt to changes in the environment. Smart fibres find application in wearable medical devices.

For point-of-care cancer diagnosis, the detection of circulating tumor cells in cancer patients, the diagnosis of malaria, and the detection of urea, glucose, cholesterol, bacteria, etc., nanofibres have been investigated as ultrasensitive biosensors.

3.6   ESSENTIAL PROPERTIES FOR MEDICAL TEXTILES

In the world of healthcare, the textiles we encounter go beyond ordinary fabrics. Medical textiles play a vital role, offering properties tailored to the unique demands of the medical field. These properties not only ensure comfort, durability, and safety but also extend to specialized attributes that empower these textiles to contribute significantly to diagnostics, therapeutics, and overall healthcare efficacy. In this context, delving into the pivotal properties that underpin the design and fabrication of medical textiles becomes paramount, ushering in an era of innovation that redefines the very fabric of healthcare. The properties required for medical textiles are driven by the specific medical application they are intended for.

Important characteristics of a medical product include:

- **Strength**: The textile substrate should possess enough strength for durability. The term "strength" refers to the ability of fibres, yarns, or fabrics to resist breaking when subjected to force. Depending on how the force is applied, the strength may be tensile, bending, or bursting strength.
- **Elasticity**: Elasticity is a quality that describes a material's capacity to recover from deformation caused by the application of force. A desirable quality of the cloth is that it shouldn't lose its shape during application. Higher elasticity means better deformation recovery. Elasticity is affected by the length of time a material is stretched.
- **Uniformity**: In order to maintain overall mechanical qualities, fibre uniformity is crucial.
- **Ability to be sterilized**: This quality pertains to the material's ability to be clean in the presence of bacterial contamination.

- **Biocompatibility**: They should not cause adverse reactions when they come into contact with the human body. This property is crucial to avoid irritation, allergic reactions, and other negative responses.
- **Absorbency**: Textiles used in wound dressing, surgical drapes, and patient bedding must possess high absorbency to effectively manage bodily fluids, exudates, and spills. It is necessary for maintaining hygiene and preventing infections.
- **Barrier properties**: Certain medical textiles such as surgical gowns, masks, and drapes need to act as a barrier to prevent transmission of micro-organisms between healthcare professionals and patients. These textiles should effectively block bacteria and viruses while remaining breathable.

To promote healing, mitigate negative side effects, and improve patient compliance, an optimal textile material utilized in the medical domain should meet certain standards. Significant characteristics of a medical product include elasticity; biocompatibility; better resistance to germs, alkaline, or acidic substances; superior dimensional stability; being free from contamination or impurities; proficient absorption or repellency properties; and commendable air permeability (Morris & Murray, 2020). The materials intended for medical textiles must fulfill stringent criteria of being non-toxic, non-allergic, non-carcinogenic, and sterilizable without undergoing any alteration to their inherent physical or chemical attributes. Numerous nanofibres fabrication techniques are available including electrospinning, melt-blown spinning, rotary jet spinning, template synthesis, bicomponent extrusion, centrifugal spinning, self-assembly, and thermal induced phase separation, etc. for producing distinctive morphological structures in accordance with medical applications. The ultimate goal is to enhance the adhesion, flexibility, and serviceability of the implantable fibrous material. Medical textiles are used in the form of fibre, yarn, fabric, and composite structures. In comparison to other biomaterials like metals and ceramics, biotextiles have thinner, stronger, more flexible, and lighter structures. They have also already shown that they are superior at withstanding compression, tension, stress, and bending forces. We observe that a wide range of innovative fibre-forming polymers with special qualities is currently being developed. Until now, antibiotics (like ciprofloxacin, sulfadiazine tetracycline, and gentamicin), metallic nanoparticles (e.g., silver nanoparticles), and/or natural items (such as honey and chitosan) have largely been used as antibacterial agents. These agents are added to the structure of the dressing to boost their antibacterial capabilities. These materials also have distinctive electroactive, elastomeric, resorbable, responsive, and "smart" capabilities. Surgical apparel needs to exhibit good wear comfort in addition to the barrier effect because healthcare staff needs to wear them for several hours while executing their occupational task. The ideal surgical attire should resist liquid intrusion while allowing excess body heat to be distributed through the movement of air and moisture. The fabric's permeability and elasticity influence comfort properties. The overall fit is a crucial factor to take into account for surgical clothing. It should not create hindrances while healthcare staff are performing their job. To boost the level of protection offered by surgical gowns without sacrificing comfort or breathability, manufacturers have adopted cutting-edge fabric production techniques and new seaming procedures. Medical gowns can be "disposable/single-use" or "reusable/multi-use."

Additional materials, such as coatings, copolymerization, laminates, composite materials, and films, are frequently used to enhance the barrier resistance, absorbency, and non-slippage performance of both single-use and reusable items. Besides this, techniques for enhancing the longevity of applied finishes on natural fibre-based products, especially antimicrobial and antifungal have been researched. These techniques include oxygen plasma treatment, ultrasonic technology, UV radiation, surface bonding, and enzymatic treatments (Karim et al., 2020). Graphene-modified textiles using various processes have recently been described by researchers. The qualities of fabrics can be improved by adding graphene or graphene derivatives to polymers or textiles. This can enhance mechanical strength, antibacterial properties, resistance to abrasion, and inhibit the transmission of heat and gases. Woven textiles made of graphene also have exceptional flexibility. PPE fabrics might incorporate all these properties in a single treatment (Bhattacharjee et al., 2019). Gloves should be comfortable, soft, flexible, and easy to put on. In recent times polymers have gained huge attraction due to their unique elasticity, durability, biocompatible, mechanical strength, non-toxic, and non-allergic features. In the ever-evolving landscape of medical textiles, these essential properties underscore the transformative impact of specialized fabrics. Table 3.1 outlines strategies for introducing/loading drugs into medical textile substrates. Medical textiles play an indispensable role in advancing patient care, diagnostics, and therapeutic intervention ultimately redefining the very fabric of healthcare (Prabhu, 2019). Figure 3.1 illustrates the key attributes of medical textiles.

3.7   STRATEGIES FOR INTRODUCING/LOADING DRUGS INTO MEDICAL TEXTILE SUBSTRATES

TABLE 3.1

Strategies for loading drug onto the medical textile substrate: techniques methodology and benefits

Method/Strategy	Definition	Applied Products	Advantages	Drawbacks
Direct Impregnation	Soaking textiles in drug solutions	Wound dressings, bandages	Easy application, targeted delivery	Uneven drug distribution, limited loading
Electrospinning	Spinning drug-polymer blends electrostatically	Scaffolds, wound dressings	Controlled release, high surface area	Complex setup, potential drug damage
Layer-by-Layer	Sequential adsorption of drug and polymers	Implants, stents	Precise control, tailored release	Time-consuming, labour-intensive
Sol-gel	Mixing drugs with gel-like matrix	Bone grafts, dressings	Controlled release, compatibility	Slow release, restricted loading
Encapsulation	Trapping drugs in protective nanocarriers	Microcapsules, textiles	Sustained release, protection	Complex process, potential toxicity

TABLE 1.1 (Continued)

Strategies for loading drug onto the medical textile substrate: techniques methodology and benefits

Method/Strategy	Definition	Applied Products	Advantages	Drawbacks
Coating	Applying a drug-coated layer on textiles	Implants, wearables	Targeted delivery, versatile use	Mechanical wear, coating detachment
Microencapsulation	Encasing drug particles in protective shells	Patches, wound dressings	Extended stability, controlled release	Large particles, limited breathability
Printing	Printing drug solutions onto textiles	Wearable drug systems	Customizable patterns, non-invasive	Limited loading, printing precision
Nanofibres	Creating drug-infused nanofibre structures	Tissue engineering, dressings	Controlled release, large surface area	Technical complexity, higher cost
Supercritical Fluid Processing	Infusing textiles with drugs using supercritical fluids	Gowns, drapes	Uniform distribution, gentle process	Expensive equipment, specialized setup

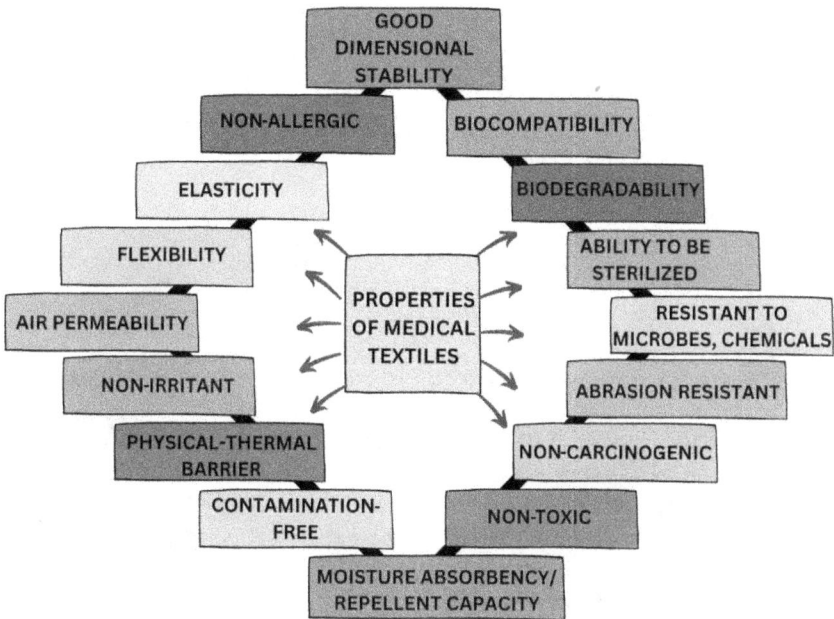

FIGURE 3.1 Key attributes of medical textiles

3.8 CLASSIFICATION OF MEDICAL TEXTILES

In the realm of healthcare and modern medical practices, textiles have transcended their conventional role as mere fabrics, emerging as sophisticated materials with tailored functionalities. The classification of medical textiles represents a systematic approach to categorizing these versatile materials based on their inherent properties, applications, and intended end use. These textile materials may be used for internal as well as external purposes. Figure 3.2 depicts the classification framework of medical textiles: exploring diverse applications and materials.

I. **Internal application of medical textiles**

   This segment consists of textile products that are intended for usage inside the human body and are biocompatible. There are numerous restorative applications for implantable materials. For cartilage repair, materials like polydioxanone and PGA/PLA (polyglactin, vicryl) copolymer are utilized (Maruf Hasan et al., 2019).

II. **External application of medical textiles**

   Washable, disposable, or single-use products are available for health and hygiene. The market for medical textiles is heavily dominated by this category.

Table 3.2 details the many types of textile materials used in this category, along with the fibres they are made of, their major method of manufacturing, their characteristics, and their uses (Anand & Kennedy, 2007) (Vaishya et al., 2018) (Parvin et al., 2020).

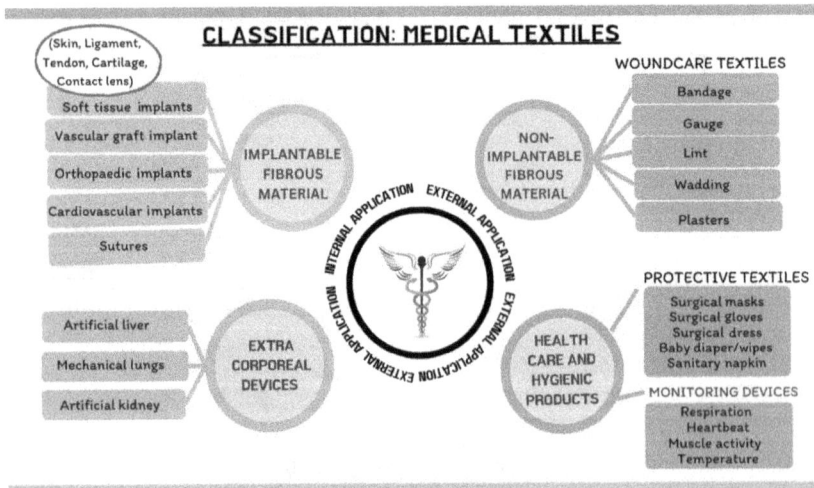

FIGURE 3.2 Classification framework of medical textiles: exploring diverse applications and materials

TABLE 3.2

Textile materials in healthcare: fibres, production techniques, properties, and applications

S. NO	Particular	Fibre	Production Technique	Properties	Application
		Internal Application			
1.	**Suture**	Monofilament/ Multifilament **Absorbable/ Biodegradable**—cotton, viscose, collagen, alginate, chromic catgut, polyamide (PA), polyglycolic acid (PGA), polylactic acid (PLA) polydioxanone **Non-absorbable/ Nonbiodegradable**— nylon, Polyester (PET), polypropylene (PP), and polytetrafluoroethylene (PTFE)	Braiding, twisting	Non-sliding, sterilizable, biocompatible, good tensile strength, flexible, re-absorbable, non-allergic, good knotting, and easy handling	Used to tie off bleeding veins, bind tissue, seal an incision, and stitch wounds
2.	**Orthopaedic implants** Artificial bones	Reinforcedcompositefibre- Polypropylene (PP), Polyethylene (PE), Polysulphone (PS), Polycarbonate (PC), Hyaluronic acid (HA), Polylactic acid (PLA), Polydioxanone (PDS), Polyglycolic acid (PGA), Polycaprolactone (PCL), Polydimethylsulphoxide (PDMS), Polyacetal, silicone	Braiding, weaving, nonwoven fabrication, moulding, 3D printing, casting	High abrasion resistance, robust toughness, light weight, ease of fabrication, biocompatible biostable, and nontoxic	Used to repair, replace musculoskeletal tissue and stabilize bones, bone fracture fixation, joint replacement, bone reconstruction
3.	**Soft Tissue implants** Artificial cornea Artificial skin Artificial cartilage Artificial ligament Artificial tendon	Composite fibre **Natural polymers**— chitin, chitosan, collagen, cellulose **Synthetic materials**— Carbon fibre, silicon rubber, polyester, polyamide polyurethane, Polymethyl methacrylate, Polymethyl methacrylate, cornea-silicone	Braiding, woven, nonwoven, 3D printing, layer-by-layer fabrication, moulding	Flexible, resistant to chemical degradation, non-irritant, bacterial resistant, non-carcinogenic biocompatible, biostable, biodegradable	Used to reconstruct artificial organs such as ears, nose, cornea replacement, skin grafts, cartilage replacement and repair, ligament reconstruction and support

TABLE 3.2 (Continued)

Textile materials in healthcare: fibres, production techniques, properties, and applications

S. NO	Particular	Fibre	Production Technique	Properties	Application
4.	**Cardiovascular implants** Artificial Heart valve Artificial Vascular graft	Polymer composites Polyurethane (PU) elastomers, expanded Polytetrafluorethylene (ePTFE), polyethylene terephthalate (PET)	Knitting, woven, coating, moulding, machining, braiding	High tensile strength, durability, flexibility, biocompatibility, resistance to infection, and ease of implantation	Heart valve replacement, vascular grafts, blood vessel replacement and repair
		Collagens, elastin, fibrinogen, Polycaprolactone (PCL)	Knitted, woven	Flexible, good dimensional stability, infection resistance, biocompatibility	Function as an artificial conduit or substitute for an abnormality in veins or arteries

External Application

S. NO	Particular	Fibre	Production Technique	Properties	Application
1. (i) a) b) c) d)	**Non-Implantable Textiles** Wound care Base Material Absorbent Pad Wound contact layer	Viscose, Cotton, viscose Silk, viscose, polyamide, polyethylene Chitosan	Woven, nonwoven Nonwoven, Woven, nonwoven, knitted Electrospun	Light weight, high air permeability, Cytocompatibility, degree of adherence, anti-bacterial, ability to be sterilized, physical and thermal barrier, drug load capacity, non-irritant, non-toxic	Offer padding to protect wounds, absorb exudate, provide moisture, and protect against germs
(ii) a) b) c) d)	Bandages Elastic crepe bandage Compression bandage Light support bandage Orthopaedic cushion bandage	Cotton, viscose, elastomers, polyamide. Cotton, elastomers, polyamide. Cotton, viscose, elastomers. Cotton, viscose, Polyester, polypropylene, polyurethane	Weaving, nonwoven Fabrication, knitting	Elasticity, extensibility, comfortable	Provides comfort and secures the dressing over the wound in place
(iii)	Gauze	Cotton, viscose	Weaving, nonwoven fabrication	Moisture absorbency, contamination-free, anti-allergic	Prevent the entry of bacteria by forming a protective barrier
(iv)	Lint	Cotton	Weaving	Lightweight, high vapor permeability	Protective dressing for minor burn treatment and in first aid
(v)	Wadding	Viscose, wood pulp	Non-woven fabrication	High absorbency	Absorbent material for wound exudate

TABLE 3.2 (Continued)

Textile materials in healthcare: fibres, production techniques, properties, and applications

S. NO	Particular	Fibre	Production Technique	Properties	Application
(vi)	Plasters	Cotton, viscose, polyester, plastic film, polypropylene, glass	Woven, nonwoven fabrication, knitted	Strength, elasticity	Prevents injured area mobility, and restricts unnecessary movements
(vii)	Optic fibres	Glass, or plastic	Drawing and deposition	Flexibility, inert to chemicals, lightweight, small-sized, durability, cost-effectiveness, and immune to electromagnetic interference	Visualization of internal organs and tissue via bodily orifices
2.	**Extra Corporeal Device** Artificial Liver	Carbon fibre, hollow viscose, poly (ether urethane)	Hollow fibre membrane	Biostable, excellent mechanical properties, Biocompatible	Support or replacement of organ functions, to filter and discard patient plasma and provide fresh blood
	Artificial Kidney/ Dialyzer	Chitin, hollow viscose, hollow polyester, cuprammonium hollow fibre, PAN, Polymethylmethacrylate.	Hollow fibre membrane, layer-by-layer fabrication	Moderate mechanical strength and permeability	To purge waste product from the blood, removing metabolic substances, adjusting pH and electrolytes, and ultrafiltering excess water
	Mechanical Lungs	Hollow silicone, silicone membrane, hollow polypropylene, Polysulphone	Microporous membrane	High permeability for gases but low permeability for liquid	To provide fresh supply of blood while removing carbon dioxide
3.	**Healthcare and Hygiene Textiles** Surgical mask Surgical cap Surgical gloves Surgical gown Surgical drape Bedding Baby diapers/sanitary napkins/wipes Surgical hosiery	Cotton, viscose, polyester, polyethylene, composites	Nonwoven fabrication, weaving, Latex dipping	Air permeability, bacterial filtration, splash resistance, lightweight, non-allergic	For hygienic precaution, provides protection against microbes, bodily liquids, and particulate material, Infection control

3.9   THE MANUFACTURING PROCESS OF MEDICAL TEXTILES

Weaving and knitting are traditional techniques used to create fabrics by interlocking yarns. Weaving involves interlacing warp and weft yarns at right angles, creating stable and structured fabrics. Knitting, on the other hand, forms fabrics through interlocking loops of yarns. Nonwoven fabrics are manufactured by bonding or interlocking fibres using mechanical, thermal, or chemical processes. For particular goods like sutures and ligament prostheses that demand superior mechanical qualities in the longitudinal direction, filaments can be braided into three-dimensional braids. Techniques such as melt blowing and spun-bonding are utilized to create nonwoven fabrics with specific properties like breathability, barrier protection, and absorbency. In addition to significantly reducing the cost of production, this technique leads to producing goods with porous and highly absorbent structures.

Medical textiles often require additional functionalities beyond their inherent properties. Functionalization involves incorporating additives or treatments to enhance properties such as antimicrobial activity, moisture management, or drug delivery. These processes extend the utility of medical textiles, enabling them to address specific medical challenges.

For the purpose of making textiles more resistant to water, stains, wrinkles, and infections like bacteria and fungi, recent developments in nanotechnology and materials science have contributed to the development of surface treatment and modification techniques imparting functional finish (Artain et al., 2011). The most typical types of coating for textile materials include electrospun nanofibres, colloidal nanoparticles, nano-capsules, metallic nanoparticles, plasma-sputtered coatings, and cold plasma polymerized coatings. Numerous coating techniques exist, including spraying, dipping, painting, rolling, etc. However, ultrasonic and microwave technologies are seen as novel approaches that can get around the limitations of conventional approaches. Plasma technology's primary function is to add hydrophilic groups to textiles that are utilized as blood filters or filtering membranes for dialysis systems. Sterilization of medical textiles is another use for plasma therapy. Recent studies have concentrated on novel structures including hydrogels, dendrimers, polymer micelles, liposomes, and polymer nanoparticles each with their distinct applications. Highly branching, star-shaped macromolecules known as dendrimers find utility in surface modification, drug delivery, enhancing dyeing process, and infusing fabric with enduring aromas. Micelles are amphiphilic polymer-based spheres with sizes between 5 and 100 nm (Yu et al., 2019). Three-dimensional polymer networks known as hydrogels are capable of absorbing large volumes of fluids. They also have numerous desirable properties, including high biocompatibility, oxygen permeability, minimal interfacial tension, non-toxic nature, effective bio-adhesion, mucoadhesion capabilities, and ease of surface modification to precisely conform to the contours of the intended application area (Atanasova et al., 2021). Nano-coatings, which comprise thin films, nanocapsules, and nanoparticles, are widely utilized in biofiltration components for extracorporeal devices, enhancement of medical implants, fabrication of textile substrates conducive to cell growth, and other medical textiles.

Quality assurance and testing are of utmost importance throughout the manufacturing process. Rigorous testing is conducted to ensure that the textile materials meet the required specifications, performance standards, and regulatory guidelines. This step is essential to verify that the textiles are safe, effective, and suitable for their intended medical applications. Once the medical textiles are manufactured and tested, they undergo sterilization, to eliminate any potential microbial contamination. After sterilization, the textiles are carefully packed to maintain their stability until they are ready for use in medical procedures. The manufacturing process of medical textiles is a complex blend of traditional techniques, cutting-edge technologies, and quality control measures. The final product ensures safety and optimal performance in medical applications.

3.10 APPLICATION OF MEDICAL TEXTILES

Medical textiles have revolutionized the healthcare textile segment by offering a diverse array of applications that extend well beyond conventional fabric functions. These specialized textiles possess properties tailored to the unique demands of various medical contexts, encompassing tissue regeneration, drug delivery, physiotherapy, healthcare applications, hygienic textiles, wearable sensors, and woundcare textiles. Figure 3.3 shows the application of Medical Textiles: Transforming Healthcare through Innovation.

3.10.1 TISSUE REGENERATION

This technology is a boon for millions of patients who suffer organ failure. Nanofibre emerged as a favorable solution that imitates the permeable topography of the extracellular matrix facilitating tissue regeneration. Due to high surface area,

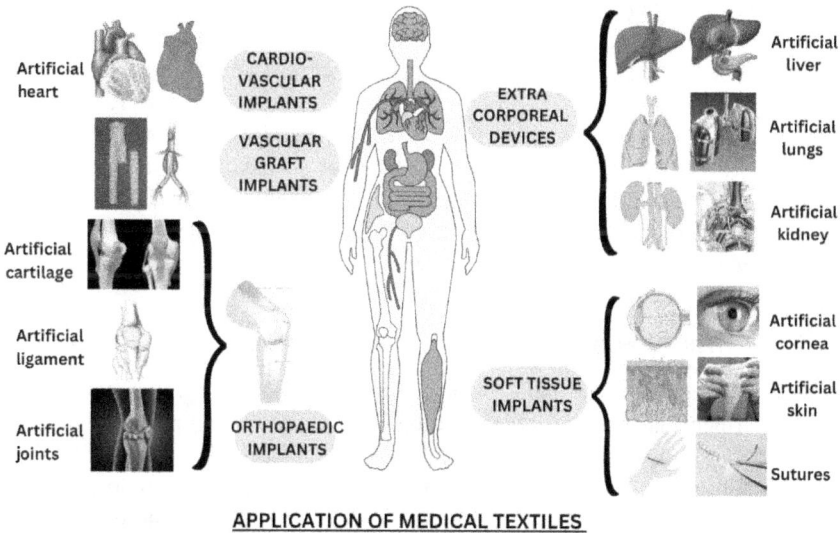

APPLICATION OF MEDICAL TEXTILES

FIGURE 3.3 Application of medical textiles: transforming healthcare through innovation

these nanofibres offer optimized absorption of exudate with adequate ventilation. Additionally, an antimicrobial finish can be imparted to the material. Different polymeric nanofibres are utilized in tissue engineering for the growth of inner cells that possess a size of less than 1μm. Polymers including polyethylene, Polyglycolic acid (PGA), polylactic acid (PLA), polydioxanone (PDO), Polycaprolactone (PCL), Polycarbonate, Polydimethylsuphoxide, and polymethacrylate are utilized in medical textiles (Vaishya et al., 2018). Nanofibrous scaffold coated with collagen helps improve restoration of denuded epithelium surface. Nowadays, matrices made of collagen and hyaluronan are among the most widely used scaffolds In medicine because they provide substrates that are typically crucial components of natural articular cartilage. A revolutionary method for producing 3D porous scaffolds for bone tissue engineering is 3D printing. Composites made of PLA have been utilized to make bone clips. The 3D-printed PLA, PLA/hydroxyapatite, and PLA/hydroxyapatite/silk composite bone clips created by Yeon et al. (2018) were successful. A biodegradable 3D-printed scaffold with high biocompatibility was produced by Grigora et al. (2023). The textile material provides a supportive structure that guides cell growth and enables the regeneration of damaged or lost tissues. Tissue-engineered constructs crafted from biocompatible and biodegradable textiles offer immense potential in fields like skin grafts, bone regeneration, and organ transplantation.

3.10.2 DRUG DELIVERY

The textiles can be engineered to encapsulate drugs and release them in a controlled manner, enhancing therapeutic outcomes. Drug carriers for current wound dressings include hydrocolloids, hydrogels, alginates, silicone gels, polyurethane foams, and films. A polydioxanone nanotextile implant containing paclitaxel was created, and the device was enhanced for continuous long-term drug administration for oncological purposes (Padmakumar et al., 2019).

A transdermal drug delivery patch is a multilayer permeable membrane that slowly releases drug solution or suspension. The earliest membrane patch structure was composed of three layers: an adhesive layer, a backing layer to regulate drug release, and a reservoir layer that holds a gel or liquid medication. Matrix patch featuring textile pad has drug within its polymer structure and is held in direct contact with skin. Later, extremely light, thin, relatively comfortable, and flexible patches that combined the drug and the adhesive into a single layer were developed (Atanasova et al., 2021).

3.10.3 PHYSIOTHERAPY

Medical textiles also contribute to the realm of physiotherapy by providing supportive garments that aid in rehabilitation and recovery. Compression garments, braces, and orthopaedic textiles offer stability and enhanced joint mobility. Knitted orthopaedic supports represent a specific category of medical compression textiles, designed to cater to a wide spectrum of anatomical needs. These textiles find application in the development of braces for various body parts, including knee, wrist, ankle, shoulder, and elbow, as well as providing support for the calf, lumbar region, and back. Additionally, by exerting significant mechanical pressure upon the targeted body area, compression products with elastomeric fibre function to stabilize, compress, and support the underlying tissues and limit mobility. Elastic crepe bandages are used to provide muscular relaxation for sprained wrists and ankles. Compression bandages, when applied at constant tension, exert the required amount of compression used to treat deep vein thrombosis, leg ulceration, and varicose veins. Orthopaedic compression bandages offer support to the fractured bones (Xiong & Tao, 2018).

3.10.4 HEALTHCARE APPLICATIONS

They form the foundation of surgical attire, including gowns, masks, and gloves, ensuring the safety of healthcare professionals and patients. Additionally, medical textiles find use in hospital bedding, patient garments, and even operating room drapes contributing to hygiene, comfort, and infection control. The textiles extensively employed for medical protection encompass a range of materials, including polymer-coated textiles, polypropylene spun bond/melt-blown/spun bond (SMS) nonwoven fabric, and polyethylene breathable film/nonwoven composite fabrics. Notably, researchers have crafted multi-layer face masks with alternate hydrophilic and hydrophobic layers.

Embedding fibre optics technology in textile material enables sensing signals and allows real-time monitoring. During surgery, the patient may be covered with specialized cloths known as surgical covers. As incise drapes, these coverings are positioned over the surgical region. The highly strong and absorbent material of the drapes protects the patient as well as any tubes or wires below, allowing the surgeon to work without restriction. Fibre optic biosensors can be used to access small or challenging-to-reach bodily parts and are electrically safe. They have also been employed as catheters and endoscopic tools, as well as applications including the analysis of tissues or biological fluids. In addition, it offers therapeutic treatment of jaundice in newborns and invigorates hair growth (Gong et al., 2019). Precast splints and supportive garments are among the variety of bandages available for healthcare applications.

3.10.5 HYGIENIC TEXTILES

Hygienic textiles are aimed at maintaining cleanliness and minimizing infection risks. They include antimicrobial linens for healthcare facilities, bedding for burn patients, feminine hygiene products, and adult/baby diapers. Diapers and sanitary napkins are designed to provide comfort, absorbency, and leak protection. PPE is regarded as an essential infection control strategy since it aims to reduce the risk of cross-infections and mitigate the hazards associated with exposure to potentially contaminated bodily fluids. Aprons, gowns, coveralls, masks or respirators, gloves, foot covers, and goggles are all examples of protective gear for healthcare or medical purposes. The medical mask is made of a three-layered nonwoven SMS structure: a spun-bonded inner layer to absorb moisture, a melt-blown middle layer of polypropylene that filters and provides protection against airborne particles, and the spun-bonded waterproof outer layer that serves as a barrier between the user and external fluids.

3.10.6 Wearable Sensors

Wearable sensors have ushered in a new era of healthcare innovation, seamlessly integrating technology into our daily lives. To this end, optical fibres have played a pivotal role in creating smart textiles with embedded sensors, redefining the possibilities of health monitoring. Real-time monitoring of physiological data like heart rate, respiration, muscle activity, temperature, and blood sugar level can be accomplished with the use of wearable nanofibre-based sensors (Dos Santos et al., 2020). Plastic optical fibres, micro-bend fibres, and macro-bend hetero-core optical fibres with multimode fibre transmission have been woven into the fabric to create smart textiles. Koyama et al. (2018) have fabricated a novel textile incorporating single mode transmission hetero core optical fibre sensor in a radius curvature of 6 mm, woven together with wool fibre into the textile substrate, placed close to the chest for monitoring respiratory and cardiac frequencies. Li et al. (2018) developed a wearable health monitoring device that resembles skin and can simultaneously monitor breathing in real-time and the blood pressure of the human radial arteries; it is created using a sensitive, flexible, and reasonably priced photonics sensor made of polydimethylsiloxane (PDMS) that incorporates hybrid plasmonic microfibre knot resonator (HPMKR). Also, Electronic footwear has been developed to keep track of body posture and movement patterns. Elderly people with lumbar spinal stenosis have had their walking capacity evaluated using electronic shoes. Additionally, electronic socks have been created to monitor and track the body's important functions. Electronic socks composed of polyamide, silver-coated cotton, and piezoresistive fibres were developed to prevent pressure ulcers in the feet of diabetic patients (Koyama et al., 2018).

3.10.7 Wound Care Textiles

The specialized wound care dressing manages moisture, promotes wound healing, prevents infection, and minimizes scarring. Effective wound care is essential for ensuring the timely and hygienic healing of wounds, particularly when dealing with chronic or compromised cases. Patients with a compromised immune system, particularly those suffering from diabetes and burn cases are more prone to the risk of infection. In response to these challenges, medical textiles have emerged as a critical solution offering a range of wound dressing materials. To facilitate the early healing process, wound dress material from woven pad to hydrogel dressing is available. It aims at tissue regeneration along with providing comfort, protection against dust particles, and shock absorption. Depending on the depth of the wound, the type of wound, and the exudate a judicious selection of bandage should be made (Dhivya et al., 2015). New wound care strategy focuses on moist wound healing, in which wound exudates are permitted to remain in contact with the wound area rather than being wicked away by conventional dressing.

Healing agents are microencapsulated on the textile material surface, releasing loaded drugs to repair damaged cells. Furthermore, nanostructured scaffolds create a continuous filament structure that offers a platform for regenerating damaged tissues and organs. The suspended nano-sized particle serves the purpose of treating injured body parts. The high porosity of nanofibre exhibits capillary effect to a higher degree. Oxygen and nutrients are supplied through interconnected pores of nanofibres enabling cell growth and regeneration of tissue. Hydrocolloids are applied on lightly to moderately exuding wounds and have the ability to debride wounds and absorb wound exudates. In addition to being bacteria-resistant but permeable to water vapour, these dressings are also suggested for treating paediatric wound, due to the fact that they don't hurt when removed.

Alginate dressings are suitable for wounds with higher fluids discharge but not for dry wounds, third-degree burn wounds, or severe injuries. Furthermore, these dressings necessitate supplementary dressing due to the existent risk of wound area dehydration that slows down the healing process. In addition to its barrier function of inhibiting the entry of microbes at the wound site, the antimicrobial dressing also promotes the immune system and fibroblast/keratinocyte migration, which aids in the healing process (Kalantari et al., 2019). A composite wound dressing made of PLGA, Aloe Vera, and lipid nanoparticles was created by Garcia-Orue et al. (2019) for treatment of chronic wounds. In another research study, Baghersad et al. (2018) biodegradable electrospun Gelatin/Aloe-vera/Poly(-caprolactone) hybrid nanofibrous scaffolds that were developed with improved drug delivery, biodegradability, and antibacterial activity, for use as skin substitutes. Perumal et al. (2017) used electrospun PLA/HPG nanofibres loaded with curcumin, which exhibited high hydrophilicity, swelling, and drug uptake and promoted better cell viability, adhesion, and proliferation, to assess wound healing in vitro. Fereydouni et al. (2019) also synthesized curcumin nanofibres for wound healing applications which demonstrated that curcumin accelerates the epidermis's re-epithelialization process and promotes neovascularization and collagen deposition at lower concentrations in the in vitro and in vivo models. Additionally, it stimulates the migration of a variety of cells, including myofibroblasts, fibroblasts, endothelial cells, and macrophages in the wound bed.

3.11 ADVANTAGES OF ADVANCED TECHNOLOGY

One of the standout advantages of advanced technology in medical textiles is the significant reduction in required drug dosage. Modern systems enable precise drug release at specific sites, thereby minimizing unnecessary dosing. The targeted approach ensures that therapeutic agents are delivered directly to the intended area, optimizing treatment efficacy and minimizing potential side effects. Advanced technology empowers medical textiles to achieve site-specific drug release. This approach maximizes the therapeutic impact while minimizing the risk of adverse reactions. The increased bioavailability not only accelerates the healing process but also potentially reduces the frequency of required dose administrations. Additionally, it has enhanced the possibilities of integrating diverse kinetics with different local and systematic medications, increasing the duration of drug release. The prolonged-release capability is particularly beneficial in scenarios where sustained therapy is required. It also provides precise control over the toxicity and bioavailability of drugs (Aggarwal et al., 2022).

3.12   FUTURE APPLICATIONS AND CONCLUSION

The future prospects lie in the effort of scientists and professionals to open new avenues for monitoring, creating, and upgrading miniaturized value-added products. This is likely meant to stimulate healing and counteract infection with cost-effective, functionalized, sophisticated nanofabricated structures. Future research will use nanotechnology to construct Smart and Interactive Textiles (SMIT) that can detect electrical, thermal, chemical, magnetic, or other inputs. Structural nanocomposites are expected to make products smaller and lighter with cost-effective benefits. The future development of materials for effective local or transdermal treatments may be enabled by the loading of polymeric micelles with intelligent responsiveness to various stimuli onto textile materials. Invariably, recommendations are made that the plethora of scientific and application advancement studies regarding nanomaterials be complemented by comprehensive studies on the future impact on human health and the environment. Both private and public sectors are promoting research in these many areas. In general, we can anticipate that as more nano-based products will enter the market, many pressing health problems faced by a large segment of the population will be reduced to a minimum. While the opportunities appear promising, current challenges that need to be addressed include improving the lifetime of implants, developing therapies that promote cell repair, and creating versatile nanodevices. The commercialization of novel nano-products through extensive research and industry collaboration is vital for accelerating the growth of nanotechnology within clearly defined and ethically responsible boundaries of the medical field to ensure proper healthcare.

REFERENCES

Aggarwal, D., Kumar, V., Sharma, S. (2022). Drug-loaded biomaterials for orthopedic applications: A review. *Journal of Controlled Release*, 344, 113.

Anand, S., Kennedy, J. (2007). Medical and healthcare textiles. In *Proceedings of the Fourth International Conference on Healthcare and Medical Textiles*. Oxfordshire, UK: Taylor & Francis, FL.

Artain, F.S., Reader, A., Fisher, M., Park, B., Kemp, M., Johnstone, J., NanoKTN, U.K., McCarthy, B.J. (2011). Nanotechnology and its application to medical hygiene textiles. *Textiles for Hygiene and Infection Control* (pp. 14–26). London: Woodhead Publishing.

Atanasova, D., Staneva, D., Grabchev, I. (2021). Textile materials modified with stimuli-responsive drug carrier for skin topical and transdermal delivery. *Materials*, 14(4), 1–18.

Baghersad, S., Hajir Bahrami, S., Mohammadi, M.R., Mojtahedi, M.R.M., Milan, P.B. (2018). Development of biodegradable electrospun gelatin/aloe-vera/poly(ε-caprolactone) hybrid nanofibrous scaffold for application as skin substitutes. *Materials Science and Engineering C*, 93, 367–379.

Bhattacharjee, S., Joshi, R., Chughtai, A.A., Macintyre, C.R. (2019). Graphene modified multifunctional personal protective clothing. *Advanced Materials Interfaces*, 6(21), 1–27.

Chen, S., Liu, B., Carlson, M.A., Gombart, A.F., Reilly, D.A., Xie, J. (2017). Recent advances in electrospun nano fibres for wound healing. *Nanomedicine*, 12(11), 1335–1352.

Chen, X., Cheng, L., Li, H., Barhoum, A., Zhang, Y., He, X., Yang, W., Bubakir, M.M., Chen, H. (2018). Magnetic nano fibres: Unique properties, fabrication techniques, and emerging applications. *Chemistry Select*, 3(31), 9127–9143.

Dhivya, S., Padma, V.V., Santhini, E. (2015). Wound dressings—A review. *BioMedicine (Netherlands)*, 5(4), 24–28.

Dos Santos, D.M., Correa, D.S., Medeiros, E.S., Oliveira, J.E., Mattoso, L.H.C. (2020). Advances in functional polymer nano fibres: From spinning fabrication techniques to recent biomedical applications. *ACS Applied Materials & Interfaces*, 12(41), 45673–45701.

Fereydouni, N., Darroudi, M., Movaffagh, J., Shahroodi, A., Butler, A.E., Ganjali, S., Sahebkar, A. (2019). Curcumin nano fibres for the purpose of wound healing. *Journal of Cellular Physiology*, 234(5), 5537–5554.

Garcia-Orue, I., Gainza, G., Garcia-Garcia, P., Gutierrez, F.B., Aguirre, J.J., Hernandez, R.M., Delgado, A., Igartua, M. (2019). Composite nanofibrous membranes of PLGA/Aloe vera containing lipid nanoparticles for wound dressing applications. *International Journal of Pharmaceutics*, 556, 320–329.

Gong, Z., Xiang, Z., OuYang, X., Zhang, J., Lau, N., Zhou, J., Chan, C.C. (2019). Wearable fibre optic technology based on smart textile: A review. *Materials*, 12(20).

Grigora, M.E., Terzopoulou, Z., Baciu, D., et al. (2023). 3D printed poly(lactic acid)-based nanocomposite scaffolds with bioactive coatings for tissue engineering applications. *J. Mater. Sci.*, 58, 2740–2763.

Kalantari, K., Afifi, A.M., Jahangirian, H., Webster, T.J. (2019). Biomedical applications of chitosan electrospun nano fibres as a green polymer—Review. *Carbohydrate Polymers*, 207, 588–600.

Karim, N., Afroj, S., Lloyd, K., Oaten, L.C., Andreeva, D.V., Carr, C., Farmery, A.D., Kim, I. D., Novoselov, K.S. (2020). Sustainable personal protective clothing for healthcare applications: A review. *ACS Nano*, 14(10), 12313–12340.

Koyama, Y., Nishiyama, M., Watanabe, K. (2018). Smart textile using hetero-core optical fibre for heartbeat and respiration monitoring. *IEEE Sensors Journal*, 18(15), 6175–6180.

Li, J. H., Chen, J. H., Xu, F. (2018). Sensitive and wearable optical micro fibre sensor for human health monitoring. *Advanced Materials Technologies*, 3(12), 1–8.

Lin, K., Zhang, D., Macedo, M.H., Cui, W., Sarmento, B., Shen, G. (2019). Advanced collagen-based biomaterials for regenerative biomedicine. *Advanced Functional Materials*, 29(3). https://doi.org/10.1002/adfm.201804943.

Maruf Hasan, S.M., Shahjalal, M., Mridha, J.H., Alam, A.M.R. (2019). Medical textiles: Application of implantable medical textiles. *Global Journal of Medical Research*, 19, 17–24.

Mohandas, A., Luo, H., Ramakrishna, S. (2021). An overview on atomization and its drug delivery and biomedical applications. *Applied Sciences (Switzerland)*, 11(11). https://doi.org/10.3390/app11115173.

Morris, H., Murray, R. (2020). Medical textiles. In *Textile Progress* (Vol. 52, Issues 1–2). LTD. https://doi.org/10.1080/00405167.2020.1824468.

Padmakumar, S., Paul-Prasanth, B., Pavithran, K., Vijaykumar, D.K., Rajanbabu, A., Sivanarayanan, T.B., Kadakia, E., Amiji, M.M., Nair, S.V., Menon, D. (2019). Long-term drug delivery using implantable electrospun woven polymeric nanotextiles. *Nanomedicine: Nanotechnology, Biology, and Medicine*, 15(1), 274–284.

Pamu, D., Tallapaneni, V., Karri, V.V.S.R., Singh, S.K. (2022). Biomedical applications of electrospun nano fibres in the management of diabetic wounds. *Drug Delivery and Translational Research*, 12(1), 158–166.

Parvin, F., Islam, S., Urmy, Z., Ahmed, S. (2020). A study on the textile materials applied in human medical treatment. *European Journal of Physiotherapy and Rehabilitation Studies*, 1, 57. https://doi.org/10.5281/zenodo.3779236.

Perumal, G., Pappuru, S., Chakraborty, D., Maya Nandkumar, A., Chand, D.K., Doble, M. (2017). Synthesis and characterization of curcumin loaded PLA—Hyperbranched polyglycerol electrospun blend for wound dressing applications. *Materials Science and Engineering C*, 76, 1196–1204.

Prabhu, P. (2019). Nano fibres for medical diagnosis and therapy. In Ahmed Barhoum, Mikhael Bechelany,abdel Salam Hamdy Makhlouf (Eds.), *Handbook of NanoFibres.* Springer, New York. https://doi.org/10.1007/978-3-319-53655-2_48.

Rasouli, R., Barhoum, A., Bechelany, M., Dufresne, A. (2019). Nano fibres for biomedical and healthcare applications. *Macromolecular Bioscience*, 19(2), 1–27.

Sahu, T., Ratre, Y.K., Chauhan, S., Bhaskar, L.V.K.S., Nair, M.P., Verma, H.K. (2021). Nanotechnology based drug delivery system: Current strategies and emerging therapeutic potential for medical science. *Journal of Drug Delivery Science and Technology*, 63, 102487.

Singhvi, M.S., Zinjarde, S.S., Gokhale, D.V. (2019). Polylactic acid: Synthesis and biomedical applications. *Journal of Applied Microbiology*, 127(6), 1612–1626.

Vaishya, R., Agarwal, A.K., Tiwari, M., Vaish, A., Vijay, V., Nigam, Y. (2018). Medical textiles in orthopedics: An overview. *Journal of Clinical Orthopaedics and Trauma*, 9, S26–S33.

Xiong, Y., Tao, X. (2018). Compression garments for medical therapy and sports. *Polymers*, 10(6), 1–19.

Yeon, Y.K., Park, H.S., Lee, J.S., Lee, Y.J., Sultan, M.T., Seo, Y.B., Lee, O.J., Kim, S.H., Park, C.H. (2018). New concept of 3D printed bone clip (polylactic acid/hydroxyapatite/silk composite) for internal fixation of bone fractures. *J. Biomater. Sci. Polym. Ed.*, 29(7–9), 894–906.

Yu, G., Ning, Q., Mo, Z., Tang, S. (2019). Intelligent polymeric micelles for multidrug co-delivery and cancer therapy. *Artificial Cells, Nanomedicine and Biotechnology*, 47(1), 1476–1487.

4 Modification of Surface Biotextiles Using Nanobiotechnology

Vibeizonuo Rupreo and Jhimli Bhattacharyya

4.1 INTRODUCTION

With the advent of nanobiotechnology, materials' shapes and behavioural patterns have varied when miniaturized in the scale of nanometer (Silva et al., 2020; Idumah, 2021). Breakthroughs in nanostructure development have evolved in a current type of materials with diverse functionalities. Nanotechnology is the study and application of length measurement on a scale of approximately 1–100 nanometers in at least one dimension. It can be referred to as atomically, molecularly, or macromolecularly developed materials (Idumah, 2021). Figure 4.1 portrays classification of nanomaterials (NMs). Despite being mostly unrealized, nanotechnology has a lot of potential for use in textile and garment applications (Krifa & Prichard, 2020). Nanobiotechnology is regarded as a cutting-edge method for improving the performance of functional textiles that replace traditional chemical, physical, or physiochemical alterations (Joshi & Bhattacharyya, 2011). Nanostructured materials have grains that are smaller than 100 nm, which greatly increases their surface area and increases their receptivity to surface atoms, giving them excellent physical qualities (Qiu Zhao et al., 2003). The distribution of grains, their sizes and shapes, pores, various faults and defects, second phase/dopants, stress, application duration, surface condition, impurity level, and temperature are all structural factors that affect the tensile performance of nano-crystalline materials (Padmanabhan, 2001; Lau et al., 2004). Because of this, nanotechnology has enormous potential for use in a variety of industries, including textiles, consumer goods, biomedical devices, electronics, and other innovative materials (Qiu Zhao et al., 2003; Joshi & Bhattacharyya, 2011).

Due to the incorporation of distinctive adaptive tendencies in wearable technologies, textiles are changing and developing (Sbai et al., 2020). The incorporation of nanotechnology on biotextile materials may result in the inclusion of a number of beneficial attributes to the base material. The use of silver nanoparticles, for example, exerts antimicrobial activities, whereas the combination of molecular ligands with gold nanoparticles enables the fast detection of biological substances in the environment (Figure 4.2). These nanomaterials are generally infused into textile fibres without compromising their surface or convenience (Vigneshwaran, 2009). Silver nanoparticles can then be utilized to give textiles a shiny metallic yellow to dark pink colour as well as imparting antimicrobial function. Nanoparticles metal

DOI: 10.1201/9781003331612-5

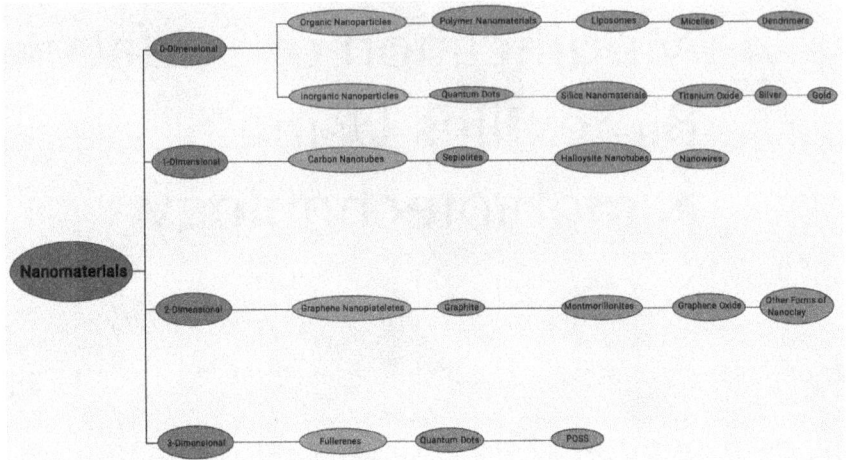

FIGURE 4.1 Classification of nanomaterials

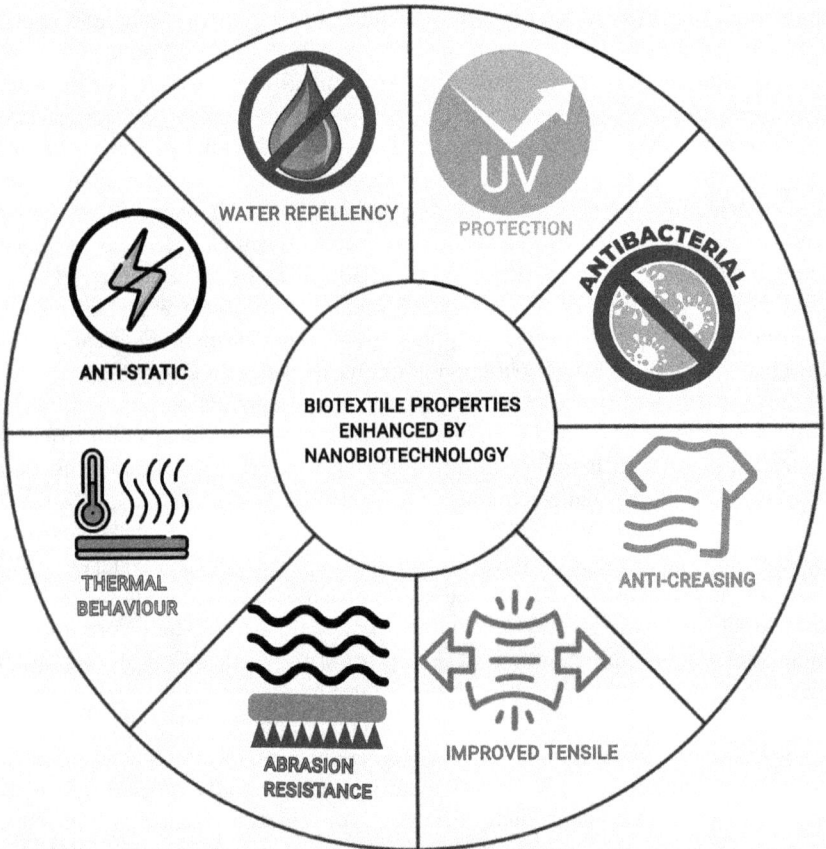

FIGURE 4.2 Biotextiles properties improved by nanobiotechnology

oxides—such as TiO_2, Al_2O_3, ZnO, MgO—acquire photocatalytic, antibacterial activity, and ultraviolet (UV) absorption characteristic properties. Textile substances incorporated with the aforementioned nanoparticles tend to deliver properties including antimicrobial, anti-bacterial, self-decontaminating, and UV blocking, which are useful for both military and civilian health products (Vigneshwaran, 2009).

In January 2020, the World Health Organization proclaimed a public health emergency of concern to the entire world; the virus was recognized as SARSCov-2 in February, and a global pandemic was announced in March. Over this time, there was a perceptible influx of people wearing face masks and face-coverings in community: it became a requisite part of daily life (Cross, 2021). As SARS-CoV-2 spreads globally, universal mask use protects the human race. The immediate explanation is to minimize viral particles from shedding into infected and asymptomatic people's noses and mouths, as validated by model simulations (Eikenberry et al., 2020) and information obtained throughout the first 100 days of 2020 (Cheng et al., 2020). Consequently, the utility of face masks in the hour of this chaotic pandemic may play an important role in population variation. If the prevalence of symptoms is proportional to viral load, masks use would gradually lower viral inoculum and hence clinical relevance by encouraging silent infections (Monica Gandhi & George W. Rutherford, 2020). Nanoengineered streamlined textiles, in which nanomaterials are incorporated into biotextiles to impart new characteristic properties without modifying the satisfaction of the substrate, comprising the cutting edge in clothing technology (Yetisen et al., 2016). Viral particles and nanomaterials have similar sizes and, due to their high surface-to-volume ratio, exhibit physical, chemical, and bioactivities distinct from larger-scale materials. Properties that vary depending on the particle's size include electrical conductivity, surface area, magnetic permeability, melting temperature, etc. With nanosized creatures like viruses and bacteria, this phenomenon specifically interacts with biological systems. The research community in the nano field has responded quickly to the Coronavirus Disease 2019 (COVID-19) pandemic in terms of individual protection gears creation due to the significance of mask-wearing health measures. Respiratory masks have been made with nanofibres and nanoparticles that have antiviral, highly breathable, and filtration capabilities (Valdiglesias & Laffon, 2020). In the following text, we will primarily focus on the potential implementation of nanobiotechnology in the modification of biotextiles and the main research results in nanotechnology-based face mask output.

4.2 METHODS

We aimed to examine the various published and compiled data on the modification of surface biotextiles using nanobiotechnology in the literature. The majority of the publications considered were those related to the title.

4.3 BIOTEXTILES FINISHING BY NANOBIOTECHNOLOGY

With revolutionary nanobiotechnology techniques, biotextile texture becomes more comprehensive, even, and concise. Nanofinishing, also known as nanotechnology finishing, is divided into two major categories: the application of nanoparticles in customary finishing constitution through the usage of a finishing constituents capable of generating nanostructures on the fabric's layer. Neither nanoparticles nor in situ nanostructures influence the feel or comfort of the fabric while exhibiting functionality or multifunctionality with extraordinary fastness. The majority of nanofinishes are available as nanoemulsions or nanosols. The term "nanoemulsions" refers to emulsions with mean droplet diameters ranging from 50 to 1000 nm. Comparatively, nanoemulsion droplet sizes are typically between 100 and 500 nm, as opposed to the micron range of regular emulsions. The nanoscale emulsions, nanomicelles, and nanocapsules that are created can cling to textile substrates more uniformly. In recent years, more and more attention has been paid to the research of fundamental and practical aspects of nano-emulsions. In studies on nanoemulsion applications, a monomer is often utilized as the disperse phase to create polymeric nanoparticles (the mini-emulsion polymerization method). Droplet nucleation is claimed to be the primary mechanism of nanoemulsion polymerization, as opposed to micro- and emulsion polymerization accounting for the persistence of each droplet's size and composition. The polymer particles in the nanoemulsion are shielded, stabilized, and functionalized using surfactants with a polymerizable group. Droplets of nanoemulsion can therefore be interpreted as little nanoreactors. The majority of commercially accessible nanofinishes use nanoemulsion processes to generate nanostructures on the fabric's surface layer. The drying and curing of the emulsions after these dispersions have been applied using a typical finishing technique results in long-lasting, high-efficiency nanofinishes on the fabric's outer layer (Joshi & Bhattacharyya, 2011).

4.3.1 Oil and Water Resistant Nanofinishes

To acquire the properties of oil and water-resistant facade, materials with low surface energy are employed in cotton fabrics. Numerous commercially available finishing compounds that repel water and oil can be categorized as fluorocarbon-based or non-fluorocarbon-formed. Silicon-build waterproofing is often utilized on its own or in accordance with fluorocarbon-based intermediaries. The most prevalent are fluorinated compounds. However, since fluorinated materials are exorbitant and frequently under threat as a result of rising environmental consciousness and strict regulations, non-fluorocarbon-form finishes are currently used in the market. In addition, maintaining the fabric's original feel and strength as well as finish durability are crucial considerations. Novel and inventive nanofinishes based on nanotechnology appear to be getting closer to meeting these market needs (Joshi & Bhattacharyya, 2011).

4.3.2 Ultraviolet-Protection Nanofinishes

Human skin cancer incidence has been found to rise as a result of prolonged and frequent exposure to UV radiation by sunlight. The greatest strategy to lower risk is to limit skin exposure to sun, particularly during peak hours. The greatest option for someone who has to work outside but cannot do so is well-designed apparel composed of UV-blocking materials (Vigneshwaran, 2009). A fabric's UV-blocking efficiency improves when it has a pigment, dye, and UV-absorbing coating that prevents ultraviolet radiation from penetrating fabrics (Dierickx & Van Den Berghe, 2004). A person's exposure to UV radiation is decreased and their skin is shielded from potential hazard by clothing made of fabric coated with UV absorbers to ensure that the garments reflect the sun's harmful ultraviolet rays. Different types of human skin may require varying levels of skin protection depending on UV radiation intensity and dispersion in relation to geographic location, time of day, and season. Sun Protection Factor (SPF) is a measure of this protection; the UV radiation defence is better when the SPF value is higher. Figure 4.3 illustrates the many stages that the incident UV light on a fabric material goes through. Here, the transmitted and dispersed light will be the central subject since it is this light that causes sunburn (Vigneshwaran, 2009). As UV blockers, metal oxides—notably zinc oxide (ZnO)—are more stable metals than organic UV-blocking substances. Nano ZnO improves UV-blocking properties due to its larger surface area and strong UV absorption. Additionally, ZnO nanoparticles outperform nano-silver in terms of affordability, whiteness, and UV-blocking ability (Lines, 2008). The wet chemical approach can be used to develop ZnO nanoparticles, stabilizing them with soluble starch while leveraging zinc nitrate and sodium hydroxide as precursors. These 40 nm-sized nanoparticles were padded onto the bleached cotton fibres by utilizing an acrylic binder. For cotton textiles treated with a negligibly small (2%) amount of ZnO nanoparticles, almost 75% UV blocking was observed. The friction when it comes to the nano-ZnO coated fabric was much lesser than that of the bulk-ZnO lubricated fabric because of its nano-size and even distribution, and as a result, the fabric with nano-ZnO coating

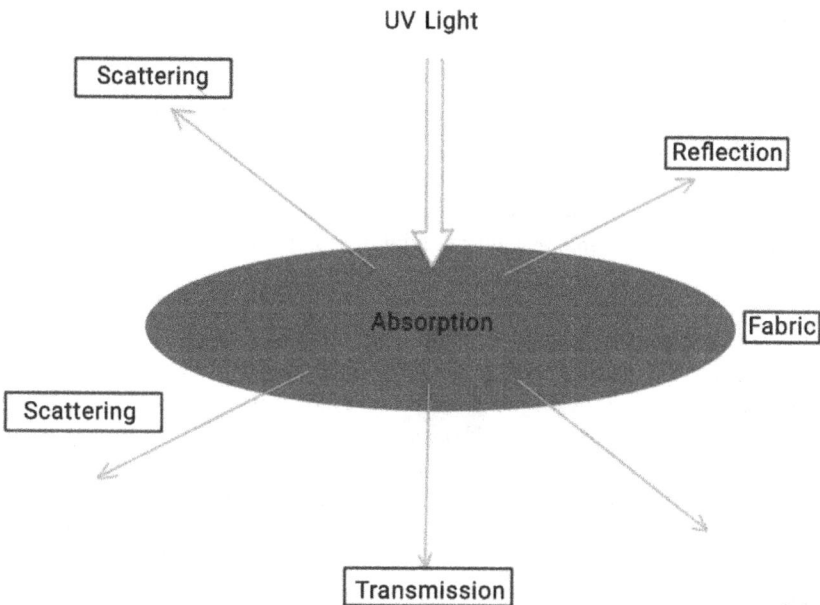

FIGURE 4.3   Characteristics of textile materials by UV-transmittance

feels superior (Yadav et al., 2006). Additional research is being conducted to assess the fabric's wash fastness, antibacterial, abrasion, and handling characteristics (Joshi et al., 2011; Vigneshwaran, 2009).

4.3.3 ANTIBACTERIAL NANOFINISHES

Whether the constituent fibres are natural or synthetic, a majority of textiles do not have the properties to resist harmful bacteria or fungi. A variety of bacteria, whether pathogenic or not, can grow on textile inner or outer wear when humidity, perspiration, and moisture are present. These may result in illnesses, an unpleasant odour for the user, and a loss of fabric characteristics like colour or strength. For all types of textiles, numerous antibacterial coatings and disinfection methods have been created. In the present era, the management of microbes on textile materials has expanded to include not only domestic items but also textiles used in health-care. Numerous bioactive components are integrated into textiles as a result of the multidisciplinary approach used in nanotechnology studies and research to deliver antibacterial, antimicrobial, or antifungal properties. The claim that conventional materials have less surface area than nanostructured materials is of primary interest to material scientists. By saturating the surface of fibres with colloidal solution, a minuscule quantity of noble metal nanoparticles can be used to prevent bacterial development (Joshi & Bhattacharyya, 2011).

The antibacterial properties of silver, which are now acknowledged by science, prevent the microbial activity and other germs in food or water when it is stored in silver containers (Vigneshwaran, 2009). Silver compounds were an important tool in World War I for preventing fungal infection before the discovery of antibiotics (Joshi & Bhattacharyya, 2011). Silver ions have a wide variety of antimicrobial effects. Utilizing metal nanoparticles has the additional benefit of the presence of surface plasmons. By adjusting the plasmons' size and shape, it is feasible to tune their strong optical extinctions to a range of colours (Vigneshwaran, 2009). The antibacterial effect and endurance of the nanoscale silver particles are outstanding, and they are generated or fragmented in colloidal solution before being applied to textile fibres. If a fibre reactive polymer such as polystyrene co-maleic anhydride is being used to encase the silver compound or nano material, it may be used to offer a long-lasting bactericidal finish. Nanosilver has been effectively applied to a variety of organic and conventional fabrics due to its potent antibacterial properties. In comparison to PP having micron-sized particles, polypropylene (PP) mixed with silver nanoparticles demonstrates higher antibacterial activity (Jeong et al., 2005). Even after numerous washing process, cotton and polyester fabrics respond favourably to the powerful antibacterial effect of nanosilver's colloidal solution (Yeo et al., 2003). When wool cloth is cushioned using ethanol-based colloids made of sulphur nanosilver, with low silver concentration, it demonstrates mothproofing, antibacterial, and antistatic capabilities (20 ppm) (Ki et al., 2007). Studies employing SEM and TEM methods demonstrate that the biocidal properties of Ag NPs are extensively explored, highlighting their antimicrobial and antioxidant activities, according to several researches. The findings demonstrated that E. coli cells have been harmed by nanosilver interaction, with pits appearing in the bacteria's cell walls and an accumulation of silver nanoparticles in their membranes. The said membrane's shape causes a dramatic increase in permeability, which eliminates the cell. Nanosilver is currently recognized for its broad spectrum anti-microbial properties in colloidal solutions; it could be applied to fabric or fibre surfaces as a nanofinishing. As a result of nanosilver exposure in the body becoming more extensive and common, silver nanoparticles have gained increased access to human body tissues, cells, and biological components. Silver is generally considered to be largely non-toxic to mammalian cells, with the exception of argyrosis and a few minor issues. Only workers with a prolonged history of exposure to silver experience silver poisoning. The perceived health risk from metallic silver was low. Although if they can be biochemically neutral and benign in bulk, several materials do show considerable susceptibility to mammalian cells once they are reduced to the nanometric scale. Silver nanoparticles can bind to and interact with proteins in the human body via phagocytosis, deposition, clearance, and translocation. However, they can also cause a wide range of tissue reactions, including cell activation, inflammation, the generation of reactive oxygen species, and cell death. Numerous reports suggest that silver nanoparticles cause toxic nanosilver to be released into freshwater ecosystems, potentially harming aquatic life (Blaser et al., 2008). Nanosilver applications' toxicity must be carefully considered as products made of nanosilver enter consumer goods like textiles (Joshi & Bhattacharyya, 2011).

4.4 IMPACT OF NANOCOATING IN BIOTEXTILES

There are many different reasons why materials are coated. A coating can improve a material's mechanical, chemical, or thermal stability; wear resistance; toughness; or longevity; as well as its general physicochemical and biological qualities. It can also minimize friction and inhibit corrosion. It has long been a practice to apply polymeric coating to substrates made of wood, metal, textile, or leather in order to add certain surface attributes like gloss, wear, hydrophobicity, gas and water barrier, conductivity, antistatic, and antibacterial, among others. However, conventional coating has a number of issues, including reduction in strength, adhesion, abrasion resistance, and decreased durability (Joshi & Bhattacharyya, 2011). Higher coat-to-weight ratios is frequently needed in order to obtain the desired quantity of surface property. Researchers concentrate their efforts on reducing the coat-to-weight ratio in an effort to solve these issues. With the development of nanotechnology, a brand-new field in the field of extremely thin (50 nm) textile nanocoating has emerged. Coating is the simple process of applying a layer to a surface, so nanocoating involves either applying a thin layer or material that is applied to a surface in the nanometer range. Despite the fact that there are currently very few acknowledged studies on nanocoatings on fibres or textiles (Hyde et al., 2005; Dubas et al., 2006), the impact of these nanostructures on the reactivity of coatings, corrosion resistance, endurance, and longevity is significant. In order to develop new kinds of highly functional systems, nanoscience and nanotechnology have the ability to challenge some of the accepted notions about coating techniques and ideal coating topologies (Joshi & Bhattacharyya, 2011). In biotextile applications, such as bio-filtration materials, medical apparel, medical fabrics, textile implants, textile substrates for cell development, and other textile products for medical systems, nanocoatings are being employed more and more (Tessier, 2013). Vapour deposition, plasma-assisted/ion-beam-assisted techniques, chemical reduction, pulsed laser deposition, mechanical milling, magnetron sputtering, self-assembly, layer-by-layer coating, dipcoating, sol-gel coating, and electrochemical deposition are a few of the commonly used nanocoating techniques. Planar substrates are coated using the majority of these processes more frequently than other types (Joshi & Bhattacharyya, 2011). Medical fabrics and equipment, as well as multipurpose filters (for ultrafine particles, germs, and viruses), may be created commercially. For textile coatings and composites utilized in biomedical applications, carbon nanofibres (Lynam et al., 2007; Yang et al., 2007) with their eminent mechanical strength, light weight, high electrical conductivity, and thermal and chemical resistance can also be employed. Nanocoatings can be used to give biotextiles additional surface qualities like liquid repulsion, resistance to stains, antibacterial activity, deodorizer, and the transport of biologically active substances (Tessier, 2013).

4.4.1 Nanocoating Using Sol-Gel

Surface nanocoating of textiles and clothing is a more recent technique for creating surfaces that are extremely active with UV-blocking, antibacterial, and innate cleaning abilities, as well as remarkable durability and minimal coat weight. A molecular framework of inorganic metal oxide nanoparticles in three dimensions is created in this sol-gel nanocoating technique where inorganic precursors, such as metal salts or organometallic compounds, are hydrolyzed and condensed.

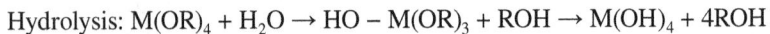

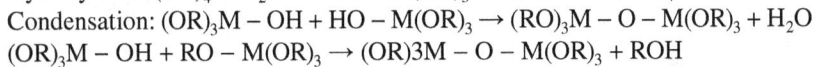

Hydrolysis: $M(OR)_4 + H_2O \rightarrow HO - M(OR)_3 + ROH \rightarrow M(OH)_4 + 4ROH$
Condensation: $(OR)_3M - OH + HO - M(OR)_3 \rightarrow (RO)_3M - O - M(OR)_3 + H_2O$
$(OR)_3M - OH + RO - M(OR)_3 \rightarrow (OR)3M - O - M(OR)_3 + ROH$

Here, M is a metal and R is an alkyl group (Caruso & Antonietti, 2001). Even though they are simple to manufacture by sol-gel processing, very fine particles (20 to 40 nm) cannot be produced through conventional grinding. For sol-gel nanocoating, dip coating is typically utilized (Xu & Cai, 2008). Convective assembly, however, gives greater precision and less expense (Prevo et al., 2007). Recently, layers of metal oxide nanoparticles, such as nano-titanium (TiO_2) for photocatalytic activity, have been deposited on textile fabric surfaces using low temperature sol-gel based nanocoatings (Bozzi et al., 2005). After employing plasma and UV irradiation to activate the cotton surface, a sol-gel nanocoating is created on the fabric's surface using a TiO_2 colloidal solution. This guarantees that nanotitanium particles will adhere well. According to research, polycarboxylic acids, a suitable chemical spacer, can also provide cotton with a long-lasting, stable performance of TiO_2's photocatalytic activity (Meilert et al., 2005). Sol-gel nanocoatings have significant difficulties in controlling inorganic coatings' adherence to surfaces and maintaining coating thickness uniformity. This effort is currently underway to a great extent, and in the not too distant future, we will see a variety of sol-gel-based nanocoated materials reaching remarkable outcomes in a variety of application areas, including textiles (Joshi & Bhattacharyya, 2011).

4.4.2 Layer-by-Layer Nanocoating

A thin film coating with molecular level control over film thickness and reactivity can be created using the layer-by-layer (L-b-L) nanocoating process. Nanocoating can be produced using the L-b-L approach without the use of any extra tools and in safe physical and chemical environments. Due to their distinctive cross-section and the variety of their surfaces' chemical and physical compositions, cotton fibres pose special difficulties for the deposition of nanolayers. Using the L-b-L technique, it has been possible to effectively coat cationic cotton surfaces with layers of polyelectrolytes that are alternately anionic and cationic, such as poly (sodium 4-styrene sulphonate) and poly (allylamine hydrochloride) (Hyde et al., 2005). According to research by W. Ali, S. Rajendran, and M. Joshi (Ali et al., 2010), the production of polyelectrolyte multi-layers on cotton surfaces is susceptible to a number of process factors, including pH, temperature, the concentration of the polyelectrolyte solution, dipping time, and salt addition. The L-b-L method can also be used to make multifunctional textile surfaces for coatings on microfluid channels and biosensors that are water-resistant, antifouling, and self-cleaning. Antimicrobial silver nanoparticles can be immobilized with this approach on nylon and silk fibres. Sequential solution dipping of nylon or silk fibres containing silver nanoparticles coated with poly (methacrylic acid) and poly (diallyldimethylammonium chloride) results in the development of a colourful thin film with antibacterial characteristics. On both silk and nylon fibres, the amount of deposition increases as the number of deposited layers increases, despite the fact that the L-b-L coating on nylon fibres is not as uniform as it is on silk fibres. The addition of bilayers to the fibres dramatically inhibits bacterial growth for both silk and nylon fibre (Dubas et al., 2006). In a work by M. Joshi et al., chitosan was used as the cationic polyelectrolyte and poly sodium 4-styrene sulfonate as the anionic polyelectrolyte to perform L-b-L nanocoating on cotton fabric. In order to deposit the bi-layers uniformly and at a very thin (few nm) thickness, ultrasonic treatment is used to aid the process. As a result, the fabric is generated with high antibacterial capabilities; nonetheless, the fabric's feel, flexibility, and breathability are unchanged (Joshi et al., 2011).

4.4.3 Plasma Polymerization Assisted Nanocoating

As a partially ionized gas with free electrons and photons, plasma is made up of highly energized atomic, molecular, ionic, and volatile species. Plasma is created when an electric field provides enough extra energy to gases. There are several simultaneous recombination mechanisms because the plasma's reactive species, produced by the ionization, disintegration, and activation processes, are powerful enough to rupture several chemical bonds. The benefits of changing the surface properties of inert materials are demonstrated using plasma surface treatments. The primary benefits of plasma polymerization techniques are comprised of: (1) broad applicability to most organic and inorganic structures; (2) reconfiguration of surface texture without modifying bulk characteristic features; (3) it requires fewer monomeric molecules, which makes it less energy-intensive; and (4) almost all organic, organometallic, and hetero-atomic organic molecules have relevance (Höcker, 2002). Compared to traditional wet chemical techniques, plasma lessens contamination of the air, water, and land. Although much of the plasma treatment process involves the discharge of hazardous waste gases, other gases including fluorine, ammonia, and nitrous oxide are incorporated to achieve particular properties. Fabrics may stiffen and degrade as a result of plasma. Four essential processes, including surface cleaning by eliminating organic pollutants, activating fabric texture by stabilizing functional groups, and grafting monomers like acrylic acid on the fabric surface are the main uses of plasma in the textile industry. Hydrophilicity, flame retardancy, surface hardness, hydrophilic-hydrophobic inclination, printability, electromagnetic radiation reflection, dirt-repellent qualities, and antistatic properties are all enhanced by plasma treatments. Even for fluoropolymers, the surface energy of polymeric surfaces improves after plasma treatment, producing improvements in hydrophilicity and stickiness. Vacuum-UV light irradiation, microwave plasma, and radio frequency plasma can all be used to activate textiles made of bleached and mercerized cotton. Plasma or UV treatment process can be used to put negatively charged functional groups onto the surface of textiles (Figure 4.4). TiO$_2$ nanoparticles are often used to

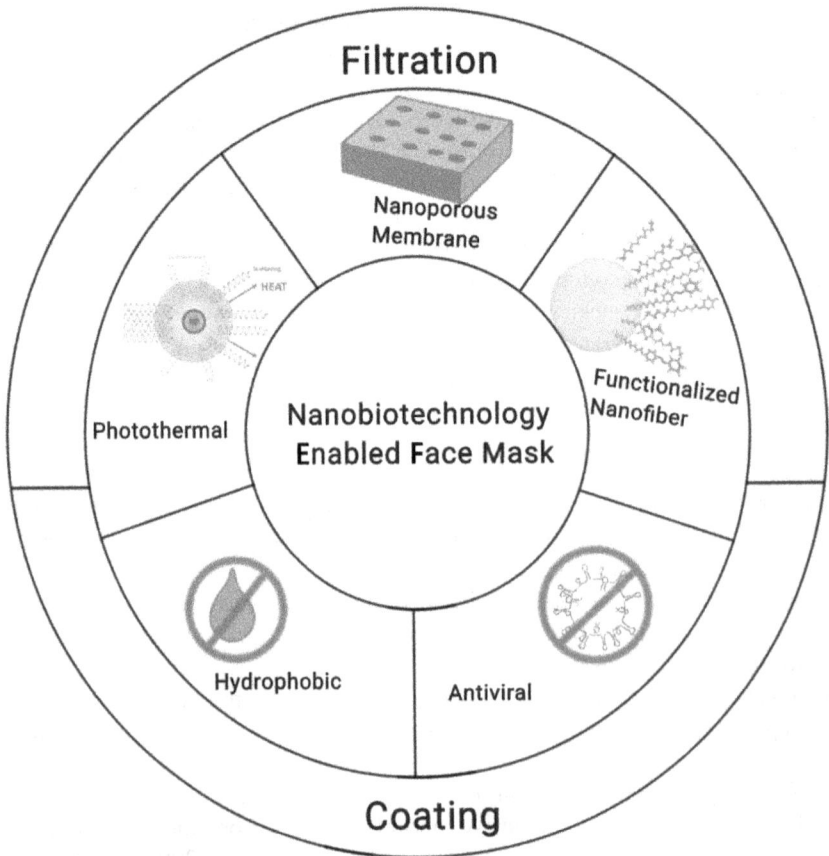

FIGURE 4.4   Properties of nanobiotechnology enabled face mask

establish textile surfaces that are negatively charged and UV activated. This TiO_2 implanted fabric has a self-cleaning quality, rapidly fading wine and coffee stains when exposed to sunlight (Joshi & Bhattacharyya, 2011).

4.5 FACE MASKS AND NANOBIOTECHNOLOGY

Universal mask use is significantly protecting the worldwide population as SARS-CoV-2 spreads aggressively on a global scale. They have prevented the viral shedding from infected and asymptomatic people from passing to other healthy individuals as supported by model simulations (Eikenberry et al., 2020). Based on epidemiological evidence of the substantial positive association between mask use and pandemic control, the public was urged to use facial coverings in places with high rates of community transmission by the Centres for Disease Control and Prevention in April 2020. Nanomaterials have been used in textiles to provide additional functionality while maintaining the substrate's comfort which has led to nanoengineered functional textiles getting represented as the frontier in clothing technology. Nanoparticles have a huge surface-to-volume ratio also having the same size as the viral particles. Therefore, they differ from other bigger sized particles in terms of their physical, chemical, and biological characteristics (Valdiglesias & Laffon, 2020; Valentina Palmieri et al., 2021). Surface area, melting temperature, electrical conductivity, fluorescence qualities, and other characteristics fluctuate depending on the particle's size. This characteristic of nanoparticles leads to specific interactions, particularly with bacterial and viral biological systems (Figure 4.4). Given the importance of wearing a mask health precaution in containing the pandemic of Coronavirus Disease 2019 (COVID-19), the nano science community has been quick to respond in the creation of personal protective gear. Respiratory masks have incorporated nanofibres and nanoparticles which have provided antiviral properties with high filtration and breathability properties (Valdiglesias & Laffon, 2020).

An ideal face mask should be effective in removing bioaerosols while yet offering the user a high level of comfort. External elements, such as humidity, temperature, and frequency of breathing, have an impact on the mask's quality (which in turn is influenced by comfort). The pattern and speed of airflow, the charge and size of incoming particles, and the amount of loading time are some additional external factors that affect the filtration by masks. The effectiveness of face masks depends on two key elements: external conditions and material characteristics, including chemical composition, fibre thickness and packing, the number of layers on the mask, fibre diameter, and charge density (Tcharkhtchi et al., 2021). Of all the aforementioned parameters particle charge, size, and rate of flow are the most crucial factors which are to be taken into consideration. For small particles like viruses, diffusion and electrostatic mechanisms are known to predominate at low flow rate settings. The interception of viral particles occurs when the flow rate is increased. Copper dioxide, carbon, graphene, nanodiamonds, nano-silver, and titanium dioxide are just a few of the nanoparticles that can be found in commercial face masks. A list of antiviral patents held by Campos and colleagues has also been made public (Palmieri et al., 2021). CuO possess both antiviral and antibacterial properties. Respiratory surgical face masks (SFMs) with a CuO coating have been developed which enables the user protection from viral droplets.

For both the aerosolized viruses of the human influenza virus (H1N1) and the avian influenza virus (H9N2), which were done using simulated breathing settings, CuO and control together with integrated SFMs' filtering effectiveness was assessed and found to be same. For H1N1 viruses, the treated SFMs showed viral titers retention of zero after 30 minutes, whereas for H9N2 viruses, it was reduced by five times in control masks. Antiviral air filtering fabrics with a SiO_2/Ag NPs layer have been shown to reduce virus load by up to 99.9%. Confirmed advanced air purifiers in hospitals include composites of Ag NPs/TiO_2 (Idumah, 2021). Polypropylene is a polymer that is used in masks and does not absorb moisture and is easy to charge. Polyethylene, polyesters, polyamides, and polycarbonates are other examples (Tcharkhtchi et al., 2021). Nanoparticles have been used to modify the physical properties of masks to improve its performance. An illustration is the requirement for face masks to be optimized for thermal comfort, which is required by healthcare professionals for long-term usage as well since damp, warm circumstances make it easier for germs to survive (Yang et al., 2017). The addition of nanofibres to nano-porous polyethylene can give the masks a cooling effect and effective particle filtration. In contrast, adding a layer of silver to these materials results in a significant increase in infrared reflectance and a warming effect. Given that silver has antibacterial properties and is used in surgical masks, this characteristic is especially important (Li et al., 2006; Kharaghani et al., 2018). The cloth of the masks can become perforated by virus particles that reach the surface but are not destroyed. When placed in a warm, moist milieu, this can start to accumulate microorganisms (Tcharkhtchi et al., 2021). Because of this, by cleaning the exhaled and inhaled droplets beforehand, nanoparticles may be able to inactivate the virus particles as they travel through the mask (Huang et al., 2020). The virulence of solutions containing SARS-COV-2 can be reduced with graphene and graphene oxide when passed through materials functionalized with these nanoparticles, such as cotton and polyurethane fabrics (Palmieri et al., 2021). The incorporation of graphene into fabrics is also found to improve the mechanical strength, resistance to flame, conductivity, resistance to abrasion, and protection from ultraviolet rays (Bhattacharjee et al., 2019). Pathogen mucopolysaccharides can be recognized by antiviral polysaccharide coatings which can be developed as a more sustainable way to enhance the antiviral action of mask (Otto & de Villiers, 2020). The introduction of broad-spectrum antimicrobial compounds to functionalize textiles has led to their commercialization (Yetisen et al., 2016; Campos et al., 2020). Graphene and materials based on it, quantum dots, nanodiamonds, and multiwall or single wall carbon nanotubes are examples of carbon materials that have been tested against various sorts of microbes, including viruses (Weiss et al., 2020; Palmieri & Papi, 2020). Several phases of the viral reproduction cycle can be hampered by well-known antibacterial species including silver, zinc, and copper. Textile fibres have incorporated some of these elements successfully (Palmieri et al., 2021). The best defense out against SARS-CoV-2 virus invading the human body in the recent COVID-19 pandemic is reported to be N95 face masks (Figure 4.5). Face masks made of nanofibre have drawn a lot of interest since they are inexpensive and easy to manufacture. More specifically, nanofibres have found extensive usage in the fields of energy storage, medicine, and the environment due to their superior morphological and functional properties (El-Atab et al., 2022).

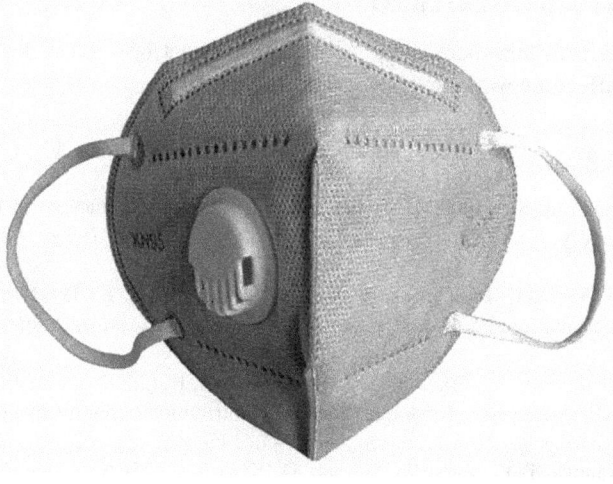

FIGURE 4.5 Reusable N95 face mask

4.6 CONCLUSION

Due to its capacity to manipulate metals into their nanometric scale, which also effectively switches their chemical, optical, and physical characteristics, nanobiotechnology is gaining significant traction in the biotextile field. When giving textile materials different functional qualities, it gets around the restrictions of traditional procedures. The wearer's comfort and maintenance are significantly improved by these functional qualities, which are of the utmost importance. When nanoparticles and nanofinishes are utilized, traditional textiles can generate and increase advanced performance features in areas like anti-microbial, anti-bacterial, water repellency, anti-infrared, and flame-retardant qualities. The method can be used to create fibres, yarns, and fabrics with the desired textile properties, such as resilience, flexibility, sturdiness, comfort, and breathability. Medical textiles are crucial in the worldwide fight against the COVID-19 virus in this age of pandemic. The creation of COVID-19 personal protection equipment requires the use of woven, knitted, and nonwoven textile materials. Ultimately, this study reviews that nanotechnology can have a substantial impact in the combat against the current public health crisis when used in the crucial area of face masks, especially since this area is not closely correlated with some of the stringent policies and procedures typically associated with vaccines, which could lead to quicker technology transcription.

4.7 ACKNOWLEDGEMENT

JB expresses gratitude for the financial assistance from NER-Twinning Project Scheme, Department of biotechnology, Govt. of India (sanction order No. BT/PR25026/NER/95/963/2017), and DRDO, Govt. of India (Project no. DFTM/07/3603/NESTC/EWM/P-04) under North East Science & Technology Center, Mizoram University.

4.8 CONFLICT OF INTEREST

The authors affirm that there is no recognized conflict of interest that could have appeared to affect the work described in this chapter.

REFERENCES

Ali, S.W., Rajendran, S., Joshi, M. (2010). Effect of process parameters on layer-by-layer self-assembly of polyelectrolytes on cotton substrate. *Polym. Polym. Compos.*, 18(5), 237–249.

Bhattacharjee, S., Joshi, R., Chughtai, A.A., Macintyre, C.R. (2019). Graphene modified multifunctional personal protective clothing. *Adv. Mater. Interfaces*, 6(21), 1900622.

Blaser, S.A., Scheringer, M., MacLeod, M., Hungerbühler, K. (2008). Estimation of cumulative aquatic exposure and risk due to silver: Contribution of nano-functionalized plastics and textiles. *Sci. Total Environ.*, 390(2–3), 396–409.

Bozzi, A., Yuranova, T., Guasaquillo, I., Laub, D., Kiwi, J. (2005). Self-cleaning of modified cotton textiles by TiO2 at low temperatures under daylight irradiation. *J. Photochem. Photobiol. A Chem.*, 174(2), 156–164.

Campos, E.V.R., Pereira, A.E.S., de Oliveira, J.L., Carvalho, L.B., Guilger-Casagrande, M., de Lima, R., Fraceto, L.F. (2020). How can nanotechnology help to combat COVID-19? Opportunities and urgent need. *J. Nanobiotechnology*, 18(1), 125.

Caruso, R.A., Antonietti, M. (2001). Sol–gel nanocoating: An approach to the preparation of structured materials. *Chem. Mater.*, 13(10), 3272–3282.

Cheng, V.C.-C., Wong, S.-C., Chuang, V. W.-M., So, S. Y.-C., Chen, J. H.-K., Sridhar, S., To, K. K.-W., Chan, J.F.-W., Hung, I.F.-N., Ho, P.-L., Yuen, K.-Y. (2020). The role of community-wide wearing of face mask for control of coronavirus disease 2019 (COVID-19) epidemic due to SARS-CoV-2. *J. Infect.*, 81(1), 107–114.

Cross, B.D.J. (2021). The use of nanotechnology in face masks against airborne pathogens nanotechnology in face masks. *Azo Materials*, 1–4.

Dierickx, W., Van Den Berghe, P. (2004). Natural weathering of textiles used in agricultural applications. *Geotext. Geomembranes*, 22(4), 255–272.

Dubas, S.T., Kumlangdudsana, P., Potiyaraj, P. (2006). Layer-by-layer deposition of antimicrobial silver nanoparticles on textile fibers. *Colloids Surfaces A Physicochem. Eng. Asp.*, 289(1–3), 105–109.

Eikenberry, S.E., Mancuso, M., Iboi, E., Phan, T., Eikenberry, K., Kuang, Y., Kostelich, E., Gumel, A.B. (2020). To mask or not to mask: Modeling the potential for face mask use by the general public to curtail the COVID-19 pandemic. *Infect. Dis. Model.*, 5, 293–308.

El-Atab, N., Mishra, R.B., Hussain, M.M. (2022). Toward nanotechnology-enabled face masks against SARS-CoV-2 and pandemic respiratory diseases. *Nanotechnology*, 33(6), 062006.

Höcker, H. (2002). Plasma treatment of textile fibers. *Pure Appl. Chem.*, 74(3), 423–427.

Huang, H., Fan, C., Li, M., Nie, H.-L., Wang, F.-B., Wang, H., Wang, R., Xia, J., Zheng, X., Zuo, X., Huang, J. (2020). COVID-19: A call for physical scientists and engineers. *ACS Nano*, 14(4), 3747–3754.

Hyde, K., Rusa, M., Hinestroza, J. (2005). Layer-by-layer deposition of polyelectrolyte nanolayers on natural fibres: Cotton. *Nanotechnology*, 16(7), S422–S428.

Idumah, C.I. (2021). Influence of nanotechnology in polymeric textiles, applications, and fight against COVID-19. *J. Text. Inst.*, 112(12), 2056–2076.

Jeong, S.H., Yeo, S.Y., Yi, S.C. (2005). The effect of filler particle size on the antibacterial properties of compounded polymer/silver fibers. *J. Mater. Sci.*, 40(20), 5407–5411.

Joshi, M., Bhattacharyya, A. (2011). Nanotechnology—A new route to high-performance functional textiles. *Text. Prog.*, 43(3), 155–233.

Joshi, M., Khanna, R., Shekhar, R., Jha, K. (2011). Chitosan nanocoating on cotton textile substrate using layer-by-layer self-assembly technique. *J. Appl. Polym. Sci.*, 119(5), 2793–2799.

Kharaghani, D., Khan, M., Shahzad, A., Inoue, Y., Yamamoto, T., Rozet, S., Tamada, Y., Kim, I. (2018). Preparation and in-vitro assessment of hierarchal organized antibacterial breath mask based on polyacrylonitrile/silver (PAN/AgNPs) nanofiber. *Nanomaterials*, 8(7), 461.

Ki, H.Y., Kim, J.H., Kwon, S.C., Jeong, S.H. (2007). A study on multifunctional wool textiles treated with nano-sized silver. *J. Mater. Sci.*, 42(19), 8020–8024.

Krifa, M., Prichard, C. (2020). Nanotechnology in textile and apparel research—An overview of technologies and processes. *J. Text. Inst.*, 111(12), 1778–1793.

Lau, K.-T., Chipara, M., Ling, H.-Y., Hui, D. (2004). On the effective elastic moduli of carbon nanotubes for nanocomposite structures. *Compos. Part B Eng.*, 35(2), 95–101.

Li, Y., Leung, P., Yao, L., Song, Q.W., Newton, E. (2006). Antimicrobial effect of surgical masks coated with nanoparticles. *J. Hosp. Infect.*, 62(1), 58–63.

Lines, M.G. (2008). Nanomaterials for practical functional uses. *J. Alloys Compd.*, 449(1–2), 242–245.

Lynam, C., Moulton, S.E., Wallace, G.G. (2007). Carbon-nanotube biofibers. *Adv. Mater.*, 19(9), 1244–1248.

Meilert, K.T., Laub, D., Kiwi, J. (2005). Photocatalytic self-cleaning of modified cotton textiles by TiO2 clusters attached by chemical spacers. *J. Mol. Catal. A Chem.*, 237(1–2), 101–108.

Monica Gandhi, M.D., M.P.H., George W. Rutherford, M. (2020). Facial masking for Covid-19—Potential for "variolation" as we await a vaccine. *N. Engl. J. Med.*, 101(1), 1969–1973.

Otto, D.P., de Villiers, M.M. (2020). Layer-by-layer nanocoating of antiviral polysaccharides on surfaces to prevent coronavirus infections. *Molecules*, 25(15), 3415.

Padmanabhan, K.A. (2001). Mechanical properties of nanostructured materials. *Mater. Sci. Eng. A*, 304–306(1–2), 200–205.

Palmieri, V., De Maio, F., De Spirito, M., Papi, M. (2021). Face masks and nanotechnology: Keep the blue side up. *Nano Today*, 37, 101077.

Palmieri, V., Papi, M. (2020). Can graphene take part in the fight against COVID-19? *Nano Today*, 33, 100883.

Prevo, B.G., Kuncicky, D.M., Velev, O.D. (2007). Engineered deposition of coatings from nano- and micro-particles: A brief review of convective assembly at high volume fraction. *Colloids Surfaces A Physicochem. Eng. Asp.*, 311(1–3), 2–10.

Qiu Zhao, Q., Boxman, A., Chowdhry, U. (2003). Nanotechnology in the chemical industry—Opportunities and challenges. *J. Nanoparticle Res.*, 5(5/6), 567–572.

Sbai, S.J., Boukhriss, A., Majid, S., Gmouh, S. (2020). The recent advances in nanotechnologies for textile functionalization. In *Advances in Functional and Protective Textiles* (pp. 531–568). Amsterdam, NY: Elsevier. https://doi.org/10.1016/B978-0-12-820257-9.00020-5.

Silva, M., Ferreira, F.N., Alves, N.M., Paiva, M.C. (2020). Biodegradable polymer nanocomposites for ligament/tendon tissue engineering. *J. Nanobiotechnology*, 18(1), 23.

Tcharkhtchi, A., Abbasnezhad, N., Zarbini Seydani, M., Zirak, N., Farzaneh, S., Shirinbayan, M. (2021). An overview of filtration efficiency through the masks: Mechanisms of the aerosols penetration. *Bioact. Mater.*, 6(1), 106–122.

Tessier, D. (2013). Surface modification of biotextiles for medical applications. In A. (M.W. King), B. (B.S. Gupta), C. (R. Guidoin) (Eds.), *Biotextiles as Medical Implants* (pp. 137–156). Amsterdam, NY: Elsevier.

Valdiglesias, V., Laffon, B. (2020). The impact of nanotechnology in the current universal COVID-19 crisis: Let's not forget nanosafety! *Nanotoxicology*, 14(8), 1013–1016.

Vigneshwaran, N. (2009). Modification of textile surfaces using nanoparticles. In Q. Wei (Ed.), *Surface Modification of Textiles* (pp. 164–184). Amsterdam, NY: Elsevier. https://doi.org/10.1533/9781845696689.164.

Weiss, C., Carriere, M., Fusco, L., Capua, I., Regla-Nava, J.A., Pasquali, M., Scott, J.A., Vitale, F., Unal, M.A., Mattevi, C., Bedognetti, D., Merkoçi, A., Tasciotti, E., Yilmazer, A., Gogotsi, Y., Stellacci, F., Delogu, L.G. (2020). Toward nanotechnology-enabled approaches against the COVID-19 pandemic. *ACS Nano*, 14(6), 6383–6406.

Xu, B., Cai, Z. (2008). Fabrication of a superhydrophobic ZnO nanorod array film on cotton fabrics via a wet chemical route and hydrophobic modification. *Appl. Surf. Sci.*, 254(18), 5899–5904.

Yadav, A., Prasad, V., Kathe, A.A., Raj, S., Yadav, D., Sundaramoorthy, C., Vigneshwaran, N. (2006). Functional finishing in cotton fabrics using zinc oxide nanoparticles. *Bull. Mater. Sci.*, 29(6), 641–645.

Yang, A., Cai, L., Zhang, R., Wang, J., Hsu, P.-C., Wang, H., Zhou, G., Xu, J., Cui, Y. (2017). Thermal management in nanofiber-based face mask. *Nano Lett.*, 17(6), 3506–3510.

Yang, W., Thordarson, P., Gooding, J.J., Ringer, S.P., Braet, F. (2007). Carbon nanotubes for biological and biomedical applications. *Nanotechnology*, 18(41).

Yeo, S.Y., Lee, H.J., Jeong, S.H. (2003). Preparation of nanocomposite fibers for permanent antibacterial effect. *J. Mater. Sci.*, 38(10), 2143–2147.

Yetisen, A.K., Qu, H., Manbachi, A., Butt, H., Dokmeci, M.R., Hinestroza, J.P., Skorobogatiy, M., Khademhosseini, A., Yun, S.H. (2016). Nanotechnology in textiles. *ACS Nano*, 10(3), 3042–3068.

5 Nano-Enhanced Biotextile Sterilization Techniques for Medical Applications

Pallerla Naveen Reddy, Vivek Dave, and Prashansa Sharma

5.1 INTRODUCTION

This chapter focuses on various sterilization methods which help in sterilizing nano-enhanced biotextiles and medical devices. Nano-enhanced biotextiles is a new field of technology in science, which combines the textile technology with the medical sciences which helps in providing various applications in the field of medical sciences. The increase of hazards to human life such as accident traumas (bleeding due to accidents), human activities, chemical injury, sports injury, chronic wounds, unhygienic conditions (feminine hygiene), blood vessel damages, damaged heart valves, several new infections, new diseases, and several other conditions has raised the use of nano-enhanced biotextiles in recent years. So, the preparation of these medical textiles and their sterility should have to be taken as an utmost priority in their production.

Biotextiles are defined as, "the fibrous structures which are specifically designed to use in biological environment for the treatment of any medical condition, where their performance depends on biostability and biocompatibility with the cells and biological fluids". Nano-enhanced biotextiles are defined as, "the induce of nano particles into the biotextile structures which helps in the treatment and delivery of drugs and also helps in increasing the integrity and biocompatibility of the textiles with the cells and biological fluids". Based on their use and polymeric structure, nano-enhanced biotextiles are manufactured by various methods as mentioned in Figure 5.1 and there is a chance of increase in the bioburden and contamination based on the selection of manufacturing method.

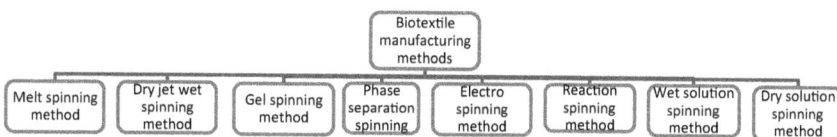

FIGURE 5.1 Various methods by which biotextiles are manufactured for medical uses.

DOI: 10.1201/9781003331612-6

As mentioned in Figure 5.1, these are the different types of biotextile manufacturing methods used for the production of biotextiles, which are meant for various types of uses, based on their biocompatibility and mechanical strength of the polymeric structure. So, the method of sterilization is based on the type of polymeric structure of the biotextiles and also on the absorbable nature of the polymer, technique, and the method of sterilization also varies among them. Sterilization is defined as "the process that removes, kills or deactivates the any form of viable microorganisms and also decreases the bioburden present on the materials".

5.2   PRINCIPLE OF STERILIZATION AND BIOBURDEN

The main motive of any sterilization technique is to decrease the amount of bioburden present on any material. Bioburden is defined as the number of contaminated or harmful viable microorganisms present on any material or device before going under sterilization process (or) bioburden is the state of cleanliness of any material or product before it is sterilized. The amount of bioburden present on any material is compared and determined by using sterility assurance levels (SAL). The accepted level of bioburden on any material after sterilization is 10^{-6} SAL (ISO 20857:2010; ANSI/AAMI/ISO 11135–1:2007). Based on the SAL levels of bioburden present on the material or product, the type of sterility method is selected, and also it is a contributory factor for the selection of sterilization dose. Various types of sterilization techniques are mentioned in Figure 5.2.

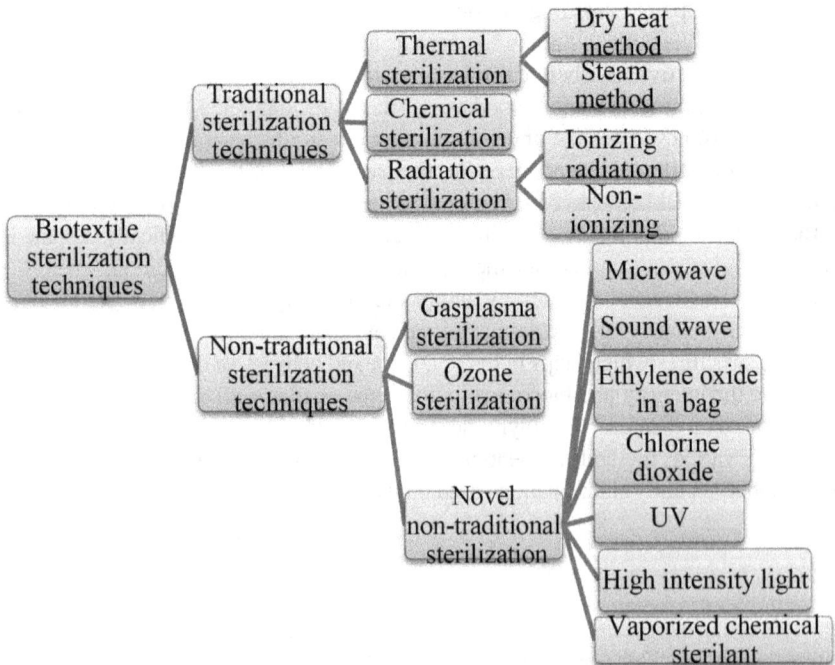

FIGURE 5.2   Various types of nano-enhanced biotextile sterilization techniques approved by the FDA.

There is a very long history of traditional sterilization methods, and these are established techniques having safe and effective use as demonstrated by ample literature, clearances, and validation. They include chemical sterilization—ethylene oxide [EO] gas sterilization, formaldehyde sterilization, thermal sterilization—moist and dry heat sterilization, and radiation sterilization (gamma, electron beam) (Hooper et al., 1997). Moist and dry heat sterilization is selected on the thermal resistance of the biotextile. Gamma radiation is also widely used and the recommended dose is 25kgy which can be used for sterilization of biotextile; however, the dose parameter can be optimized based on the biotextile material from 10 to 40kgy (Augustine et al., 2015). The advantage of gamma radiation is that it can be used in large-scale sterilization of biomaterials and its disadvantage is cost (Rutala et al., 2008).

Non-traditional sterilization techniques are the recently developed sterilization techniques, so these are also known as modern sterilization techniques. The FDA, present in the USA, has newly suggested to partition the non-traditional sterilization techniques into two different types, i) non-traditional sterilization techniques, and ii) novel non-traditional sterilization techniques (CRDH, 2008). These methods don't have any past history of safe and adequate use; there is little published information available on validation of instruments, but no standards approved by the US FDA are available.

The appropriate method to carry out sterilization is selected based on different types of factors (Rogers, 2005). They are:

- Type of microorganism to be targeted
- Thermal resistance of microorganism
- Materials needing to be sterilized
- Volume of material to be sterilized
- Thermal resistance of the material
- Bioburden present on the material
- Types of spores to be sterilized

5.3 TRADITIONAL STERILIZATION TECHNIQUES

There is a very long history of the sterilization methods which are mentioned in Figure 5.3, and these are established techniques having safe and adequate use as manifested by abundant literature, certifications, and validation. Traditional sterilization methods are defined as, "methods that have long history of safe and effective usage as demonstrated by extensive literature, clearances of 510(k)s approval and satisfactory QS inspections, and for which there are voluntary consensus criteria for verification approved by the FDA". A premarket approval review & submission form for sterility data for premarket submissions for devices labelled as sterile is termed as "510(k) form" under the Drugs and Cosmetics Act. Traditional sterilization techniques that are frequently used are "Thermal sterilization, Chemical sterilization and Radiation sterilization". Thermal sterilization is mainly used for the biomaterials which are resistant to their specific temperature. Chemical sterilization method is used for the nano-enhanced biotextiles which are difficult to sterilize and heat sensitive polymers. Radiation sterilization doesn't involve high heat and chemicals,

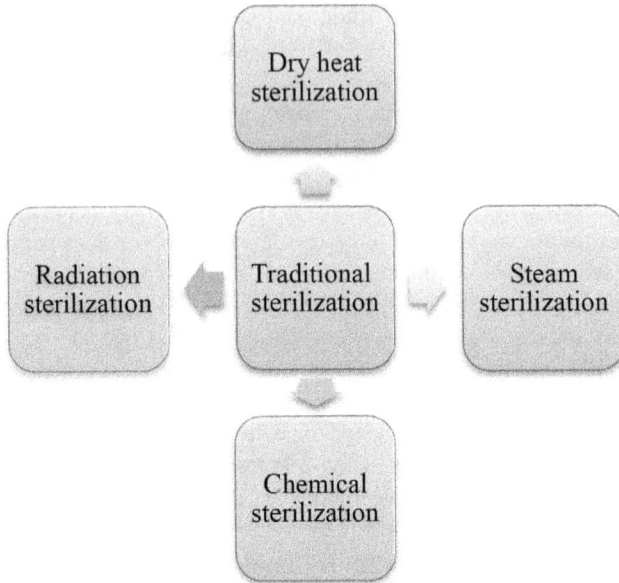

FIGURE 5.3   Different types of traditional sterilization methods classified by the FDA.

but it has its own challenges for sterilization (Hemmerich, 2000). Table 5.1 provides a summary of various techniques, encompassing their parameters, advantages, disadvantages, and the mechanisms of sterilization. Additionally, Table 5.2 outlines the selection of sterilization methods for various examples of biotextile materials.

5.3.1 THERMAL STERILIZATION TECHNIQUES

It is the oldest method of sterilization (Joslyn, 2001; Rutala et al., 2008). Thermal sterilization can be carried out on materials like glass, metals, and high thermal resistant polymers. Thermal sterilization is defined as the process of destroying the DNA proteins and enzymes in the cells by the aid of high temperature. Dry heat and steam sterilization have so many similarities like low cost, ease of control and monitoring, and absence of wastes and toxic residues. Thermal sterilization is divided into two types. They are:

- Steam sterilization
- Dry heat sterilization

5.3.1.1   Steam Sterilization Technique

Traditional steam sterilization technique is economical, non-hazardous, sporicidal, microbicidal, and also diffuses along the fibres of biotextiles very easily (Adler et al., 1998; Joslyn, 2001). This steam sterilization technique is also called moist-heat sterilization technique. In this method, heat is used as a saturated steam by the aid of pressure which kills the microorganism or denaturation

TABLE 5.1

Summary of different techniques and their parameters, advantages, disadvantages, and mechanism of sterilization.

Technique	Main parameters	Advantages	Disadvantages	Mechanism of sterilization
Dry heat sterilization	160–170°c for 1–2 hours	Simple, cost-effective. Generally, avoids metal corrosion, and depyrogenation.	It is completely dependent on the thermal resistance of materials. Long processing times.	By the aid of high temperature, it destroys the bacteria and bacterial endotoxins.
Steam sterilization (autoclave)	i) 121°c for 5–20 minutes. Other options: ii) Low-temperature steam sterilization, 110–115°c for 35–40 minutes, iii) Flash autoclave 134°c for 3–6 minutes, steam pulses in the presence of vacuum.	Simple, safe, fast, and efficient, no hazardous residues. Able to sterilize effectively. Economical, easy to monitor.	Excessive heat and moist content. Some thermosensitive materials were incompatible with it and also hydrophobic materials.	High-temperature stream de-naturates the proteins and DNA in the cells.
Ethylene oxide gas sterilization	EO: 400–1500mg/l, 2–4hour with aeration at 25–65°c (generally 55°c), high humidity (40–80%).	It has good efficiency and relatively good permeability. It is compatible with most of the materials. It will not damage heat sensitive materials. Highly flexible.	Gases being used as alkylating agents are potentially carcinogenic and mutagenic. It is a long, time taking process. It can cause potential hazards to patients, staff, and personnel.	EO gas molecules react with and destroy microorganisms.
Radiation sterilization	25kgy is the recommended radiation dose, but 10–40 dose can be used.	Large product volumes can be sterilized. Excellent efficiency, reliability, and penetrability. Dosimetric release. No toxins. No interactions with any materials. Can be compatible with many materials. Except for the dispose of radioactive materials, it is environmentally safe. Nano-enhanced biotextiles can be sterilized very effectively.	Polymers may get damaged with increased dose of radiation. Equipment and process is costly. Isotope containers and storage containers need expensive instruments and accessories for safety reasons. These facilities are available in some industries.	Ionization of nucleic acids.

TABLE 5.1 (Continued)

Summary of different techniques and their parameters, advantages, disadvantages, and mechanism of sterilization.

Technique	Main parameters	Advantages	Disadvantages	Mechanism of sterilization
Hydrogen peroxide gas plasma sterilization	Concentration of 6mg/ml at 300 watts of radio-frequency energy and 0.5torr pressure.	No toxic residues. No aeration is required. Broad range of micro-organisms can be killed effectively. Low temperature. Compatible with most medical devices. Simple to operate.	A major disadvantage is that it converts hydrophobic materials into hydrophilic materials by oxidizing of polymers. Increased exposure of hydrogen peroxide gas may be harmful to the workers.	Hydroxyl or hydropropoyl free radicals inactivate the micro-organisms by attacking lipids, DNA, and other components of the cells.
Ozone gas sterilization	Concentration varies based on the bio-burden and type of biotextile, usually carried out at 30–35°c and total cycle takes up to 4.5hours to complete.	High oxidation potential. Safe, easy to use. Economical. No toxic residues.	Till now less devices got approved by the FDA. Humidity present in the chamber may causes oxidation of the polymers.	Oxidizes the micro-organisms.
UV light sterilization	210–380 nm wavelength is used for sterilization.	Easy to handle. Environment friendly. Does not produce corrosive materials. No chemicals required. Minimal operating costs. No by-products. Effective technique.	Low penetration into deeper layers of biotextile. Can only be used for surface sterilization. Fouling of UV lamps. Energy intensive. No residual effect. Manufacturing equipment is relatively expensive.	Photons released from the radiation areused to prevent and make the bacteria incapable of carrying out cellular functions by destroying their nucleic acids and damaging their DNA/RNA.
Chlorine dioxide gas sterilization	Concentration of 10–30mg/ml, humidity of 65–90%, and at 25–30°c temperature.	Non-explosive. Non-flammable. Non-carcinogenic. Does not form trihalomethanes. More effective than chlorine.	Highly unstable. High chemical hazards. Expensive. Immediate use required.	Amino acids and RNA in the cells directly react with the chlorine dioxide and cause the death of virus, spores, microorganisms, and bacteria.

Technique	Parameters	Advantages	Limitations	Mechanism
High intensity light sterilization	High-power electric pulses (20–80kv/cm).	It shows good compatibility with the thermosensitive polymers for sterilization. No thermal effects. Intensity lasts for few seconds. Faster processing time. No toxins are released.	Folded structures of biotextile show less penetration. Not suitable for products which are having novel geometrics.	Through electroporation process it causes the cells to get swollen and leads to distortion of membrane.
Microwave radiation sterilization	Operates at 2,450MHZ.	Rapid. Inexpensive. Speed. Simple. Environment friendly.	It cannot sterilize from endospores. High initial costs for industry scale sterilization. No standard or approved FDA data are available. Heat inducing microwave radiation may cause damage to the biotextile materials.	Radiation causes apoptosis of the cell and leads to death.
Vaporized chemical sterilant technique	Example: hydrogen peroxide vapour concentration ranges from 30–35%, temperature at 25–50°c, and cycle lasts for about 1.5 hours.	Fast cycle. No toxic residues. Larger chambers enable to sterilize the large quantity of materials. Safe for environment and for workers. Safe by-products.	Sterilization efficacy is based on lumen diameter and lumen length. It converts hydrophobic materials into more hydrophilic materials.	Depends on the chemical sterilant used.

TABLE 5.2

Selection of method of sterilization for different types of examples of biotextile material.

Method of sterilization	Biotextile material that can be sterilized
Combination of gamma radiation, ethylene oxide, and dry heat.	• Dressings that include: Polyurethane foam, • Paraffin gauze, • Framycetin gauze, • Perforated film absorbent, • Sodium fusidate gauze, • Semi-permeable adhesive coating, • Knitted viscous primary, • Chlorohexidine gauze.
Any traditional sterilization method.	• Gauze pads, • Absorbent cotton gauze, • Viscose wadding that adheres, • Absorbent cotton wool.
Gamma radiation and ethylene oxide.	• Plastic wound dressing, • Elastic adhesive dressing.

makes the proteins, enzymes, cell components present in the organism irrepa-
rable for the microorganism and spores to recover. Saturated steam sterilization
requires specific temperature, pressure, and time (Mancini et al., 2005). At the
same temperature of 121°C, steam produces at least seven times as much heat
(on an equimolar basis) as dry heat, utilizing its specific heat of vaporization.
Therefore, compared to the dry heat method, the steam offers a heat-up duration
that is approximately at least 12 times faster (Ernst Robert, 1973) and the time
required to carry out sterilization is also required, because the temperature and
time at which denaturation of proteins occurs is different for different organisms. The time at which maximum sterilization can be achieved is considered
as the lowest sterilization period (Viveksarathi & Kannan, 2015). Steam sterilization is recommended for materials which are not susceptible to heat. If the
correct amount of temperature and pressure is applied, any prions, spores, and
microorganisms can be killed effectively (Rutala & Web, 2010).

The equipment used to carry out steam sterilization is autoclave, but the method
of steam sterilization varies based on the nature and thermal resistance of the biotextiles (Young, 1993). Various types of steam sterilization equipment are mentioned
in Figure 5.4:

- Gravity air displacement method
- Pressurized pulsing or vacuum method
- Dynamic-air removal method—pre-vacuum, high vacuum
- Flash sterilization technique and immediate use sterilization method
- Superheated steam sterilization method
- Novel combining steam sterilization

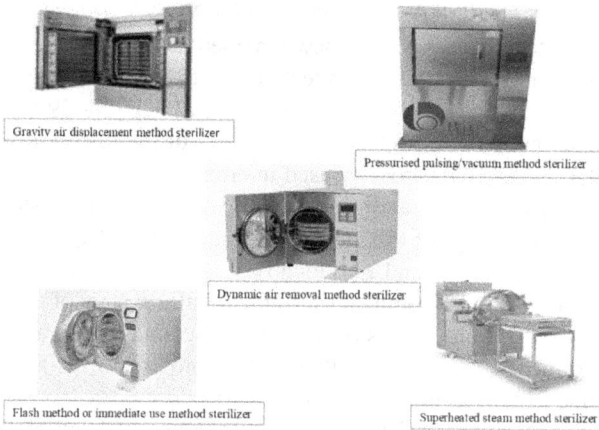

FIGURE 5.4 Different models of sterilizers that work on different principles.

5.3.1.1.1 Gravity Air Displacement Method

Gravity air displacement is a simple method, which is economical and non-toxic and requires less equipment when compared with vacuum sterilization method. In this method, heavier air is evacuated from the chamber's bottom due to gravity, so air is replaced by the steam's flow from the vent's top. The biotextile materials which are porous in nature tend to prolong the sterilization process due to the entrapped air between the pores and thus require longer durations of time to achieve sterilization (Rutala et al., 1982; Lauer et al., 1982). This methodology can be used for "sterilising bio-medical polymers, vascular poly tetrafluoroethylene prosthetics, hematic poly vinyl chloride circuit, and pacemaker cables made by polyurethanes (PU), catheters and ventricular-assisted devices".

5.3.1.1.2 Pressurized Pulsing Method and Dynamic Air Removal Method

These methods are identical to the gravity air displacement methods except that they are fixed with the help of vacuum pumps. For the pressure pulsing method, vacuum is applied, which removes the entrapped air in the chamber. A series of vacuum and steam pressurizations are applied before the steam reaches the loaded material. This drives out the entrapped air in the loaded material and allows the uniform heating. Air removal can be checked by a Bowie-Dick test. This removal of air allows the immediate penetration of steam into the loaded material.

The dynamic air removal method, also known as the pre-vacuum method, actively removes the vacuum through a series of pressure cycles before introducing steam. This method is not effective like pressure pulsing method because of the lack of pressure pulsations. AAMI recognized both SFPP cycle and pre-vacuum as a dynamic air removal method and AMSCO steam sterilizers cleared FDA approval in 1998 to carry out steam sterilization by dynamic air removal method and SFPP cycle.

5.3.1.1.3 Flash Sterilization and Immediate Use Sterilization Method

Flash sterilization technique has been newly named as immediate use steam sterilization and it is a very rapid sterilization technique. It is carried out at very high temperatures like 132°–138°c and also at high pressure (2.02bar or 29.41psig) typically with pre-vacuum and without packaging or barriers of the material (Rogers, 2006; ANSI/AAMI ST79, 2010). It is mainly used in order to process cleaned patient care products that cannot be stored and packaged and thus need to be sterilized before use. The main disadvantage of this method is removing package and exposing the material to high temperatures and additionally, this approach also excludes biological indicators. It is also not recommended as the regular system of sterilization. The immediate use sterilization process demonstrates the smallest duration betwixt the sterilization and the transfer of biotextile material into aseptic chamber. This sterilization technique demonstrates that this product has not been exposed to contaminated air or other environmental factors. The materials sterilized by this technique cannot be stored for long-term usage, so this sterilization is useful for the materials which are used immediately. The medical implants which are meant for immediate use can be sterilized by using flash sterilization.

5.3.1.1.4 Superheated Steam Sterilization and Other Novel Steam Sterilization Techniques

In the superheated steam sterilization, steam is used whose temperature is more than the vaporization point, at which the temperature is measured at the absolute pressure. The saturated steam (100°c, 1bar, 2690kJ kg^{-1}) is after heated to a superheated state at 110°c gains 30kJ kg^{-1} (2720KJ kg^{-1}) at 1 bar pressure, and this process is detailly explained in schematic Figure 5.5. Superheated steam can be used for microbial deactivation, inactivate enzymatic reaction, and denature microbial proteins at higher temperatures for sufficient duration of time is exposed to inactivate microorganisms.

In the novel steam sterilization techniques, propylene oxide may be used in the place of ethylene oxide and formaldehyde. Propylene oxide is non-toxic and non-explosive. It can be applied with steam, resulting in a non-toxic end product preservative glycol. Propylene oxide is more stable in water when compared with formaldehyde or ethylene oxide. Exposure of biotextiles and medical devices to the steam can be reduced by combining the steam along with the propylene oxide at higher temperatures. As mentioned in Table 5.3, low-temperature steam sterilization can be carried out at <100°c; other techniques, such as combining steam with either acidic or basic pH, typically reduce the duration required to sterilize biotextiles at lower temperatures for an extended period. Additionally, methods like combining low-steam with chemicals such as formaldehyde (Rogers, 2005) facilitate shorter-duration sterilization processes.

5.3.1.2 Dry Heat Sterilization Technique

It is the oldest method of sterilization which is used for inactivation and preservation. In this method, sterilization is achieved by exposure of dry heat for a longer period of time than the steam sterilization. It is not as effective as steam sterilization (Rhodes &

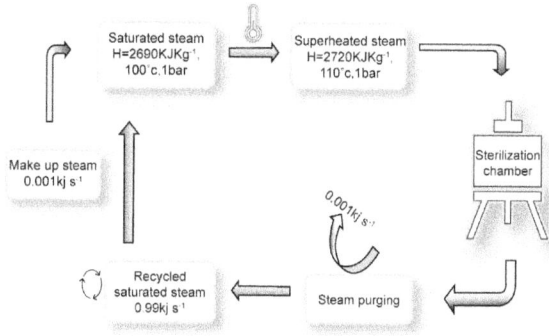

Schematic representation of working of superheated sterilization

FIGURE 5.5 Schematic representation of the working of superheated sterilization technique.

TABLE 5.3
Parameters involved in different types of steam sterilization techniques.

Method of sterilization	Parameters	
	Temperature	Time
Gravity air displacement method	121°c	15 minutes
Gravity air displacement method	121°c	60 minutes for killing prions
Gravity air displacement method or flash sterilization	121°c	10 minutes
Pre-vacuum	132°–134°c	18 minutes for killing prions
Pre-vacuum	132°–134°c	4–20 minutes
Pre-vacuum or flash	132°–138°c	3 minutes for unwrapped items
Superheated steam sterilization	≥100°c	Time varies based on material

Note: The preceding exposure parameters may differ depending on the sterilizer, bioburden, test instruments, amount of material to be sterilized, time for heating and cooling, as well as time for penetration into material, overall kill.

Fletcher, 1996). Unlike steam, dry heat sterilization uses high temperatures (160–190°c) for a longer period of time. As mentioned in Table 5.4, the time required for exposure to dry heat also plays a crucial role (Ram Mohan & Gupta, 2016). This method mainly involves the oxidation of viable cell components, proteins, enzymes, DNA, spores, and prions by the aid of high temperature. Due to the high temperature, the materials which are thermal resistant can only be sterilized. The major advantages of this technique are that it is inexpensive, doesn't cause harm to the environment, doesn't corrode with the metals, and doesn't produce any toxic end by-products. Major disadvantages of this method are that most of the biotextile materials cannot tolerate the high temperatures in the dry heat sterilization and penetration of heat into the materials takes a longer duration of time. Some examples of biotextile materials are given in Table 5.5.

TABLE 5.4
Different parameters of temperature and time at which sterilization can be carried out.

Sterilization method	Time	Temperature (°c)
Dry heat sterilization	≥8 hours	105–135°c
Dry heat sterilization	180 minutes	150°c
Dry heat sterilization	2 hours	160°c
Dry heat sterilization	1 hour	170°c
Dry heat sterilization	30 minutes	180°c
Dry heat sterilization	12 minutes with package	190°c
Dry heat sterilization	6 minutes	190°c
Dry heat sterilization	1.15 minutes	330°c

Note: The time and temperature may vary based on the bioburden, type of instrument, type of biomaterial, type of microorganism, sterility assurance level, and other factors.

TABLE 5.5
The potential dry heat of the materials at which they can be sterilized.

Polymer or material	Temperature at which can be sterilized
Glass	> 190°c
Ethylene-chlorotrifluoroethylene	Up to 150°c
Poly ether ketone (PEI)	Up to 250°c
Ethylene-tetra fluoroethylene ETFE	Up to 150°c
Polyetherimide	Up to 134°c
Fluoropolymers (most Teflon)	Varies (see polymers)
Poly methyl pentene (PMP or TPX)	Up to 170°c
High-density polyethylene (HDPE)	Up to 120°c
Polypropylene (PP)	Up to 135°c (no stacking)
Instruments	Up to 190°c
Poly propylene co-polymer (PPCO)	Varies between 120–135°c
Metals	Up to 190°c
Poly phenyl oxides (PPO)	Varies between 100–148°c
Muslin	Up to 160°c
Poly urethane (PU)	Varies depending on grade and loads
Nylon (polyamide—heat-stabilized grades)	Up to 130°c
Poly vinyl chloride	Up to 120°c
Needles	Up to 190°c
Polyethylene (HDPE and XLP)	Up to 120°c
Polyethylene terephthalate copolymer (PETG)	Up to 134°c
Polyvinylidene fluoride (PVF)	Up to 125°c

There are different models in dry heat sterilizer instruments—ovens are the most basic dry heat sterilizers. In gravity convection ovens, hot air is displaced by gravity, but this method is not adequate. In a mechanical air displacement oven or forced convection, heated air is displaced all over the area and it is one of the quickest sterilizers. Heated up air is moved at 2500–3000feet/min at 190°c for three to six minutes (Wood, 1993) in this oven. Modern dry heat sterilization techniques include continuous belt system and infrared radiation. Continuous belt sterilizer works by forced air convection, in which items pass along the belt and get sterilized. The biotextile materials or medical devices should have direct contact with infrared radiation to get sterilized uniformly.

5.3.1.3 Chemical Sterilization Technique

Chemical sterilization is a very old method which is completely reliable on chemicals. It is defined as the process of sterilizing of materials by the aid of chemical sterilant. The most commonly used chemicals for sterilization are ethylene oxide and formaldehyde. This method of sterilization has its own limits, however; they are:

i) The harmful effect of chemicals remains over the materials
ii) User protection concerns due to exposure to the gases
iii) Chemicals might react with the polymers
iv) Environment pollution
v) Toxic residues

5.3.1.3.1 Ethylene Oxide (EtO) Sterilization Technique

Ethylene oxide (EtO) gas is a colourless, extremely skin irritant, and highly flammable gas; despite many disadvantages of the ethylene oxide gas, it has many advantages like microbicidal and sporicidal. It is a very dominant sterilization method used till now and also known as low heat sterilization method. Ethylene oxide gas sterilizes by acting on the proteins, nucleic acid, and amino groups, and the sulfhydryl, amino, hydroxyl, and carboxyl groups which are present in cells are also alkylated. The sterilization efficacy of this gas relies on the relative humidity, temperature, exposure time, bioburden, and gas concentration (Freeman, 2014). The sterilization process includes the removal of gases by vacuum in autoclave and then injection of ethylene oxide gas in the concentration ranging from 600–1200mg/l, relative humidity ranging from 40–50% at a constant temperature of 30–50°c (preconditioning, humidification, gas exposure, evacuation, and air washes), and the exposure period should be two to eight hours based on the bioburden and the type of material. Various advantages of this method are: excellent microbicidal activity, moisture or heat sensitive materials can be sterilized, ideal gas sterilant, high diffusivity through materials, virucidal, fungicidal, and sporicidal. The main disadvantages of this method are carcinogenic property of gas; by product formation and alkylation reactions were observed with urea and urethane groups (Abraham et al., 1997); a high humidity level can initiate chain deterioration and have a negative impact on the mechanical characteristics of biotextiles; extra time is required to remove the EO gas (aeration) out of the material; and potential hazards to patients, staff, and environment (Hermanson et al., 1997).

5.3.1.3.2 *Formaldehyde Sterilization*

Formaldehyde is a colourless, strong smelling, and flammable gas that causes irritation to skin. For a very long time, it has been utilized as a sterilizing agent. This method is economical in nature, but it has several drawbacks like ethylene oxide gas. Formaldehyde mostly is used as a surface sterilant. The formation of formaldehyde gas is difficult and it has potential for the polymerization of the gaseous monomers (Clough & Shalaby, 1996).

5.3.1.4 Radiation Sterilization Technique

Radiation sterilization method utilizes both ionizing and non-ionizing radiation to carry out sterilization, and it is also a widely used method for sterilization. It is a quick and effective method of sterilization, but higher capital expenditures are a significant drawback. The sources of ionizing radiation are gamma radiation, x-ray sources, and high-energy electron sources. Commercially, high energy electrons as well as high energy photons are utilized to sterilize medical products.

The most frequently used gamma radiation sources are Cobalt-60 (^{60}co) and caesium-137 (^{137}cs). The minimum recommended dose is 25kgy, and it can also be modified based on the biotextile (Augustine et al., 2015). However, use of gamma radiation on biotextile polymers causes physical changes, discolouration, odour generation, stiffening, and decrease in molecular weight. Gamma radiation also has the potential to produce toxic products as by-products; when high molecular weight polyurethane material irradiates with gamma radiation it produces 4,4'-methylenedianiline toxic product (Shintani & Nakamura, 1991). Temperature generated due to radiation depends on the design and cobalt activity, and maximum temperature can go up to 45–50°c.

X-ray sterilization has high penetration characteristics when compared with gamma radiation and high energy electrons. The penetration efficacy of x-ray, gamma, and electron radiation are represented graphically in Figure 5.6. X-ray is an electromagnetic (photon) energy that is generated from the electron cloud of an atom. X-rays are generally produced in two forms: characteristic x-rays and Bremsstrahlung radiation. Bremsstrahlung radiation contains high-energy x-rays which are high-frequency short wavelength electromagnetic radiations. Temperature generated depends on design and power, and typically reaches maximum from 35–40°c. X-rays generation is much costlier than the gamma radiation energy, but it will decrease exposure times and shorten turnaround times, and requires less shielding. It requires less dose for sterilization of biotextiles when compared with gamma and electron radiations.

Up to 7Mev, high energy photons can be generated using either gamma irradiators or X-ray machines, but its production is relatively high cost. There are three mechanisms by which these photons interact with the matter: i) photoelectric-effect, ii) Compton scattering/Compton effect, and iii) pair formation process and causes ionization of the electrons in the atom/cell. The high penetration of these photons helps in the sterilization of many biotextiles. Electron accelerators such as DC-accelerator and radio frequency-accelerator are used to produce high energy electrons. By using radio frequency-accelerator, up to 10MeV energy can be reached. The radiation limits are currently 10MeV for electrons and 7MeV for photons. Temperature generated mainly depends on electric power and can reach maximum of 50°c. It is extensively used in industries for sterilizing various medical products and biotextiles because of its penetration nature and no toxic residues.

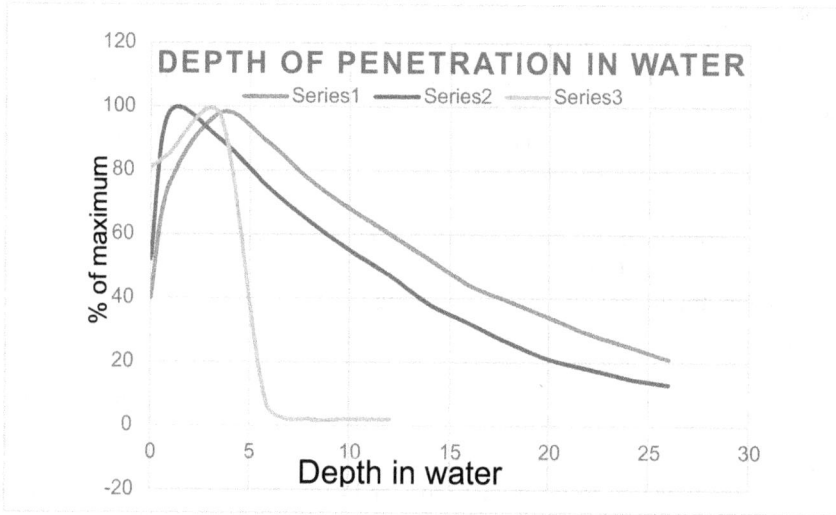

FIGURE 5.6 Graphical representation of the penetration efficacy of various radiations in water.

Series: 1–7.5MeV x-ray
Series: 2–10MeV electrons
Series: 3–Cobalt 60

5.4 NON-TRADITIONAL STERILIZATION TECHNIQUES

Methods like thermal heat, steam, radiation, and chemical sterilization were developed and have been followed for a very long time, yet there is no perfect sterilization technique to sterilize the biotextiles effectively, and toxic residues are also produced from these methods. The toxicity of ethylene oxide gas sterilization and the increased use of thermal sensitive polymers in clinical applications have resulted in the creation of novel sterilization techniques. So, for the past 25 years research developments were mainly focused on developing the most effective sterilization techniques for sterilizing biotextiles. These methods are known as non-traditional sterilization techniques. Non-traditional sterilization technique is defined by FDA as,

> The methods that do not have a long history of safe and effective usage and no standards approved by the FDA, but information is available to validate those methods, and for which the FDA had previously evaluated the data as a part of the QS review-510(k) and method turned out to be efficient.

A premarket approval review & submission form for sterility data for premarket submissions for devices labelled as sterile is termed as "510(k) form" under the Drugs and Cosmetics Act. The US FDA has recently divided these techniques into two different categories (CDRH, 2008). This separation has been initiated by FDA, because it had started receiving many (510k) applications for medical devices labelled as using a sterile technique that uses a non-traditional sterilization method for manufacturing biotextile medical instruments. While the FDA has information about a few non-traditional sterilization techniques, it has identified that some methods are very new and these can cause substantial risk to human life because of inadequate sterility assurance. Thereupon, the FDA has decided to examine the production site before approving the 510(k)'s for devices sterilized by novel non-traditional sterilization technique. Then FDA has recognized sterilization techniques into three different groups: a) traditional sterilization techniques, b) non-traditional sterilization techniques, and c) novel non-traditional sterilization techniques.

Non-traditional sterilization techniques are: i) hydrogen peroxide (H_2O_2) gas plasma, and ii) ozone (O_3).

Novel non-traditional sterilization techniques are defined by FDA as, newly developed methods for which there are no FDA approved standard criteria or there is no FDA inspectional history, or there is little or no published information on validation, and for which there is no history of comprehensive FDA evaluation of sterilization validation data.

A novel non-traditional sterilization method is one that uses sterilization techniques that the FDA has not examined and found sufficient to offer reasonable assurance of safe and effective use. It has also not been analysed by FDA as part of a QS evaluation. Novel non-traditional sterilization techniques are:

i) Chlorine Dioxide (ClO_2)
   Ethylene Oxide-in-a-Bag (EtO-in-a-Bag, Diffusion method, or Injection method). This method differs from traditional EtO methods in that Ethylene Oxide-in-a Bag specifies a volume of EtO instead of a concentration (e.g., 7.2 grains instead of 500–600 mg/L), uses an EtO cartridge or capsule, uses humidichips, or uses a long gas dwell time (e.g., greater than 8 hours).
ii) High Intensity Light or Pulse Light
iii) Microwave Radiation
iv) Sound Waves
v) Ultraviolet Light
vi) Vaporized Chemical Sterilant Systems (e.g., hydrogen peroxide or peracetic acid)

5.4.1   Hydrogen Peroxide (H_2O_2) Gas Plasma Sterilization

The hydrogen peroxide gas plasma sterilization is also known as "low temperature hydrogen peroxide gas plasma sterilization". Plasma, which is considered as a fourth state of matter, could be generated by using higher electric or magnetic or temperature, although low temperature sterilization is easily compatible with many medical devices (Okpara-Hofmann et al., 2005). For materials and gadgets that are sensitive to moisture and temperature, this technique is often commonly utilized. Low temperature plasma is an appropriate method for heat sensitive materials because of these plasmas' unique ability to destroy covalent bond while the product is kept at normal temperatures (Jacobs & Lin, 2001; Holler et al., 1993). Plasma can be generated by two methods—hot and cold method. Hot method is not widely used due to its damaging nature to the thermally sensitive materials. Hydrogen peroxide gas plasma (concentration-6mg/l) is generated by cold plasma method. Cold plasma consists of a partially ionized gas, encompassing ions, electrons, ultraviolet photons, and reactive neutrals, including radicals, excited molecules, and ground-state molecules. It is produced by exposing a hydrogen peroxide (H_2O_2) or peracetic acid to an electric (or) magnetic field (Lerouge et al., 2002). Peracetic acid is an organic solution that produces acetic acid as a by-product in the oxidation process. One method accommodates a 45-minute cycle during which vapourised H_2O_2 is dispersed via the treatment compartment, and then the plasma is produced by applying 300 watts of radio frequency energy at a pressure of 0.5 Torr. The plasma is kept for long enough to ensure complete sterilization, with a regular period that will last 15 minutes. Overall, the process lasts about a one hour (Bathina et al., 1998). Another method uses hydrogen peroxide and peracetic acid vapor treatment, which is replaced with the subsequent plasma treatment by microwave activation of the low-pressure gaseous mixture, consisting of O_2, H_2, and Ar. The device works via vaporizing the chemical substances and dispersing the vapor into the compartment, fluctuating with the plasma. When sterilization is finished, the chemical agents combine to form oxygen and water which are non- toxic, removing the need for aeration as like traditional ethylene oxide sterilization, along with that plasma chemical activated components immediately vanishes once the device is turned off. The sterilized biotextile materials can be safely handled, whether for immediate use or storage. The procedure operates within the range of 37–44°c and has a cycle time of 75 minutes. If there is any moisture present on the objects, the vacuum will not be achieved, and the cycle will abort.

The plasma sterilization process combines the use of hydrogen peroxide gas with the free radicals—hydroxyl or hydroproxyl radicals— and helps to inactivate microorganisms by attacking DNA, membrane lipids, and other cell elements (Rutala et al., 1999). Peracetic acid, also known as peroxyacetic acid (PAA), operates as an oxidizing agent, functioning similarly to hydrogen peroxide. It induces denaturation of proteins, disrupts cell wall permeability, and oxidizes sulfhydryl and sulfur bonds in proteins, enzymes, and other metabolites (Rutala et al., 1999). Plasma sterilization has the potential to destroy or deactivate a wide spectrum of bacterial spores, bacteriums, vegetative bacteria, yeasts, fungi, and viruses. Like all sterilization processes, method effectiveness depends on time, temperature, lumen diameter and length, concentration, organic substances, and inorganic salts. The main disadvantage of this method is, via the oxidation of the polymer it causes the hydrophobic materials to turn into hydrophilic materials. Consequently, this technique isn't really appropriate for extremely hydrophilic materials, biological tissues, paper, cotton, and linen.

5.4.2 OZONE (O_3) STERILIZATION

Ozone (O_3) gas is a highly reactive gas which is used as a drinking water disinfecting agent, as well as for food and air sterilization (Dufresne et al., 2008; Murphy, 2006) from the past. It has a strong pungent odour and is highly oxidative in nature which can be used for chemically altering and inactivating a variety of chemical toxicants and microorganisms (Kim et al., 1999). This sterilization technique can be used as an alternative to the low temperature hydrogen peroxide gas plasma sterilization. For sterilization of reusable medical gadgets, this method is cleared by the FDA under 510(k) submission form (Kyi et al., 1995).

It is composed of three oxygen atoms in its structure which can be obtained naturally or synthetically. Ozone can be produced by splitting the diatomic oxygen (O_2) molecules into two monoatomic oxygen (O_2) molecules by supplying sufficient energy. Produced monoatomic oxygen molecules are allowed to colloid with the diatomic oxygen molecules to form ozone (O_3) as represented in Figure 5.7. The oxidation potential of ozone (O_3) is E^O −2.07 is greater than the oxidation potential of hydrogen peroxide (H_2O_2) −1.78v and chlorine dioxide (ClO_2) −1.57v. The STERIZONE 125L which is schematically represented in Figure 5.8 is an ozone sterilizer instrument merchandized by technologies of sterilization with ozone incorporated and was approved by Canada in 2002 and by the FDA in 2003. Internally, the sterilizer produces its own sterilant using its USP-grade oxygen, water, and electricity. Oxygen gas is passed through an ozone generator and via electric field which converts the oxygen gas (O_2) into ozone gas (O_3) sterilant. This process is separated into two

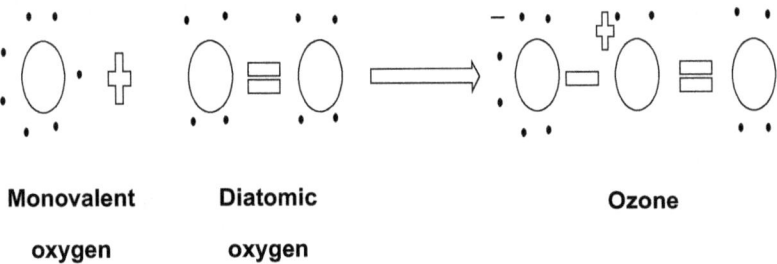

Monovalent   **Diatomic**   **Ozone**

  oxygen   **oxygen**

FIGURE 5.7 Representation of generation of ozone by chemical reaction by using Lewis dot structure.

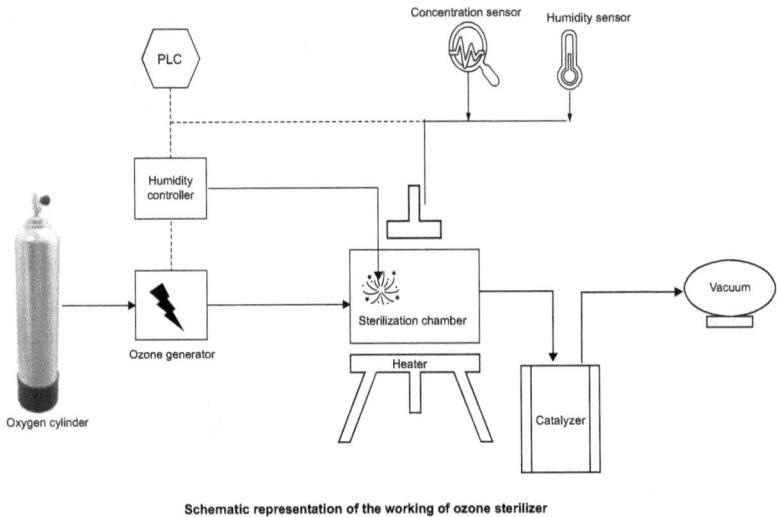

Schematic representation of the working of ozone sterilizer

FIGURE 5.8 Schematic representation of the working procedure of ozone gas sterilizer.

equivalent half sterilization phases: in the first phase vacuum is generated and in the second phase devices are humidified and then ozone (O_3) gas is generated and this sterilization cycle lasts for about 4.5 hours in a 125L system and it occurs at 30–35°c. The ozone gas concentration is monitored by an internally presented ozone monitor to induce the correct dose of sterilant to attain proper sterilization of the material. At the termination of the process, the sterilant is transformed back into water vapour and oxygen by passing via a catalyst before being expelled into the room.

Microbial effectiveness has been proven by obtaining a SAL of 10^{-6} on a variety of bacteria, microorganisms, Geobacillus stearothermophilus, and also including the most resistant microorganism. Exposure to any sterilant for a prolonged period of time causes toxicity and health hazard. That's why the Occupational Safety and Health Administration (OSHA, US) created a short-term exposure restriction of 0.3parts or less per million (ppm) in 15 minutes and a vulnerability limit of 0.1ppm or less as average throughout time of 8 hours. The main advantages of this technique are safety, ease of use, lower cost, absence of toxic by-products, and also potential inactivation of prions.

The biggest drawback of this method is the small number of sterilization instruments that have been approved till the date to carry out this sterilization process. The humidity present in the chamber and highly oxidative ozone may interact with the materials like natural rubber, textile fabrics, and latex and may also cause corrosion with metals like copper, zinc, nickel, bronze, and brass. The STERIZONE ozone sterilizer, constructed from stainless steel with specific lumen diameter and length, has received FDA approval. The approved specifications include an internal diameter (ID) of >4 mm and a length of ≤60 cm; an ID of >3 mm and a length of ≤47 cm; and an ID of >2 mm and a length of ≤25 cm. Until now, no sterilizer has received clearance for the sterilization of glass, ampoules, and medical implant devices that will be in contact with human skin for more than 24 hours. Due to these reasons, sterilizers like the STERIZONE 125L, which utilize pure ozone, have ceased production. To overcome these difficulties, a new system has been developed by TSO_3, combining hydrogen peroxide (H_2O_2) in the place of water and ozone, which shows that the synergistic effect between hydrogen peroxide and ozone facilitates penetration of sterilant into the narrow, long lumens (Wallace, 2010) and it is marketed as "3M™Optreoz™125-Z" low temperature sterilization device by 3M™ in Europe and Canada. Therefore, ozone (O_3) gas and hydrogen peroxide gas may also lead to a synergetic reaction on deterioration of biotextile materials. A standard procedure and data are not available because it has not been authorized by any governing bodies. Novel non-traditional techniques help in the generation of ozone by cold plasma, coronary discharge, and ultraviolet light at two wave lengths (185 and 254 nm photons) but the system produces less ozone and substantially requires a longer period of exposure to attain sterilization (Vig, 1985).

5.4.3 Ultraviolet Light Sterilization Technique

Ultraviolet light radiation is also known as electromagnetic radiation. The radiated waves are in the range of 210–380 nm which shows the electromagnetic spectrum. Short-wavelength waves emitted from UV light are employed for disinfection and sterilization. In general UV spectrum consists of three different ranges—UVA:(315–400 nm), UVB:(280–315 nm), and UVC:(100–280 nm). UVC is the short-wavelength ultraviolet light, which has the properties of disinfection (Rutala et al., 2008). By damaging their nucleic acids and altering their DNA and RNA, the photons emitted by the radiation are utilized to destroy or deactivate the bacteria, leaving them incapable to carrying out cellular functions. Mercury based lamps-253.7 nm, pulsed-xenon lamps-230 nm and light emitting diode lamps-255 to 280 nm are used for the generation UV light radiation (Kowalski, 2019; Messina et al., 2015).

When compared with the other radiation techniques, UV radiation has very low permeation into the inner layers of the biotextiles and medical devices. The main disadvantage of this technique is that it can be used only for surface sterilization. By placing the scaffold in a UV decontamination device, the scaffold was subjected to UV radiation at 40 watts, wavelength 254 nm, average density 15 kJ/cm^2 for three hours (Naderi et al., 2016).

5.4.4 Chlorine Dioxide Gas Sterilization Technique

Chlorine dioxide (ClO_2) gas is a potent oxidizer which is a reddish to yellowish green colour gas. This gas is applied for sterilization of medical gadgets, same as like ethyleneoxide (EtO) gas, which is most efficient at ambient temperatures 25 to 30°c (Kowalski & Morrissey, 2004). It is a non-explosive and non-flammable gas when used at specific concentrations for sterilization and it is also not carcinogenic. It can sterilize effectively from viruses, bacteria, spores, and also inactivated microorganisms; unlike chlorine it may doesn't form trihalomethanes and chloramines. Chlorine dioxide (ClO_2) is produced from sodium hypochlorite ($NaclO_2$) and sodium chlorate ($NaclO_3$), and this is stored as a liquid at 4°c. Chlorine dioxide cannot be stored for a long time, because it is highly unstable and converts back into chlorine and oxygen. Chlorine dioxide gas is generally more soluble in water up to 10 times faster than chlorine and will remain as a dissolved gas in water.

The FDA has approved ClorDiSys—sterilizer (ISO 13485–2016) in the year 2014, for carrying out sterilization of medical devices by using chlorine dioxide gas under (510k)'s submission form (US Environmental protection agency) which is schematically represented in Figure 5.9. This alternative provides a new approach for sterilization of various medical devices for manufacturers and also answers the need for new medical devices and biotextiles which are sensitive to temperature and harsh chemicals and introduces environmentally safe sterilization techniques. The airtight chamber is filled with chloride gas at a concentration of 10 to 30 mg/L along with the humidity (65–90%) to sterilize the materials in the chamber. The chlorine dioxide gas concentration is easily monitored by using built in UV-visible spectrophotometer to ensure the concentration range of gas acquires enough sterilization. Aeration is rapid (1.5–3 hours) and it can be simply exhausted into the environment without the need to scrub with hazardous chemicals, though sometimes scrubbing is also carried out. Amino acids and RNA in the cells react directly with the chlorinedioxide gas which causes the death of virus, spores, bacteria, and microorganisms, and sterility assurance level (SAL) of 10^{-6} is also achieved.

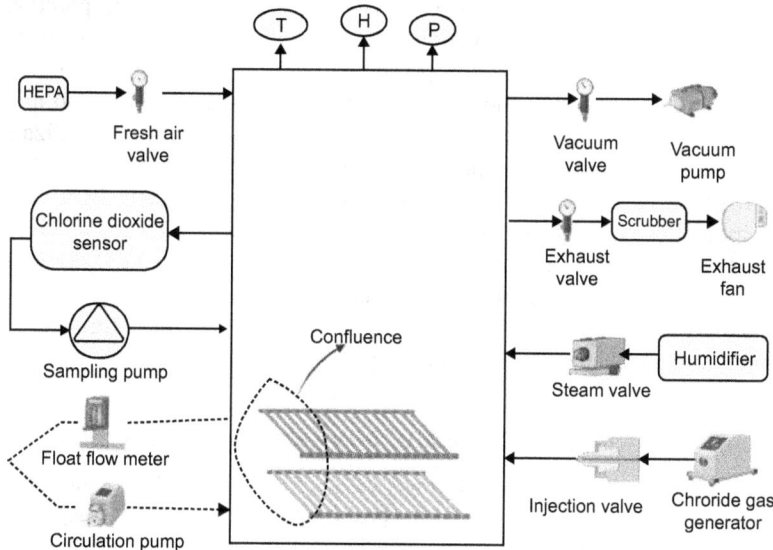

FIGURE 5.9 Schematic representation of the working procedure of chlorine dioxide gas sterilizer.

HEPA-High efficiency particulate matter, P-Differential pressure sensor, H-Relative humidity sensor, T-Temperature sensor.

5.4.5 High Intensity Light Sterilization Technique

High Intensity Light sterilization is as well as known as pulsed light (or) white light and it had been approved by the, FDA in the year 1996 for processing and handling of food. This sterilization technique is capable of only surface sterilization because it cannot penetrate into the layers of biotextiles and medical devices. This technique has its own limitations like UV-sterilization, specifically the deficiency of permeation into deeper layers that causes the researchers' loss of interest for sterilization of nano-enhanced biotextiles and new medical devices. However, several studies have shown the potential of pulsed light to decontaminate surfaces (Demirci & Panico, 2008; Oms-Oliu et al., 2012). This is one of the reasons why it is not used in large scale sterilization. This technique is considered to be promising to sterilize the biomaterials and medical gadgets with the usage of high intensity electric field. It is an innovative method which uses flashlamp for the creation of small duration and high-power electric pulses (20–80kv/cm) for carrying out sterilization like in ultraviolet sterilization.

It primarily involves producing higher power electric pulses as in Figure 5.10, which are subsequently converted into high-power light pulses using electric lamps with gas in them (quartz lamp) (Rowan et al., 1999; Dunn et al., 1997) and then allowed to fall on the target materials to inactivate or kill the microorganisms by disrupting or breaking the membrane of the cells. Bacterial membrane rupture is reached at a membrane potential of approximately 1v. In *E.coli*, this is similar to around 10kv/cm (Castro et al., 1993). This process is called electroporation and causes swelling of cells and destruction of the membrane. No specific standard procedures and parameters have been approved by the FDA. So, very less information is available about the sterilization of biotextiles, but its compatibility and minimal alteration of food characteristics indicate the good suitability with the sterilization of temperature sensitive polymers and also with biotextiles.

Sterilization can be enhanced by combining the high intensity light with any other physical or chemical stresses used for sterilization of biotextiles. There is a proposed combination of high intensity light with the supercritical CO_2 for inactivation of microorganisms at temperature lower than 40°c (Spilimbergo et al., 2002), by enhancing the penetration of supercritical CO_2 liquid into the cell membrane by electroporation mechanism of high intensity light.

5.4.6 MICROWAVE RADIATION STERILIZATION TECHNIQUE

Microwave sterilization is a novel, innovative sterilization technique which is widely used for sterilization in the food industry. It is a rapid, inexpensive, simple, and environment friendly technique for sterilization of food, dental devices/instruments, soft contact lenses, biomedical waste, and urinary catheters. Sterility assurance levels for the materials that need to be sterilized can only be accomplished by rotating the materials in three dimensions for penetration of microwaves into the deeper layers of the material This process can be influenced by the presence of water in microorganisms and microwave radiation power. Most of the microwave instruments operate at 2,450MHZ. Different types of materials exhibit varying properties with magnetic waves. Metals reflect magnetic waves, while denture base acrylic resins are transparent, neither absorbing nor reflecting them, and they do not heat up.

Microwave radiation sterilization technique is carried out by two types: heat inducing low frequency radiation and non-thermal pulsed microwave radiation. The amount of water present in microorganisms alters the heat inducing characteristics of the microwaves (Wang et al., 2005). Several studies had revealed that non-thermal

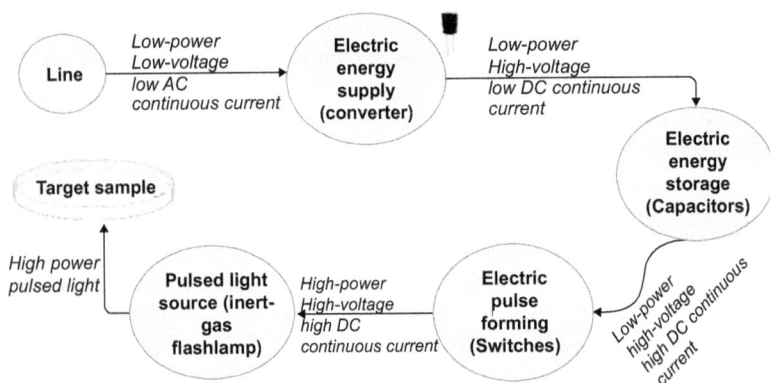

FIGURE 5.10   Flow chart of generation of high intensity pulsed light.

pulsed microwave radiation effects the metabolism of microorganisms without raising the temperature of the system (Tanner et al., 1967; Woo et al., 2000). Sterilization
is achieved by apoptosis of the cell resulting in death of the cell (Eriksson &
Stigbrand, 2010; Zhou et al., 2003). Microwave treatment at 650W for three minutes
has been shown to sterilize infected dentures from candida species as effectively as
or similar to that of chemical sterilization techniques (sterilization up to eight hours
in the 0.002% solvent of NaOCl-Sodium hypochlorite) (Klironomos et al., 2015;
Webb et al., 1998). At 2,450MHZ microwave radiation it has been reported that
hydrophilic contact lenses had been sterilized (45seconds–8minutes) from different
types of viral, bacterial, and fungal corneal pathogens (Rohrer et al., 1986). The
microwave radiation at 2,450MHZ for two minutes on bone allografts had reported
sterilization from bacteria (Singh & Singh, 2012). The main disadvantage of this
method is that it cannot sterilize the materials from endospores. Till now, no biotextile product has been sterilized and been approved by the FDA or any standards.

5.4.7   SOUND WAVES STERILIZATION TECHNIQUE

This is a very new innovative technique, which is in the initial phase of method
development. Till now no instrument or method/procedure for sterilization has been
approved by the FDA. But the use of high intensity sound waves has shown very
good progress in the killing of microorganisms and viruses. The outbreak of SARS-
COVID-19 has led to the development of theoretical research in the field of sterilization, as it has been stated that use of high intensity sound waves 100–120db has
killed the viruses in the air, on surfaces, and also on humans (Bertha Wikara, 2021).
The main disadvantage of this technique is that these waves are harmful to human
ears and also cause sound pollution. Till now no sound wave sterilization technique
has gotten approval from the FDA or any other regulatory body to carry out sterilization on biotextile materials and medical devices.

5.4.8   VAPORIZED CHEMICAL STERILANT TECHNIQUE

The new trend is to use both chemical and ideal gas/air to carry out sterilization, this
technique is known as vaporized chemical sterilant technique. A typical vaporized
chemical sterilant technique process consists of three different phases: i) vacuum
generation, ii) chemical injection, and iii) aeration. For instance, chemicals like
peracetic acid and hydrogen peroxide are used to generate chemical sterilant for
sterilization. To address the constraints of liquid sterilization, sterilization methods
employing vaporized hydrogen peroxide (VHP) were introduced in the mid-1980s.
These methods utilize various technologies to convert liquid H_2O_2 (approximately
30–35% concentration) into vapor and distribute it within the chamber. One technique involves drawing liquid hydrogen peroxide into a chamber using a disposable cartridge, passing via a heated vaporizer, and then placing it in the sterilization
chamber once it has vaporized. The second type of technique is also known as flow
through approach, by which a carrier air is used to carry vaporized hydrogen peroxide into the sterilization chamber with the help of either a slight positive pressure
or negative pressure (vacuum). Sterilization temperatures ranges from 25 to 50°c

and the entire cycle, including aeration, can last up to 1.5 hours (Tipnis & Burgess, 2018). Water and oxygen, which are also environmentally safe, are produced at the termination of the process.

The efficacy of vaporized hydrogen peroxide is verified by using *Geobacillus stearothermophillus* and *Bacillus subtilis*. For spores of *Bacillus subtilis* var. *niger* can be sterilized and sterility assurance level ($\log 10^{-6}$) can be achieved within 1.2 minutes by using saturated hydrogen peroxide vapor having a concentration of 7.6mgl⁻¹ at 70°c. In the preliminary studies vaporized hydrogen peroxide effectively sterilized the species of Clostridium botulinum spores, Clostridium difficile, MRSA, and Serratia marcescens (Boyce et al., 2006; Jeanes et al., 2005; French et al., 2004; Bates & Pearse, 2005). Further investigation of the method is required to demonstrate both safety and effectiveness and also to get approval from the FDA (Rutala et al., 2008). Various benefits of this sterilization technique are: causes no harm to the ecosystem and medical professionals, fast cycle, produces no harmful chemicals, larger chambers for sterilization of more materials at a time, and it is mainly utilized for temperature and humidity sensitive biotextile materials and medical gadgets. There are some limitations for this method: restricted sterilization based on lumen diameter and lumen length, restricted clinical application, incomplete information on the compatibility of materials, and comparable microbiological viability information is not applicable for linens, powdered materials, cellulose materials, or any liquids. It causes the transformation of hydrophobic materials into more hydrophilic materials through the oxidation of polymers. Table 5.6 presents biotextile materials that are compatible with various sterilization techniques.

5.5 FUTURE ASPECTS

The use of biotextiles in the medical industry has increased very quickly in the last five decades. Due to significant advancements in science and technology, biotextiles are increasingly employed in the manufacturing of novel medical devices. These devices are becoming more fragile, featuring complex geometrics, and are also getting much smaller. Many new polymeric biotextiles are synthesized and are also utilized for the manufacturing of several clinical gadgets which are very complicated in nature and are also used for the treatment of several disease conditions. These devices are used both topically and internally for implantation, so these ought to be compatible with the biological systems, that is, free from pyrogens, microorganisms, viruses (Anderson et al., 1996), and other contaminants. So, these biotextiles need to be sterilized properly without altering any of their physical and medical properties.

Sterilization techniques still had not been changed much even after the science and technology had developed very well. Sterilization is considered to be a very important step in the manufacturing and packaging of any product to make them safe for the use of patients for intended treatment. There are several types of traditional sterilization techniques like thermal, chemical, and radiation sterilization, and the recently developed non-traditional sterilization techniques like hydrogen peroxide gas plasma and ozone (O_3) gas sterilization and also most recently developed novel non-traditional sterilization techniques like chlorine dioxide, ultraviolent

TABLE 5.6
Biotextile materials that are compatible with different sterilization techniques.

Sterilization technique	Compatible materials with the technique
Steam sterilization	Canvas
	Chinese cotton
	Crepe
	Fluoro polymers
	Instruments
	Liquid crystal polymer
	Muslin
	Nylon
	Polyethylene
	Polyesters
	Polycarbonate
	Polyethylene
	Polyketones
	Polymethyl pentene
	Polyvinyl chloride
	Silica
	Syndiotactic polystyrene
	Some wraps
	Some acetals
	Cellophane
	Varies-butyl rubber
	Cotton
	Ethylene propylene diene monomer elastomers
	Glass
	Kraft polymer
	Most metallic instruments
	Nitrile elastomers
	Varies-paper
	Varies-polyamide
	Polyallomer
	Polyimides
	Polypropylene
	Polyurethane
	Varies-Polyvinyl chloride
	Silica
	Syndiotactic polystyrene
	Some wraps
Dry heat sterilization	Glass
	Ethylene-chlorotrifluoroethylene
	Ethylene-tetra fluoroethylene (ETFE)
	Fluoropolymers (most Teflon)
	High-density polyethylene (HDPE)
	Instruments
	Metals
	Muslin
	Nylon (polyamide—heat-stabilized grades)

TABLE 5.6   (Continued)

Biotextile materials that are compatible with different sterilization techniques.

Sterilization technique	Compatible materials with the technique
	Needles
	Polyethylene (HDPE and XLP)
	Polyetherimide
	Poly ether ketone (PEI)
	Polyethylene terephthalate copolymer (PETG)
	Poly methyl pentene (PMP or TPX)
	Polypropylene (PP)
	Poly propylene co-polymer (PPCO)
	Poly phenyl oxides (PPO)
	Polyvinylidene fluoride (PVF)
Radiation sterilization	Most of the materials are compatible
Hydrogen peroxide sterilization	Polyvinyl chloride
	Polyurethane
	Poly ethylene
	Natural rubber
	Metals
	Silicone
	95% of the medical devices are compatible
	Polytetrafluoroethylene
Ozone sterilization	Stainless steel
	Polyethylene
	Polypropylene
	Glass
	Teflon
	Acrylic
	Silica
	Ceramic
	Titanium
	Polyvinyl chloride
	Poly-L-lactic acid
	Silicone
	Anodized aluminium
	Polylactic-co-glycolic acid
Chlorine dioxide sterilization	Polypropylene
	Polysulfones
	PEEK
	PET/PETG
	Polyethylene
	Polyetherimide
	Polycarbonate
	Cyclic Olefins
	PVC
	Hypalon
	Fluoropolymers
	Most gasket materials
	Thermoplastic Elastomers

light, pulsed light, sound waves, and vaporized chemical sterilization are available. Sterilization technique is selected based on the properties of biotextiles and the amount of bioburden present on the material. But most of the times, sterilization techniques are selected based on the past similar product, which leads to the improper sterilization of the biotextiles and damage to the product.

Generally, sterilization is achieved by killing the microorganisms either by chemically or physically acting on them. In the same way biotextiles may also get effected and toxic (Lelah & Cooper, 1986) by-products are also produced, if the technique is not selected properly. We can conclude that no single sterilization technique is applicable for the sterilization of all the biotextile products.

Steam sterilization has been used since very ancient times, but it still cannot be used for most of the novel biotextile products due to their thermal sensitive nature. Several tests and research data need to be developed on novel low-temperature steam sterilization methods to carry out sterilization for novel biotextile products. The most commonly used gas for sterilization is ethylene oxide (EtO), but the end products formed are toxic in nature. However, recent developments have shown a decrease of the toxic end products. Radiation sterilization has the fixed dose of 25kGy, but sterilization with D_{10} value cannot be achieved all the time on all types of microorganisms, so ISO has revised their standards-ISO 2006a, 2006b & 2006c to alter the dose of radiation based on the bioburden and type of material. Radiation sterilization is mostly used nowadays, but the limitation of permeation into the inner layers, damage to biotextiles, discolouration, and toxic products can be decreased by replacing the radioactive metal sources with the high-energy electrons. Non-traditional sterilization techniques and novel non-traditional sterilization techniques are designed for specific applications and their limitations are also not studied and developed very well. Non-traditional sterilization techniques like hydrogen peroxide gas plasma have shown very good effect on sterilization of biotextiles, but it converts hydrophilic materials into more hydrophilic materials. Ozone gas sterilization has shown very good sterilization properties, but the only drawback is that the number of instruments approved is much less. The very new techniques known as novel non-traditional sterilization techniques have shown proper sterilization on a limited number of biotextile products, and many more biotextile products are still in developing stage. So, these sterilization techniques can be considered for sterilization of modern biotextile products.

None of these sterilization techniques is considered to be ideal to carry out sterilization on all types of biotextile products and medical devices. Any method to be considered as an ideal sterilization technique should have the following properties: very rapid; inexpensive; easy to handle; environment friendly; lethal to unwanted microorganisms, viruses, and pyrogens; safer to workers, customers, and technicians; good penetration efficacy; no alteration of properties of the biotextile products; no toxic residues; no by-products; compatible with all types of materials; no damage to any thermal sensitive materials; stable; necessary sterility assurance level; wide range of adjustable parameters; and no limitations.

In the future, steam and dry heat sterilization techniques will be used widely at low-temperatures along with another agent (combining with acids/bases to modify pH, etc.) (Stewart, 1974), to be compatible with all types of biotextile products and medical devices. These two techniques can be considered as ideal sterilization techniques for most of the materials at low temperatures. Also, the trend to use thermal resistant biotextile materials has been increased.

5.6 CONCLUSION

Sterilization has an essential role in the manufacturing of any product which is intended for use with sterile tissues and biological systems. So, a suitable sterilization technique should be selected and planned before manufacturing any product. The growing use of biotextile materials in the medical industry on one hand and no ideal sterilization technique, however, has led to the advancement of novel (innovative) non-traditional sterilization techniques, but every technique has its own limitations. The selection of appropriate biotextile components that are well compatible with radiation, thermal resistance, and also medical devices should be manufactured in simple geometries to carry out sterilization easily. Because of the limitations, no ideal sterilization technique is applicable to carry out sterilization for all types of nano-enhanced biotextiles. So, when no proper standard data or sterilization technique is available, it is better to select the low-temperature steam or dry heat sterilization technique, which is compatible with almost all types of materials. Carrying out sterilization on the products by following the regulatory guidelines builds trust and ensures the customer or patient is satisfied to use the product without fear of any contamination. Many research activities still need to be carried out on developing and establishing the standard data of any ideal sterilization technique.

REFERENCES

Abraham, G.A., Frontini, P.M., Cuadrado, T.R. (1997). Physical and mechanical behavior of sterilized biomedical segmented polyurethanes. *Journal of Applied Polymer Science*, 65(6), 1193–1203.
Adler, S., Scherrer, M., Daschner, F.D. (1998). Costs of low-temperature plasma sterilization compared with other sterilization methods. *J. Hosp. Infect.*, 40, 125–134.
Anderson, J.M., Bevacqua, B., Cranin, A.N., Graham, L.M., Hoffman, A.S., Klein, M., Kowalski, J.B., Morrissey, R.F., Obstbaum, S.A., Ratner, B.D., Schoen, F.J., Sirakian, A. Whittlesey, D. (1996). Implants and devices. In B.D. Ratner, A.S. Hoffman, F.J. Schoen, J.E. Lemons (Eds.), *Biomaterials Science* (pp. 415–420). London: Academic Press.
ANSI/AAMI/ISO 11135–1. (2007). Sterilization of health care products—Ethylene oxide—Part 1: Requirements for development, validation, and routine control of a sterilization process for medical devices, 4th edition.
Association for the Advancement of Medical Instrumentation. (2010). ANSI/AAMI ST79: 2010 & A1: 2010—Comprehensive Guide to Steam Sterilization and Sterility Assurance in Health Care Facilities. Arlington, VA: Association for the Advancement of Medical Instrumentation.
Augustine, R., Saha, A., Jayachandran, V.P., Thomas, S., Kalarikkal, N. (2015). Dose-dependent effects of gamma irradiation on the materials properties and cell proliferation of electrospun polycaprolactone tissue engineering scaffolds. *Int. J. Polym. Mater. Polymer Biomater,* 64, 526–533.
Bates, C.J., Pearse, R. (2005). Use of hydrogen peroxide vapour for environmental control during a Serratia outbreak in a neonatal intensive care unit. *J. Hosp. Infect.*, 61, 364–366.

Bathina, M.N., Mickelsen, S., Brooks, C., Jaramillo, J., Hepton, T., Kusumoto, F. M. (1998). Safety and efficacy of hydrogen peroxide plasma sterilization for repeated use of electrophysiology catheters. *Journal of the American College of Cardiology*, 32(5), 1384–1388.

Bertha, W. (2021). Sterilization of human-filled public spaces by using sound waves: A hypothesis for suppressing sars-cov-2 and its variants spreading.

Boyce, J.M., Havill, N.L., Otter, J.A., et al. (2006). Impact of hydrogen peroxide vapor room bio-decontamination on environmental contamination and nosocomial transmission of Clostridium difficile. *The Society of Healthcare Epidemiology of America*, 155, 109.

Castro, A.J., Barbosa-Canovas, G.V., Swanson, B.G. (1993). Microbial inactivation of foods by pulsed electric fields. *J. Food Process. Pres.*, 17, 47–73.

CDRH, C.F.D.A.R.H. (2008). *Draft Guidance for Industry and FDA Staff—Submission and Review of Sterility Information in Premarket Notification (510(k)) Submissions for Devices Labeled as Sterile*. FDA.

Clough, R., Shalaby, S. (Eds.). (1996). *Irradiation of Polymers: Fundamentals and Technological Applications*. Washington, DC: ACS Books.

Demirci, A., Panico, L. (2008). Pulsed ultraviolet light. *Food Science and Technology International*, 14, 443–446.

Dufresne, S., Leblond, H., Chaunet, M. (2008). Relationship between lumen diameter and length sterilized in the 125L ozone sterilizer. *American Journal of Infection Control*, 36, 291–297.

Dunn, J., Salisbury, K., Bushnell, A., Clarke, W. (1997). Sterilization using pulsed white light. *Medical Device Technology*, 8, 24–26.

Eriksson, D., Stigbrand, T. (2010). Radiation-induced cell death mechanisms. *Tumor Biol.*, 31, 363–372.

Ernst Robert, R. (1973). The control of sterilization procedures. In M.S. Cooper (Ed.), *Quality Control in the Pharmaceutical Industry*. Cambridge, NY: Academic Press.

Freeman, A. (2014). Sterilization methods for medical devices. Google Patents.

French, G.L., Otter, J.A., Shannon, K.P., Adams, N.M.T., Watling, D., Parks, M.J. (2004). Tackling contamination of the hospital environment by Methicillin-Resistant Staphylococcus Aureus (MRSA): A comparison between conventional terminal cleaning and hydrogen peroxide vapour decontamination. *J. Hosp. Infect.*, 57, 31–37.

Hemmerich, K.J. (2000). Polymer materials selection for radiation-sterilized products. *Medical Device and Diagnostic Industry Magazine*.

Hermanson, N.J., Navarette, L., Crittendon, P. (1997). The effects of high-energy and EtO sterilisation on thermoplastics. *Medical Device and Diagnostic Industry Magazine*, Available from mddionline.com/news/effects-high-energy-and-eto-sterilisaton-thermoplastics.

Holler, C., Martiny, H., Christiansen, B., Ruden, H., Gundermann, K.O. (1993). The efficacy of Low Temperature Plasma (LTP) sterilization, a new sterilization technique. *Zentralbl. Hyg. Umweltmed*, 194, 380–391.

Hooper, K.A., Cox, J.D., Kohn, J. (1997). Comparison of the effect of ethylene oxide and gamma-irradiation on selected tyrosine-derived polycarbonates and poly (L-lactic acid). *Journal of Applied Polymer Science*, 63(11), 1499–1510.

ISO 20857:2010 Sterilization of health care products—Dry heat: Requirements for the development, validation and routine control of a sterilization process for medical devices.

Jacobs, P.T., Lin, S.M. (2001). Sterilization processes utilizing low-temperature plasma. In S.S. Block (Ed.), *Disinfection, Sterilization, and Preservation* (pp. 747–763). Philadelphia, NY: Lippincott Williams & Wilkins.

Jeanes, A., Rao, G., Osman, M., Merrick, P. (2005). Eradication of persistent environmental MRSA. *J. Hosp. Infect.*, 61, 85–86.

Joslyn, L. (2001). Sterilization by heat. In S. Block (Ed.), *Disinfection, Sterilization, and Preservation* (5th ed., p. 669). Philadelphia, NY: Lippincott Williams & Wilkins.

Kim, J.G., Yousef, A.E., Dave, S. (1999). Application of ozone for enhancing the microbiological safety and quality of foods: A review. *Journal of Food Protection*, 62, 1071–1087.

Klironomos, T., Katsimpali, A., Polyzois, G. (2015). The effect of microwave disinfection on denture base polymers, liners and teeth: A basic overview. *Acta Stomatol. Croat*, 242–253.

Kowalski, J.B., Morrissey, R.F. (2004). Sterilization of implants. In B.D. Ratner, A.S. Hoffman, F.J. Schoen, J.E. Lemons (Eds.), *Biomaterials Science: An Introduction to Materials in Medicine*. New York, NY: Academic Press.

Kowalski, W. (2019). *Ultraviolet Germicidal Irradiation Handbook: UVGI for Air and Surface Disinfection*. New York: Springer Science & Business Media.

Kyi, M.S., Holton, J., Ridgway, G.L. (1995). Assessment of the efficacy of a low temperature hydrogen peroxide gas plasma sterilization system. *J. Hosp. Infect.*, 31, 275–284.

Lauer, J.L., Battles, D.R., Vesley, D. (1982). Decontaminating infectious laboratory waste by autoclaving. *Appl. Environ. Microbiol*, 44, 690–694.

Lelah, M.D., Cooper, S.L. (1986). *Polyurethanes in Medicine*. Boca Raton, NY: CRC Press.

Lerouge, S., Tabrizian, M., Wertheimer, M.R., Marchand, R., Yahia, L. (2002). Safety of plasma-based sterilization: Surface modifications of polymeric medical devices induced by Sterrad and Plazlyte processes. *Biomed. Mater. Eng.*, 12, 3–13.

Mancini, G., Lopes, R.M., Clemente, P., Raposo, S., Gonçalves, L., Bica, A., et al., (2005). Lecithin and parabens play a crucial role in tripalmitin-based lipid nanoparticle stabilization throughout moist heat sterilization and freeze-drying. *Eur. J. Lipid Sci. Technol.*, 117(12), 1947–1959.

Messina, G., Burgassi, S., Messina, D., Montagnani, V., Cevenini, G. (2015). A new UV-LED device for automatic disinfection of stethoscope membranes. *American Journal of Infection Control*, 43(10), e61–e66.

Murphy, L. (2006). Ozone—The latest advance in sterilization of medical devices. *Canadian Operating Room Nursing Journal*, 24, 28–38.

Naderi, N., Griffin, M., Malins, E., et al. (2016). Slow chlorine releasing compounds: A viable sterilisation method for bioabsorbable nanocomposite biomaterials. *Journal of Biomaterials Applications*, 30(7), 1114–1124.

Okpara-Hofmann, J., Knoll, M., Durr, M., Schmitt, B., Borneff-Lipp, M. (2005). Comparison of low-temperature hydrogen peroxide gas plasma sterilization for endoscopes using various Sterrad models. *J. Hosp. Infect.*, 59, 280–285.

Oms-Oliu, G., Martín-Belloso, O., Soliva-Fortuny, R. (2012). Pulsed light treatments for food preservation: A review. *Food and Bioprocess Technology*, 3, 13–23.

Ram Mohan, S., Gupta, N.V. (2016). Qualification of tunnel sterilizing machine. *Int. J. ChemTech Res.*, 9(3), 400–405.

Rhodes, A., Fletcher, D. (1966). Principles of sterilisation, sterility tests and asepsis. In *Principles of Industrial Microbiology* (pp. 45–57). Oxford, NY: Pergamon Press.

Rogers, W.J. (2005). *Sterilisation of Polymer Healthcare Products* (p. 282). Shawbury, UK: Smithers Rapra Publishing.

Rogers, W.J. (2006). Steam: Uses and challenges for device sterilization. *Medical Device & Diagnostic Industry News* (pp. 80–87), Available from https://www.mddionline.com/sterilization/steam-uses-and-challenges-for-device-sterilization.

Rohrer, M.D., Terry, M.A., Bulard, R.A., Graves, D.C., Taylor, E.M. (1986). Microwave sterilization of hydrophilic contact lenses. *Am J. Ophthalmol.*, 49–57.

Rowan, N.J., Macgregor, S.J., Anderson, J.G., Fouracre, R.A., Mcilvaney, L., Farish, O. (1999). Pulsed-light inactivation of food-related microorganisms. *Applied Environmental Microbiology*, 65, 1312–1315.

Rutala, W.A., Gergen, M.F., Weber, D.J. (1999). Sporicidal activity of a new low-temperature sterilization technology: The Sterrad 50 sterilizer. *Infect. Control Hosp. Epidemiol.*, 20, 514–516.

Rutala, W.A., Stiegel, M.M., Sarubbi, F.A. (1982). Decontamination of laboratory microbiological waste by steam sterilization. *Appl. Environ. Microbiol*, 43, 1311–1316.

Rutala, W.A., Web, D.J. (2010). Guideline for disinfection and sterilization of prion-contaminated medical instruments. *Infection Control & Hospital Epidemiology*, 31(2), 107–117.

Rutala, W.A., Weber, D.J., The Healthcare Infection Control Practices Advisory Committee (HICPAC). (2008). *Guideline for disinfection and sterilization in healthcare facilities*, Available from https://stacks.cdc.gov/view/cdc/47378.

Shintani, H., Nakamura, A. (1991). Formation of 4, 4'-methylenedianiline in polyurethane potting materials by either gamma-ray or autoclave sterilization. *Journal of Biomedical Materials Research*, 25(10), 1275–1286.

Singh, R., Singh, D. (2012). Sterilization of bone allografts by microwave and gamma radiation. *Int. J. Radiat. Biol.*, 661–666.

Spilimbergo, S., Dehghani, F., Bertucce, A., Foster, N.R. (2002). Inactivation of bacteria and spores by pulse electric field and high-pressure $CO2$ at low temperature. *Biotechnol. Bioeng*, 82, 118–125.

Stewart Jr., A. [cited 10.08.1974]. Acid steam sterilization, United States Patent 3839843.

Tanner, J., Romero-Sierra, C., Davie, S. (1967). Non-thermal effects of microwave radiation on birds. *Nature*, 216, 1139.

Tipnis, N.P., Burgess, D.J. (2018). Sterilization of implantable polymer- based medical devices: A review. *International Journal of Pharmaceutics*, 544(2), 455–460.

Vig, J. (1985). UV/ozone cleaning of surfaces. *Journal of Vacuum Science & Technology A. 2010*, 3, 1027–1034.

Viveksarathi, K., Kannan, K. (2015). Effect of the moist-heat sterilization on fabricated nanoscale solid lipid particles containing rasagiline mesylate. *Int. J. Pharm. Investig.*, 5(2), 87.

Wallace, C. (2010). *RE: Optreoz™ 125-Z Low Temperature Sterilization System*. 3M Publication.

Wang, H., Takashima, H., Miyakawa, Y., Kanno, Y. (2005). Development of catalyst materials being effective for microwave sterilization. *Science and Technology of Advanced Materials*, 921–926.

Webb, B.C., Thomas, C.J., Harty, D.W., Willcox, M.D. (1998). Effectiveness of two methods of denture sterilization. *J. Oral Rehabil*, 25, 416–423.

Woo, I.-S., Rhee, I.-K., Park, H.-D. (2000). Differential damage in bacterial cells by microwave radiation on the basis of cell wall structure. *Appl. Environ. Microbiol.*, 66, 2243–2247.

Wood, R.T. (1993). Sterilization with dry heat. In R. Morrissey, C.B. Phillips (Eds.), *Sterilization Technology: A Practical Guide for Manufacturers and Users of Health Care Products* (pp. 100–110). New York, NY: Van Nostrand Reinhold.

Young, J. (1993). Sterilization with steam under pressure. In R. Morrissey, C.B. Phillips (Eds), *Sterilization Technology: A Practical Guide for Manufacturers and Users of Health Care Products* (p. 134). New York, NY: Springer.

Zhou, L., Yuan, R., Lanata, S. (2003). Molecular mechanisms of irradiation-induced apoptosis. *Front. Biosci.*, 8, d9.

Part 2

Applications of Medical
Textiles for Non-Implants

6 Advancement of Nanomedical Biotextiles for Infection Control and Protection Materials

Shovan Ghosh, Vivek Dave,
Prashansa Sharma, and Pranay Wal

6.1 INTRODUCTION

The term "biotextile" has been used for a long time and can be defined as a natural or synthetic fiber textile structure used to benefit life. When their application is primarily for medical purposes, they are referred to as "medical biotextiles," (Figure 6.1) and their use has increased dramatically due to the introduction of advanced fabrication technology. Despite the fact that they cover a wide range of topics, this chapter focuses solely on infection control and protective materials. Personal protective equipment (PPE) made from medical textiles reduces cross-infection as well as direct exposure to harmful substances. The use of specific PPE is determined by a variety of factors, including the risk of a specific body part (the face, eye, hand, etc.), the number of exposures, the type of exposures (aerosols, droplets, liquids, etc.), the duration of exposure, and so on (Sun, 2011).

Nanomedical biotextile-based products in the medical field are implants, artificial body parts, orthopedic implants, and various personal protective equipment, and their use is widening due to their various advantages over normal textiles, like biocompatibility, biodegradability, and high mechanical properties with controlled permeability. The term "medical biotextile" refers to an organized textile fiber structure used in healthcare and other biological applications where the term "biotextile" is used because biosafety and biocompatibility determine their effectiveness.

Personal protective equipment (PPE) is that which acts as a protective barrier between users and harmful substances and is specially intended for individual use. Different types of PPE are used according to the need for protection; for example, for respiratory protection, air purifying devices like masks are used, and the selection of a particular mask depends upon the presence of hazards (Singh et al., 2016; Prasad et al., 2008). Along with PPE, another similar term is PPE kit, which is the assembly of a few pieces of PPE. A medical PPE kit contains a respirator and surgical mask, a pair of surgical gloves, a medical bonnet, a long-sleeve fluid-resistant gown, a face shield, wipes, etc. The use of biotextile in those PPE preparations made them more

DOI: 10.1201/9781003331612-8

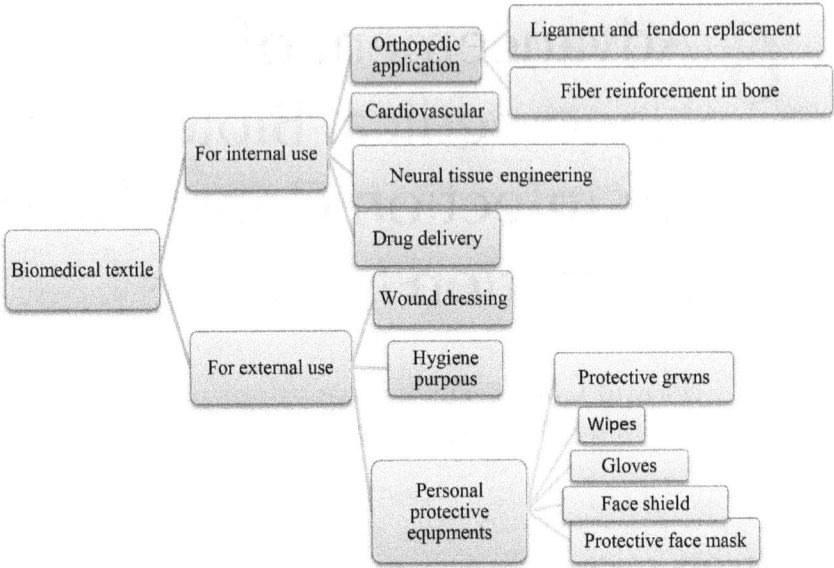

FIGURE 6.1   Application area of biomedical textile in PPE

sustainable, durable, protective, and comfortable. Among all of them, this chapter will focus on the few most important ones.

Because of the ongoing pandemic, masks have recently become a hot topic. The availability of different types of masks prepared by using different microfabrication technologies with different materials provides a distinct level of protection. They further classified them into different categories according to their level of protection as well as preparation materials. Surgical gloves are another important piece of PPE that medical professionals commonly use during surgery to protect themselves and patients from contamination. Nanocare wipes are one of the more modern approaches in the field of PPE. Those wipes are coming out in different forms for different types of uses. For total body protection, protective gowns are used.

6.2   DIFFERENT POLYMERS ARE USED FOR INFECTION CONTROL AND PROTECTIVE MATERIALS

Various polymers are used in medical biotextiles to get the desired benefits. Properties like biodegradability, mechanical strength, durability, non-toxicity, and other properties of polymers are used. Polymers are mainly of two types: natural and synthetic. Natural polymers are those that are collected from either an animal or plant source (Sionkowska, 2011). Natural polymers have less thermal stability, inertness, low mechanical properties, and resistivity than synthetic polymers, but they are still biodegradable and contain various bioactive molecules that can be helpful in the fabrication process as well as provide biofunction, such as cellulose's high thrombogenic property, which is very helpful in the wound healing process. Those polymers are converted into fibers by using different fabricating procedures. Though there are few limitations, all polymers cannot be fabricated due to their chemical structure. Polymer molecular weight should be between intermediate and high (approximately 20,000 to 250,000 Dalton) for fabrication. Linear chain polymer makes the fabrication process easier. The process was hampered by the presence of bulky side chain groups or side chains. They should have rapid crystal structure formation ability. Levels of entanglement and intermolecular bonding should have been kept to a minimum to allow for easy structure modification.

The fiber used in biomedical textiles can be divided into two types: natural fiber and man-made fiber. According to their source, natural fibers can be separated into animal source fiber (ex. silk) and plant source fiber (ex. cotton). Man-made fiber is further classified into three categories: i) artificial fiber, which is prepared by transforming natural polymers (ex. Chitosan, polylactide fiber), ii) synthetic fiber, made from synthetic polymers (ex., polyester, polypropylene), and iii) inorganic fiber, made from inorganic material like carbon or glass.

6.3 DIFFERENT MEDICAL BIOTEXTILE PRODUCTION METHODS

Fabrication is an important aspect in the preparation of medical biotextiles from various types of polymers using various spinning techniques, which can reduce the spun size to 1 m. Fabric characteristics (texture, size, and cross-section shape) can vary along with the spinning process. There are a few important spinning techniques, which we discuss next.

6.3.1 Wet Spinning

This process is more suitable for fabric formation from non-thermoplastic polymers. Polymers are dissolved in an aqueous or organic solvent, then extruded using a spinneret, and then transferred into a coagulating solution or a cross-linking solution, from which precipitate fibers are collected (Mather & Wardman, 2011). Chitosan fiber, polylactide fiber, alginate fiber, etc. can be prepared by this technique (Knaul et al., 1999; Razal et al., 2009).

6.3.2 Melt Extraction

Fiber formation is quicker than wet spinning, and the solvent is not required for this process. Polymers are heated to temperatures above their melting points in this process, and then extruded by spinneret to produce polymer resin. Then cold air is used for solidification as filament, and after that, lubrication is done to improve texture and reduce friction. The characteristics of filaments depend on the design of the spinneret (holes, size, shape, length), just as the number of holes determines the type of filament (single hole produces monofilament, and multihole produces multifilament).

6.3.3 Electrospinning

This is the most versatile as well as commonly used technique. This process is capable of producing nanometer range fiber with controlled diameter, morphology, and distribution at a very low cost. In this process, polymers are dissolved or melted by a high-voltage electrostatic field. And with the continuous flow, they formed fiber through splitting jet ejection and Taylor cone formation. After that cool, solidified fiber are collected on a grounded rotating drum (Ma et al., 2021; Lannutti et al., 2007; Haider et al., 2015). This widely used process can be further modified, like co-electrospinning where hollow structures or core cell fiber are prepared by coaxial electrospinning and centrifugal electrospinning developed to minimize the limitation (low yield, limited scalability) of the original process.

6.3.4 BICOMPONENT SPINNING

This process is used for multicomponent fiber preparation where the properties of different polymers (more than one) are used in a fiber. A cross-section of fiber prepared by using this process shows different individual polymers used in the preparation. This fiber is created by introducing multiple polymers into the spinneret at the same time.

After the fiber formation, surface functionalization is done on those fibers to avoid any kind of adverse reaction or other beneficial purposes. Physical functionalization like plasma treatment (O_2 and N_2), physical vapor deposition, and chemical functionalization like cross-linking are used.

6.4 DIFFERENT TYPES OF TEXTILES ARE USED AS INFECTION CONTROL AND PROTECTIVE MATERIALS

Various techniques are used to convert prepared fibers into textiles. Medical textiles are further divided into different categories according to their porosity, strength, permeability, fixability, stability, etc. They are categorizable as follows:

6.4.1 WOVEN TEXTILES

They are dimensionally stable and strong textiles that display sufficient elongation with low permeability and porosity. In the case of woven textile yarns that are present at a 90-degree angle with each other, this interlacing primary structure of yarns is formed by using an orthogonal position between warp and weft, where warp is the machine direction and weft is the cross direction.

6.4.2 NONWOVEN TEXTILES

They can be prepared directly from fiber without involving the production of yarn. In the case of nonwoven textiles, where fibers are bonded together by mechanical, thermal, or adhesive mechanisms, the presence of fiber is random. Pore size and pore size distribution can be maintained by selecting the right bonding method and other variables such as web orientation and fiber length and diameter.

6.4.3 KNITTED TEXTILE

That structure is prepared by the continuous interconnection between the wale (rows) and the course (columns). This textile is softer, and more fixable than woven fabric. This type of fabric must be coated with gelatin or collagen for surgical application because they have high water permeability. They also need some special processing to minimize their porous structure. This fabric can be classified as weft knit, where courses are formed by a single yarn, or warp knit, where wales are formed by a series of yarns.

6.4.4 BRAIDED TEXTILE

This type of textile is commonly prepared by introducing three or more yarns at different angles and frequencies. These structures are mostly used as sutures because of their strong and highly flexible nature. They are also used as ligament prostheses due to their expanding ability and low bending rigidity.

6.5 PROTECTIVE FACE MASK

A protective face mask is one of the most effective respiratory protective devices. This is an important piece of PPE that protects the wearer from airborne pathogens and other health hazards by acting as a protective barrier and expelling infectious droplets from the wearer. These devices cover the front of the face and protect against breathable hazard inhalation. Masks became a symbol of our daily lives during this COVID-19, as government agencies in many countries issued guidelines making mask use mandatory in the fight against this disease. Those PPE can be classified in a variety of ways. For any kind of mask, it has to fulfill some basic properties like resistance to fluid, high filtration efficiency, air permeability, and a few wearing properties like comfort, fittings, etc.

They are classified according to their length as follows: i) full masks, which cover the entire face; ii) quarter masks, which cover the area between the top of the chin and the top of the nose; and iii) half masks, which cover from above the nose to under the chin. According to their level of protection and filtration efficiency, they can be classified as follows:

Single-use face masks and cloth masks are both single-layer masks, usually homemade and made of cloth that can protect against large droplets. Those masks can be classified as cloth mask 1, cloth mask 2, and cloth mask 3 according to their protective nature, where symbols 1 and 2 suggest better protection.

Surgical mask: As the name suggests, those masks are specially designed for the purpose of surgery to protect medical staff from the harmful chemicals of surgical smoke and protect patients from droplet infection by medical staff (Bruske-Hohlfed et al., 2008). They look like Figure 6.2. Those masks can be further categorized as level 1, level 2, and level 3 on the basis of their level of protection, where level 3 provides better protection. Surgical masks are commonly made up of three layers (generally known as 3-ply surgical masks), where the filtration layer is sandwiched between the soft, adsorbent inside layer and the hydrophobic outer layer.

Respirator: Fitting devices with high filtration efficiency and the ability to filter out particles in the micron range (for example, an N95 respirator that can filter out 95% of particles in the 0.3-m range). Because of their high bacterial and viral filtration efficiency, their acceptance is much higher than other types of masks. They are typically four or five-layered spun bond or melt-blown

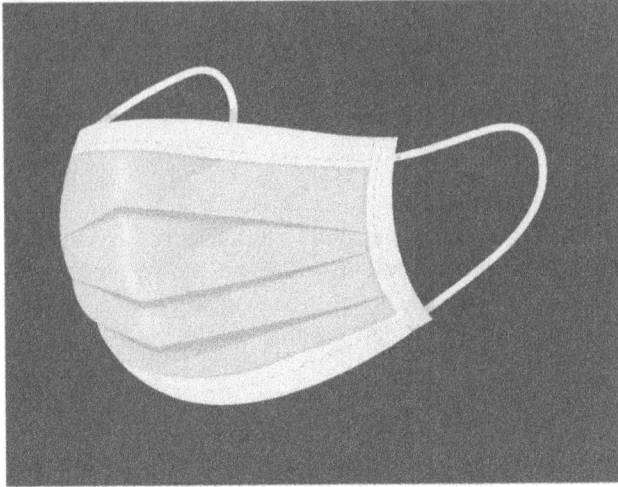

FIGURE 6.2   Surgical mask

structures with charged hydrophobic layers on the outside that are usually coated with an antimicrobial or antiviral substance. Inside are comfortable absorbent layers, with a filter layer and an activated carbon layer in the middle to protect against organic gas. Except those layers of the respirator contain a strap for holding it in place, an adjustable nose clip, and nose foam for proper fit and comfort, and sometimes a valve to keep it cool from the inside and reduce breathing resistance as well. Those respirators are available in different shapes (oval, cone, and cup) and sizes (Das et al., 2021).

6.5.1   Mechanism of Filtration in the Mask

The mask prevents particles from moving in both directions, and the filtration efficiency is determined by the fiber dimension. Nanotechnology plays an important role in the formation of low-dimensional fibers (1–10µm). The use of nanomaterials and nanotechnology improved mask quality by improving filtration, breathability, comfort, viral and bacterial protection, and so on. Filtration of any mask is based on the different principles as shown as Figure 6.3.

Electrostatic attraction occurs when an oppositely charged particle comes into contact with a charged fiber. The inertial impaction process aids in the capture of particles in a specific size range. Diffusion is the capture of randomly moving particles in mask layers. Interception is the capture of a small particle as a result of physical contact with the mask layer.

6.5.2   Application of Different Polymers as Mask Materials

Various polymers or their combinations are used for making the structure of the mask, including polymers like polycarbonate, polyethylene, polystyrene, polypropylene,

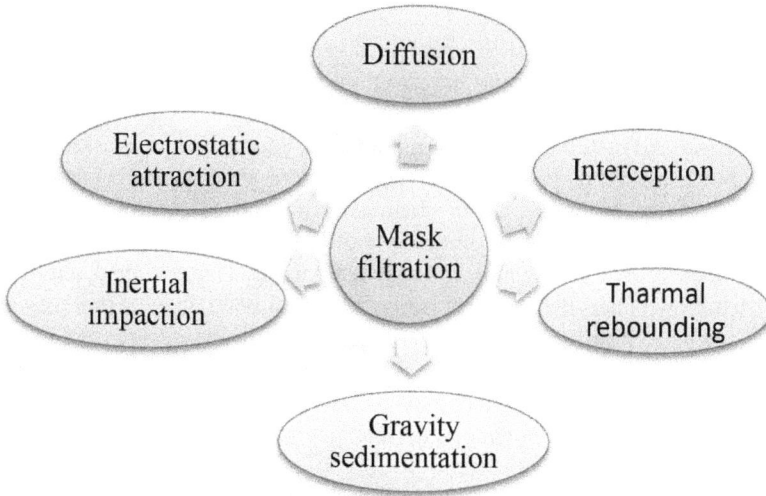

FIGURE 6.3   Mechanism of filtration

polyacrylonitrile, polyurethane, and polyester; among them, polypropylene is the most commonly used polymer because of its moisture repellant and charged capacity (Tcharkhtchi et al., 2020). Polyester also maintains a high static charge compared to other natural fibers (Konda et al., 2020).

Mask filters are mainly made of melt-blown polypropylene, which is a semicrystalline, nonpolar, thermoplastic, propylene polymerization-synthesized polymer (Cook, 2020). The exception to this is polypropylene wool felt, fiberglass paper, and other filter materials (Tcharkhtchi et al., 2020). Polymers like polyvinylpyrrolidone, polyvinylidene, polyvinyl alcohol, polystyrene, etc. are also used as filter materials. Among them, polyvinyl alcohol fiber is washable and reusable.

Natural polymers and their derivatives are also used as filter materials because of their natural protective capabilities against airborne pathogens and other properties (hydrophilicity, biofouling resistance, etc.). Polymers like cellulose, micro cellulose, and nanocellulose are commonly used. Cellulose acetate, a natural polymer derivative, can be used as a substitute for synthetic polymers. It shows high filtration efficiency, mainly for organic compounds, with good processing and water stability and high biodegradability. Combining this polymer with some synthetics shows a much better response; polyvinylidene difluoride makes fine and smooth nanofibers by electrospinning, which shows highly improved filtration (Junter & Lebrun, 2017; Akduman, 2019; Liu et al., 2012; Carpenter et al., 2015; Omollo et al., 2016).

6.5.3   Introduction of Nanotechnology and Nanomaterials in Masks

The efficiency of any mask depends upon the properties of the preparation material and some external factors. External factors include humidity, temperature, respiration frequency, velocity, the pattern of airflow, size and charge of coming particles, etc., and material properties include the number of layers, thickness, fiber diameter, charge, chemical composition, etc. The combination of those properties decides the filtration efficiency of the mask. The application of nanotechnology and nanomaterials modified those properties and improved the performance, efficiency, and safety of the mask.

Spun bond and melt blown are the main technologies used for mask production. In spun bond, melted polymers are subjected to cool air for fiber formation, which is then thermally, mechanically, or chemically bonded as nonwoven fabric. This process mainly produces coarse filament with high tensile strength. To create soft foaming fiber from melt-blown fiber, a high temperature is maintained and hot air is used. Melt-blown fibers differ significantly from spun-bond fibers in that they have a small diameter, typically in the 1–2 μm range, a smooth surface, are light in weight, and have a high filtration efficiency. That's why melt-blown fiber is mainly used as a filter layer. The electrospinning technique is also utilized for mask fiber preparation; this is mainly done for metal, nanocomposite, nanoparticle, and polymer composite-based fiber formulation.

Another important technique that has been introduced in recent years to improve the filtration efficiency of masks is electret technology. The function of this technique involves the introduction of charge and increased charge-storing capacity of fiber, and it also improves charge stability and morphology. This process involves mainly three charging techniques: i) corona charging, which is used to develop electrostatic charge in monomers, fiber blends, or fabrics. In this process, a high electric field is introduced between two asymmetric electrodes that effectively produce ionized air, and from that electrostatic charge, a charge on the fiber surface is developed. ii) Tribocharging, also known as triboelectric charging, is used to charge polymers having electronegative dissimilarities. This process produces fiber, which shows better filtration efficiency than corona charging. iii) Electrostatic fiber spinning: by charging polymers and spinning fibers in a single step, this process can produce extremely efficient nanofibers.

The introduction of nanomaterials also improves the mask's performance by altering the physical properties. Some antiviral and antibacterial nonmaterial is also used to make antiviral and antibacterial masks. A mask with a few nanomaterials is already available on the market, like carbon, titanium dioxide, graphene, silver, copper, etc. (Borkow and Gabbay, 2012).

Synthetic metal-based nanomaterials like silver, copper, and titanium dioxide are widely suggested for their antiviral and antibacterial properties. Those materials are used in mask making in two ways: one is by surface coating or incorporation in polymeric matrices. Silver, copper oxide, cobalt, and silica coatings display their effectiveness against viral pathogens. Graphene is also an antiviral agent and very effective against SARS-CoV-2; graphene-incorporated masks exhibit high mechanical strength and conductivity with UV protection and abrasion resistance (De Maio et al., 2021; Bhattacharjee et al., 2019). Nanomaterials like TiO_2 exhibit antimicrobial activity in masks, and the combination of TiO_2 with graphene and silver shows photocatalytic activity in specific wavelengths of light.

Some natural compounds also responded well. Some essential oils, like carvacrol, eugenol, and thymol, show their antibacterial and antimicrobial effects in polymer-based filters. Curcumin and riboflavin and some other photosensitizing substances show their photodynamic killing activity against virus and bacteria in the exposure of light. Few polymers also display good response; coatings of polyethyleneimine cause viral adhesion and structural damage. Nanofibers of chitosan show surface positive charge and antiviral activity.

6.5.4 EVALUATION OF MASK PERFORMANCE

After preparation of the medical mask and respirator, their performance must be tested to know about filtration, breathing resistance, comfort, etc. Respirators are described as properly fitted devices, so a fit test is an important criterion for their evaluation, though it isn't necessary for surgical masks. Here in this chapter, we are going to discuss some important evaluation parameters.

6.5.4.1 Filtration Efficiency

The filtration efficiency of a mask is determined by particle size, shape, and size distribution, as well as the charge on the filter. The filtration efficiency of a mask is the combination of particulate filtration efficiency (PFE), bacterial filtration efficiency (BFE), and viral filtration efficiency (VFE). Whereas PFE describes the filtration of monodispersed solids in constant flow, BFE and VFE describe the filtration of viruses and bacteria, though VFE is not a required criterion.

6.5.4.2 Differential Pressure and Fluid Resistance

This test is performed to determine the breathability of the mask, which is the second-most important criterion for mask use. The differential pressure is calculated by comparing the pressures upstream and downstream. Fluid resistance gives an idea of the mask barrier's performance against fluids.

6.5.4.3 Fit Test

This is a required test for any respirator and ensures proper fit between the face and the mask surface, allowing only filtrate air to enter the mask.

6.5.5 THE EFFECT OF MASKS ON THE ENVIRONMENT AND HEALTH

Inappropriate disposal methods and the tremendous use of masks in recent times have caused an enormous increase in mask waste. There is a lack of specified methods for collecting masks or plastic waste in entire countries or specific regions. While the World Health Organization (WHO) recommends temperatures between 900°C and 1200°C for secure medical waste incineration, many are unaware of this temperature range. Masks are mostly made of polypropylene and aluminum, and the manufacturing process emits a lot of greenhouse gases (a single N95 mask emits 50 g of equivalent CO_2, while a surgical mask and cloth mask emit 59 g and 60 g of CO_2 equivalent, respectively). The majority of the mask is made of plastic, which lasts a long time in soil because it is chemically stable and is not destroyed by microorganisms or corrosion (Webb et al., 2013). A large portion of mask waste ends up as plastic pollution in aquatic environments. By adsorbing toxins and pollutants, marine plastic has the potential to form toxic surface films (Williams-Wynn & Naidoo, 2020). Ingestion of those plastics leads to death threats for marine animals by direct poisoning or indirectly by interfering with their immunity systems, reproduction, growth, etc. (Ferraro & Failler, 2020; Yang et al., 2020). Those plastics are further converted into microplastics by different biological factors (chemical, mechanical, or natural degradation) and pose a high risk of human consumption through the food chain (Wang et al., 2021; Wu et al., 2022).

The use of nanomaterials to improve mask efficiency is still controversial, both in terms of human health and the environment. Nanomaterial coating and washing processes generate massive amounts of dissolved and particulate nanoparticles, which pose health and environmental risks after disposal. Copper and silver nanoparticles have an immune-toxic effect on aquatic animals and mice; multiwall carbon nanotubes show a carcinogenic response in humans; and TiO_2 shows non-targeted organ toxicity (Adamcakova-Dodd et al., 2015; Luo et al., 2020; Valdiglesias & Laffon, 2020). Mask nanomaterials that are in direct contact with skin must be dermatologically tested; those materials have to be skin-friendly so that long-term use of a tightly sealed mask doesn't cause any dermatological concerns. Nanoparticles can enter the lungs directly through inhalation and cause health problems, such as silver nanoparticle inhalation influencing lung failure, heart rate elevation, and so on (Kutralam-Muniasamy et al., 2022).

6.5.6 POLLUTION REDUCTION STRATEGY USING MASKS

The development of biodegradable masks can be the best alternative to those plastic, petroleum-based masks from an environmental point of view. A variety of biopolymers show polypropylene-like properties: high tensile strength, ultralight weight, economics, etc. (Glukhikh et al., 2020; Samper et al., 2018; Siracusa & Blanco, 2020), which are essential for mask preparation along with their biodegradable and eco-friendly nature. Bioplastic is another term often used as an alternative to plastic because of its biodegradable nature. They are collected from natural substances and produce 30–70% less CO_2 than conventional plastic. Various polysaccharides, protein substances, and lipid content biodegradable polymers, plants like banana, avocado, bamboo, hemp, sisal, and sugar cane, all natural fiber containers with properties to fulfill all mask preparation criteria, can be prepared by using them (Ho, 2020; Layt, 2020; Staff, 2020). Natural fiber waste and raw materials can be used for biodegradable green mask preparation, and tea leaf waste can be used as filtering material because it contains polypropylene (Ferraro & Failler, 2020). There are a few biodegradable masks on the market that have high filtration efficiency and antibacterial properties, such as hemp fiber masks, sugar cane waste masks, and coffee-based face masks. Though bioplastic-made biodegradable masks show their ability as mask materials with an eco-friendly degradable nature, their use is still restricted because of their limited availability, preparation cost, and other factors like lifespan and sustainability (Vanapalli et al., 2021).

Masking waste and recycling it is another aspect of environmental damage reduction. This process reduces landfill waste and total waste as well. In the recycling process, it is done by using mechanical or chemical recycling, incineration, and pyrolysis processes, and the extracted materials can be further used, such as extracted polypropylene, which can be used in construction sites to increase the strength of concrete.

Extracted recycle polyethylene and polypropylene derivatives can be used in road construction (Williams-Wynn & Naidoo, 2020), strong and durable sand blocks can be produced without adding water from plastic sheets of low-density polyethylene waste (Kumi-Larbi Jnr. et al., 2018), and concrete beams can be reinforced from ring-shaped polyethylene terephthalate (Khalid et al., 2018).

The use of face masks is dramatically increased due to universal masking in COVID-19, and it also causes a shortage of protective face masks along with the increase in mask waste. Shortage and waste production issues can be minimized by using strategies like reuse, extended use, and decontamination along with the reduction of waste. Reuse can be done through mask rotation, where used masks are kept in proper storage conditions for long enough to dry out and lose viral viability. In cases of extended use, the life span of the mask is increased by using it for a long time. Some decontamination processes are used for proper sterilization and reuse of masks, as described in Table 6.1.

6.6 FACE SHIELD

The face is the most commonly affected body part for health workers. It can be easily contaminated by disease-producing organisms from infected body fluids, splashes, etc. Face shields can protect from flying biological hazards by acting as barriers in the facial area. Because a face shield is used in conjunction with other personal protective equipment (such as a mask), it is referred to as adjunctive personal protective equipment. They can be very effective against airborne pathogens; in the recent outbreak of COVID-19, their application has also increased along with other PPE.

TABLE 6.1
Face masks decontamination.

Decontamination method	Time	Medium used	Comments
Ethylene oxide sterilization	1 hour	37°C–63°C temperature	Effective process but ETO is very harmful
UV radiation	10 min.	35°C temperature	Effectiveness is good but lower than ETO sterilization
Moist heat sterilization	15 min. in 15 lb pressure	120°C temperature	Effective one, done in autoclave
Dry heat sterilization	1 hour	160°–178°C temperature	Done by hot air oven, can change filtration efficiency of mask
Ethanol treatment	2 hours	70% ethanol	Proper drying must be done
Isopropyl alcohol dip	1 min.	70% isopropyl alcohol	Proper drying required
Plasma treatment by H_2O_2	47 min. cycle with 30 min. exposure	59% H_2O_2	Highly effective

Face shields cover a large area of the face and protect from direct contamination of any kind of body fluid, though their effectiveness is still questionable (Lipp, 2003). Some study reports also show they are capable of minimizing the risk of aerosol inhalation. Lindsley et al. (2014) reported 96% and 92% risk reduction for inhalation aerosol (containing influenza) of diameter 8.5 m from 46 cm and 183 cm, respectively, while a face shield only blocks 68% of the aerosol when the diameter is reduced to 3.4 m. This experiment clearly demonstrates that a face shield can be effective in the case of a large droplet.

6.6.1 STRUCTURE OF THE FACE SHIELD

Its content follows a very simple structure, as shown in Figure 6.4. The plastic material-based transparent shield visor is the main component, which attaches to a plastic or metal-based frame, and it also contains some spongy materials and elastic bands. The major components of this protective equipment are divided as follows:

Visors are made from materials such as acetate, polyvinyl chloride, polyethylene terephthalate glycol, polycarbonate, propionate, and others. Polycarbonate is the most commonly used material, though it has some imperfect visible quality; polyethylene terephthalate glycol is the most economical; and acetate became the best option in terms of optical visibility due to its transparency. A visor can be reusable or disposable, and it comes in different lengths (half facepiece, full facepiece) and widths (wider provides more protection). The visor was also modified with different technologies like anti-fogging, anti-glare, scratch resistance, and UV resistance to improve its life span, quality of life, and comfort as well.

The frame is a glass, plastic, or metal-based structure that is attached to a transparent visor, the attachment being permanent, semi-permanent, or temporary. Frames are available in a variety of shapes (such as oval and rectangular) and styles (adjustable and non-adjustable). In most cases, a foam cushion is attached to the frame to make it more comfortable. Some face shields include a brow cap for better accommodation and splash resistance in the forehead. It also reduces fogging and improves ventilation.

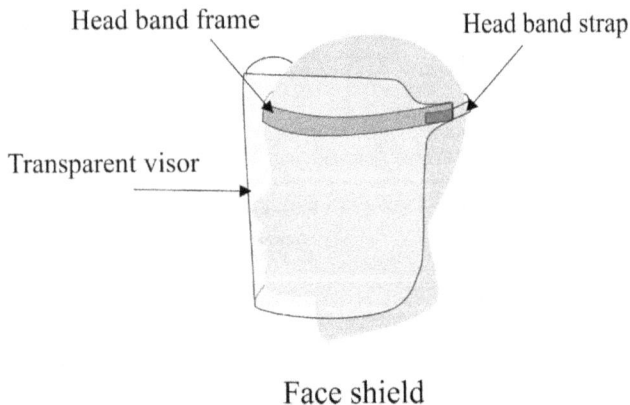

Face shield

FIGURE 6.4   Face shield

6.6.2 Benefits of a Face Shield

They have many advantages over other face-protective equipment. As with comfort, using a face shield is less claustrophobic than wearing a mask for a long time. They cover a larger face area, provide better protection against self-inoculation than other facial protective equipment, and produce very little fog when compared to goggles. Their disinfectant process is easier than a mask's, so their reuse is high. This PPE doesn't retain heat inside and doesn't hamper the normal breathing process like a mask. They are less expensive and can be used with other face and eye PPE, like masks and goggles. In the case of combined use, they extended the mask's life, though their fit test is not necessary.

Disadvantage: it causes vision problems and, in some cases, fogging. This PPE does not fit properly to the face and causes improper fitting in a few mask models. The side and bottom portions are opened in this device, so there is always the risk of a small virus entry.

6.7 PROTECTIVE GOWNS

Gowns are a common type of PPE that provides protection when the wearer comes into contact with disease-producing organisms and prevents their transmission. Gowns are named differently according to their level of protection and purpose of use, like protective gowns, isolation gowns, surgical gowns, non-surgical gowns, etc. According to their level of protection, gowns are classified in Table 6.2.

TABLE 6.2
Level of protective gowns.

Different level	Efficiency	Application
Level I	In case of minimal risk, they are used. They provide a minute barrier for fluid penetration. For ensuring protection performance single test of water impacting in the surface of gowns is done.	Standard medical unit, during basic care, standard isolation, and biopsies.
Level II	In case of low risk, they are generally used. They mainly provide a barrier from fluid penetration through soaking and splatter. Two tests are performed, one is similar to level I (spray impact) and another one by pressurizing the material.	In the intensive care unit, pathology lab, during the blood draw, suturing, and radiology.
Level III	In moderate risk, they are used. For this category spray impact and hydrostatic pressure tests are performed.	In the emergency room. Intravenous insertion, arterial blood draw, and endoscopic procedure.
Level IV	In case of high risk, they are preferable because of the highest level of fluid and viral protection they provide.	The long fluid intense procedure, for pathogen resistance, surgery. Open cardiovascular or thoracic procedure.

6.7.1 Surgical Gowns

According to the FDA, this PPE is categorized as level II and is mainly used at the time of surgery for the protection of both healthcare personnel and patients. Those protective gowns used by the surgical team must have some standard and protective qualities. Various authorized bodies have been in charge of their standards since the early 1900s. These dual-protective PPE should have the following features:

It should have properties like liquid repellent and impermeability, air permeability, tear and puncture resistance.

It must provide resistance against blood and body fluid penetration.

It should be sterile, nontoxic, comfortable, and meet an acceptable flammability standard.

It should have sufficient length to cover the exposed area.

6.7.2 Different Parts of Surgical Gowns

a) **SLEEVES AND CUFFS**: Generally, two types of sleeves are used in surgical gowns: set-in sleeves and raglan sleeves. Set-in sleeves are difficult to prepare, provide less comfort, and cause high garment pressure in the armpit as compared to raglan sleeves. Raglan sleeves provide the wearer with easy movement and comfort by creating a large space in the armpit and a better arm and shoulder fit. This most commonly used style of sleeve is easily identified by drawing a diagonal line from the neckline to the armpit (Cho, 2006; Rogina-Car et al., 2017; Liu et al., 2016).

At the very end of the sleeve's wrist cuff are attachments that help keep the sleeve in the proper place. They can be different types like elastic cuffs mainly used for disposable types, cotton or cotton-polyester blend-made knit cuffs used as disposable and reusable both, and thumb loop cuffs which are also used for both purposes.

b) **NECK CLOSURE**: Different types of closure are used in surgical gowns, like snaps, ties, hooks, loops, etc. Among them, a tie-back closure is mostly used. They contain two tie bands one at the neckline edge and another one inside present near the shoulder. The neck portion has the tendency to hang down, mainly in the case of reusable gowns, which are made up of slippery materials; this can be avoided by using the tie fastening method (Chang et al., 2020). Hook and loop neck closers are preferable because of their adjustment capabilities and availability in different sizes. The neck closer hook is generally present in the right back piece and hooks in the left neckline in this easily fixable situation with the proper fit. Snap closer is also capable to enclose the neckline; they present on the right and left sides in between 1–1.5 inches distance.

c) **SIZING AND FITTINGS**: The proper sizing of a gown is an important aspect of its use because adequate fittings and sizing not only make the put-on and take-off process easy, but also provide a better level of protection. Because different sizes (short, medium, large, and extra-large) are available, the CDC also recommends that.

d) **STITCHES-SEAM**: The barrier performance of a gown also depends upon the stitches. Joining textile pieces is conventionally done through sewing with the help of needles and threads. But this needle punching can hamper the barrier process through the creation of a small hole, which leads to the risk of unwanted penetration (Ashour et al., 2017; Rogina-Car et al., 2017). For prevention of that, technology like ultrasonic welding was introduced. A few reports also show that seams made by ultrasonic welding provide better protection than seams made by sewing processes and less leakage as well (Eryuruk et al., 2017), though tensile strength is lower in this process than in the lock and chain sewing method (Kayar, 2014). Because of that, reusable gowns are generally stitched by the conventional method, and for disposable types, mostly ultrasonic welding is used.

Different types of surgical gowns are available with different materials to minimize the chance of contamination, and they have been selected on the basis of their requirements. Their design, material, and characteristics differ depending on their intended use; they are classified in Figure 6.5.

Disposable surgical gowns are typically made of nonwoven fabrics that contain various types of polymers to make them more protective. The barrier quality of those sterile products is very high, but they are only used once, which increases production cost and environmental pollution as well.

Reusable gowns are generally made of tightly woven fabric made from cotton, polyester, or a blend for multiple uses. For reuse, those gowns are sent for washing and sterilization after every use, and those processes can change the gowns' barrier performance. Reusable gowns have properties like drape ability, high tensile strength, comfort, steam permeability, sterilizability, etc. For both disposable and reusable types, additional coating or plastic lamination is done to improve their barrier performance.

Reinforced surgical gowns are level III or IV devices that have an additional protective barrier of impermeable material over the surface (primarily the front) and are used primarily during surgery to protect both the patient and medical staff from infection (Behera & Arora, 2009; Song et al., 2011).

6.7.3 ENVIRONMENTAL IMPACT

A gown, like other surgical equipment, has a high environmental impact because it is the second most commonly used surgical item. Because of the widespread

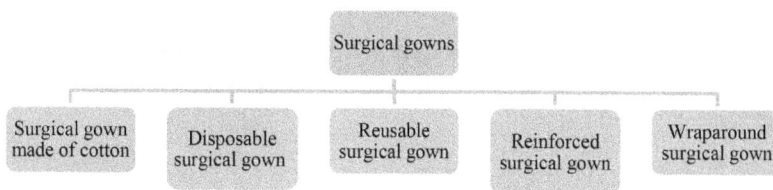

FIGURE 6.5 Classification of surgical gowns

acceptance and use of these PPE in recent years, life cycle assessment of those has become necessary to maintain environmental sustainability by understanding the environmental impact of a product.

During the manufacturing process, harmful gas emissions such as sulfur dioxide and nitrogen oxide are produced. Researchers have shown a huge amount of difference in the environmental effect by assessing raw material, manufacturing, use and reuse, and final disposal, which is known as "life cycle assessment."

Disposable gowns produce more solid waste and release a high number of toxic compounds (mercury, dioxane) compared to reusable gowns. Reusable gowns have a longer life span, so they offer extra environmental savings. But laundering and sanitizing reusable products generates more volatile organic compounds and water pollution as well. A life cycle assessment of both reusable and disposable gowns shows disposable gowns have a higher impact on eutrophication, water consumption, solid waste, global warming, carcinogens, and photochemical oxidation as compared to reusable gowns (Vozzola et al., 2020).

6.8   WIPES

Wipes are another important type of PPE whose use is tremendously increasing in modern times due to their advantages like ease of carrying, ease of use, and time savings with all those intended benefits. They are cotton, polypropylene, polyester, rayon, or synthetic fiber-made sheets available in single or bulk packaging. Those moistened sheets generally contain water along with preservatives and other ingredients according to their purpose of use.

6.8.1   COMPOSITION OF WIPES

Preservatives are one of the major constituents in wipes. Various organic acids (like benzoic acid and sorbic acid), chelating agents (like EDTA), and alcoholic substances (like benzyl alcohol and phenoxyethanol) are added to protect them from any kind of microbial growth. Emollients are another ingredient used in wipes to moisturize the skin. Buffering agents like citric acid and sodium citrate are also used to maintain the pH between 4.5 and 5.5, which is similar to the pH of healthy skin. Antioxidants like vitamin E are also added to prevent the oxidation of nutrients and oils. Different fragrances are added to make them attractive, along with moisturizers.

The activity of wipes also depends upon various factors like fiber structure and type, the absorption property of sheets, which controls the release of the required solution, and other factors like applied force, concentration of active ingredients, type of microorganism, etc. (Song et al., 2019; Edwards et al., 2017). Different types of wipes are shown in Figure 6.6.

6.8.2   CLASSIFICATION OF WIPES

According to the application purpose, they can be classified as follows:

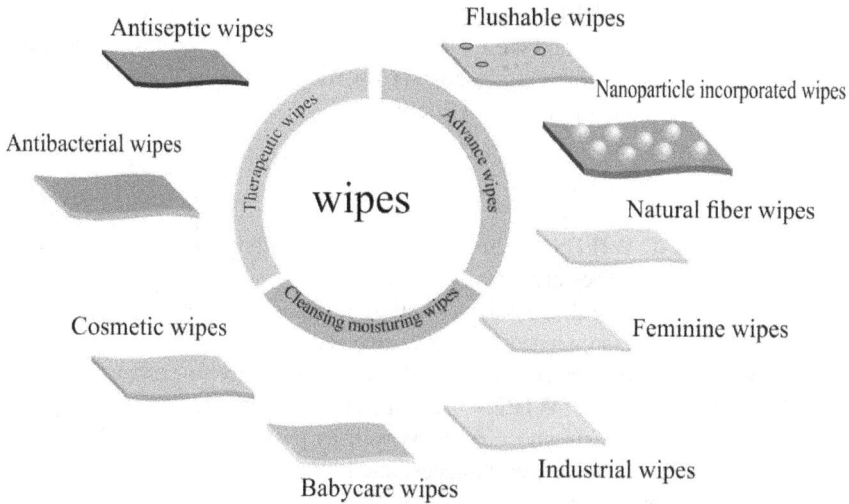

FIGURE 6.6   Different types of wipes

6.8.2.1   Cleansing and Moisturizing Wipes

a) **BABY CARE WIPES**: They are generally nonalcoholic, soap-free disposable wipes prepared by using advanced technology that is very soft and
smooth and effectively removes dirt and impurities. They contain a high
amount of moisturizing lotion, which, after use, leaves a protective barrier
over the baby's skin and protects it from rashes.

b) **CHILDCARE OR GENERAL-PURPOSE WET WIPES**: Those wipes
are generally used to maintain hand hygiene, protect from illness, and make
good hygiene habits. Those kinds of wipes reduce the workload of parents
and educational institutions to maintain child hygiene.

c) **POST-WORKOUT BODY WIPES**: Getting into the shower after a work-
out is not always possible. Those wipes come as a solution to that. They
effectively remove dirt and salt prepared during perspiration and are also
capable of removing odor and providing freshness.

d) **FEMININE HYGIENIC WIPES**: Those wipes are made for the female sensitive area. They include a cleansing agent and moisturizer, as well as some
active ingredients to reduce skin irritation and maintain sanitary conditions, as
well as a pH that is controlled between 4 and 6. The use of feminine wipes has
always been a source of concern for women because they can cause fertility
issues, allergic reactions, hormonal disruption, and, in some cases, cancer.

e) **COSMETIC WIPES**: With commercialized makeup products becoming
more water-resistant and stiffer to increase wear life, the off-the-shelf use of
cosmetic wipes as makeup removers has become a new trend. These wipes
consist of a nonwoven fabric material and a liquid component, commonly
referred to as "juice" or a solution, typically composed of water, ethanol, or
oil. The liquid component comprises 90–98% water in the wipes.

f) **INDUSTRIAL WIPES**: Those wipes contain solvents and chemicals, mainly disinfectants, and their sheets are designed with advanced technology that releases chemicals to control microorganisms in industrial construction areas and on industrial floors.

6.8.2.2   Therapeutic Wipes

a) **ANTISEPTIC WIPES**: Antiseptic wipes are typically used to kill germs and sterilize the skin. They can be very convenient for cleaning injured skin, small cuts, and other minor skin problems. Antiseptic wipes are generally individually packaged and recommended for single-time use to reduce the chance of contamination. Combining them with alcohol can be effective for coronaviruses.
b) **ANTIBACTERIAL WIPES**: Antibacterial wipes are highly capable of destroying bacteria and viruses as well as providing a certain level of hygiene in people's lives, workplaces, and homes. They can eliminate antibiotic-resistant bacteria.

6.8.2.3   Advance Wipes

a) **NATURAL FIBER WIPES**: Using natural fiber in wipes can increase hydrophilicity and moisture absorbing capacity as well as provide other activities like antibacterial activity, surface cleaning, cytotoxicity, exfoliation, anti-inflammatory activity, etc. by incorporating different herbal extracts. Natural fiber can be fabricated by using spun lace, thermal bonding, airlaid, etc. Due to their eco-friendly nature, they cause minimal environmental damage. As an example, bamboo fiber can be used as a nonwoven fabric in wipes by spinning bond technology, and the incorporation of tulsi and clove extract makes them natural antibacterial wipes (Devaki et al., 2019).
b) **NANOPARTICLE-INCORPORATED WIPES**: Different types of nanoparticles can be incorporated in wipes by using various nanotechnology techniques to get the desired action. Antiviral activity can easily be obtained by incorporating inorganic nanoparticles in wipe sheets. Among the various nanoparticles, copper, silver, and zinc are widely used for antiviral activity. Hamouda et al. prepared silver nanoparticles and incorporated them into cellulose-based wipes and observed antimicrobial and antiviral activity.
c) **FLUSHABLE WIPES ARE ENVIRONMENTALLY FRIENDLY WIPES MADE FROM BIODEGRADABLE MATERIALS**: They are generally made up of cellulose fiber, which is dispersible as well as very compatible with water systems. They easily disintegrate in the water system and do not produce any clogs in the plumbing system.

6.8.2.4   Effect on Human Health Due to Wipes Chemical

Wipes contain various formulative ingredients like preservatives, moisturizers, binders, emollients, surfactants, cleansers, penetration enhancers, and fragrances along with individual elements like antiviral agents, antibacterial agents, etc. Ingredients like siloxanes, silanes, parabens, and PEG can be harmful to humans.

Silicon compounds, siloxanes, and silanes are persistent bioaccumulative toxicants that interfere with normal endocrine function. Fragrances can sometimes be carcinogenic, a neurotoxin, a developmental toxin, or an endocrine disruptor. Polyethylene glycol, a common chemical for wipes, is prepared by ethoxylation and can be contaminated with carcinogens. Parabens used as preservatives in wipes are causing cancer and endocrine disruption. Antibacterial agents like triclosan and silver compounds are also causing toxicity in aquatic animals and affecting the human endocrine system.

6.8.2.5   Environmental Effect of Wipes

Most marketed wipes contain plastic rather than a natural substance. They are generally made up of polypropylene, polythelene terephthalate, cotton, or other materials woven with plastic resins. The majority of wipes sheets end up in the ocean and are a major source of microplastic, which endangers marine life, the aquatic environment, and drinking water. Ingestion of those harmful substances causes many problems, along with the release of various toxic chemicals. Non-flushable wipes are dangerous for the sanitary system. They don't disintegrate easily and produce clogs in sewer systems, septic tanks, and other plumbing systems, acting indirectly as flood agents.

6.9   SURGICAL GLOVES

They act as a barrier between health workers and patients during surgical procedures and prevent the transmission of disease. In 1758, the obstetrician Johann Julius Walbaum documented a partial glove design that predominantly covered the fingers. This glove was crafted from sheep cecum to prevent adherence to the vaginal wall during delivery, but now in more modern days, sterile personal protective equipment has become an essential feature of medical practice, and they are made by using natural or synthetic ingredients. Surgical gloves are classified into several types based on the material used in them. Table 6.3 displays the pros and cons of different surgical glove types.

The quality of those gloves is regulated by the FDA. Medical gloves must have certain characteristics such as leak resistance, tear resistance, biocompatibility, and be power-free, according to the FDA. Surgical gloves are classified as class 1 medical devices by the FDA for various characteristics of surgical gloves.

6.9.1   Ideal Characteristics of Surgical Gloves

a) **Gloves thickness**: This is determined in mils (1 mil = 0.001 inches). They typically range from 2 to 15 mils. Higher thickness is proportional to protection power but inversely proportional to sensitivity.

b) **Resistance against chemicals**: Gloves are capable of providing protection against chemicals. It may be accidental or extended.

c) **Elongation**: This parameter determines the stretching ability of gloves without breaking. Gloves used for medical purposes must have a minimum of 300% elongation capacity.

d) **Tensile strength**: Tensile strength is defined as the power that is needed to break a glove. It is determined in megapascal units. Medical gloves must have a minimum tensile strength of 11 mPa.

TABLE 6.3

Advantages and disadvantages of various types of surgical gloves.

Type	Latex gloves	Nitrile gloves	Vinyl gloves	Neoprene gloves	Polyisoprene gloves
	Natural	Synthetic	Synthetic	Synthetic	Synthetic
Material and character	Latex rubber	Nitrile butadiene rubber (a copolymer of acrylonitrile and butadiene)	Plasticized poly vinyl chloride	Cross-linked polymer of carbon, hydrogen, and chlorine by using sulphur	Polyisoprene
Merits	High level of protection against virus, biodegradable, durable, excellent sensitivity, elasticity, and comfort	Provide better protection against chemical, acid oil. Extract strength and thickness, puncture resistant and good enough for viruses. Best choice among medical professionals	They are inexpensive, non-allergenic, mainly used in non-pathogen sensitive area.	Provide protection against chemical and body fluids, and can withstand ultimate change of temperature. High strength	Similar properties like Latex gloves elasticity, sensitivity, strength, and comfort
Demerits	Highly allergic, effect of hydrocarbon and petrolatum-based emollient is high (weaken the rubber)	Low elasticity, comfort, and sensitivity	Poor resistance against many chemicals, less flexibility and elasticity	More expensive than Latex gloves, and elasticity and comfort level is lower than Latex gloves	Most expensive

6.9.2 PREPARATION OF SURGICAL GLOVES

A ceramic or aluminum hand mold is used in the preparation of surgical gloves, as Figure 6.7 shows. Those molds have to be clean enough so that they don't contain any previous residue because the slightest contamination can cause holes in a new one. So those hands are subjected to washing with soap water, chlorine water, and hot water. The molds are then dried. After that, they are dipped into a chemical because rubber molding materials don't adhere to molds. Chemical adhesives contain a mixture of calcium carbonate and calcium nitrate; this mixture helps in the coagulation and sticking of the adhesive material. Then those molds were again dried and dipped in a tank of glove material (PVC, NBR, NR, etc.) according to their needs. The deepening time was very important because increasing the deepening time increased the thickness of gloves, and vice versa. Then those molds are spun to

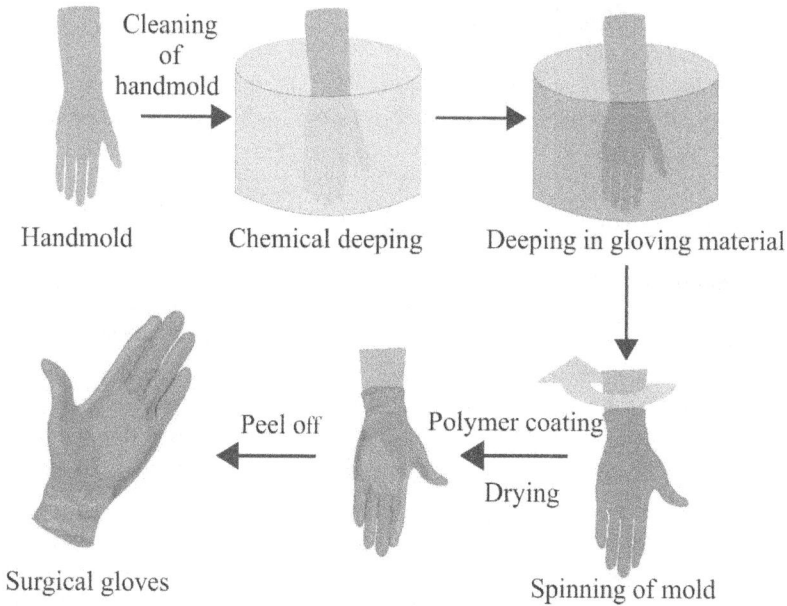

FIGURE 6.7 Preparation of surgical gloves

reduce extra materials, and the molds are transferred to an intense temperature for drying, which forms gloves sometime later. The polymer coating is also done, which makes utilization easier. After that, those gloves peel off the molds and are sent for evolution. Latex gloves can be removed very easily, but synthetic gloves are stickier, so they are mostly removed by workers.

Nitrile butadiene rubber (NBR) is used as a polymer in nitrile gloves, and it is made by copolymerizing acrylonitrile and butadiene. This material provides chemical resistance and flexibility to the gloves. Polyvinyl chloride (PVC) is combined with a plasticizer in vinyl gloves.

Latex glove material is prepared from natural rubber, which is obtained by tapping the rubber plant, which is known as *Hevea brasiliensis*. Latex is prepared by mixing chemicals like accelerator, stabilizer, pigment, vulcanizing agent (sulfur), and antioxidants with natural rubber and processing it for 24 to 30 hours, which makes it ready for dipping (Posch et al., 1997; Sussman et al., 2002). Neoprene glove material is made up of a cross-linked polymer of carbon, hydrogen, chlorine, and sulfur (Sussman et al., 2002; Yip & Cacioli, 2002).

6.9.3 EVALUATION

Surgical gloves must maintain all the parameters (like thickness, chemical resistance, biocompatibility, etc.) described by the Food and Drug Administration (FDA) before marketing; those have to be maintained. And for the whole and weak spot testing, this worker stretches and inflates each glove, and they take a sample from each batch and fill it with a liter of water. If the gloves are watertight, which ensures the outer fluid doesn't reach the wearer's hands, and then they approve the entire batch, except all gloves must pass a dimensions test, a thickness test, and an ageing test (Tlili et al., 2018).

6.9.4 ENVIRONMENTAL ASPECT OF GLOVES

Synthetic surgical gloves are also one of the major PPE components, and due to the application of various synthetic substances, they became tremendously harmful for the environment, so safe disposal of those is also an important aspect. This pandemic also increases 40% of their production, along with other PPE, based on the WHO's recommendation and application (Adyel, 2020). Among various synthetic gloves, a 0.2% addition of Nitryl gloves can increase the compressive strength of concrete by 22%, thereby reducing pollution in the environment (Kilmartin-Lynch et al., 2022).

6.10 CONCLUSION

Biomedical textiles are a broad area in the medical field, and the application of nanotechnology enhances their further growth. Textile applications in the medical field are classified into two categories: personal protective equipment (PPE) and external use biomedical textiles. Different polymer and nanotechnology-based textiles are classified according to their fiber arrangement and nature, and they show functional variation as well. Because of their excellent properties and ease of processing, synthetic polymers are preferred in the preparation of masks, gowns, gloves, wipes, face shields, and many other PPE items, but they pose a significant environmental risk. The preparation of synthetic polymer-based PPE produces an excessive amount of greenhouse gas, and their improper disposal and random use cause landfill pollution as well. The majority of those found in marine water become toxic to aquatic animals, and those plastics degrade into microplastics that enter human systems via the food chain. Utilization of natural and biodegradable polymers in those PPE can be the best option to minimize the environmental damage from plastics.

REFERENCES

Adamcakova-Dodd, M.M., Monick, L.S., Powers, K.N., Gibson-Corley, P.S. Thorne. (2015). Effects of prenatal inhalation exposure to copper nanoparticles on murine dams and offspring. *Part Fibre Toxicol.*, 12.

Adyel, T.M. (2020). Accumulation of plastic waste during COVID-19. *Science*, 369(6509), 1314–1315.

Akduman, C. (2019). Cellulose acetate and polyvinylidene fluoride nanofiber mats for N95 respirators. *J. Ind. Text.*, 1528083719858760.

Ashour, S., Gabr, B., Abdel, M.J.I. (2017). Mint: Investigating the effect of joining techniques on waterproof and comfort properties. *International Journal of Scientific & Engineering Research*, 11, 1319–1327.

Behera, B.K., Arora H. (2009). Mint: Surgical gown: A critical review. *Journal of Industrial Textiles*, 38, 205–231.

Bhattacharjee, S., Joshi, R., Chughtai, A.A., Macintyre, C.R. (2019). Graphene modified multifunctional personal protective clothing. *Adv. Mater. Interfaces*, 6, 1900622.

Borkow, G., Gabbay, J. (2012). Copper, an ancient remedy returning to fight microbial, fungal and viral infections. *Current Chemical Biology*, 3, 272–278.

Bruske-Hohlfeld, I., Preissler, G., Jauch, K.W., et al. (2008). Surgical smoke and ultrafine particles. *J. Occup. Med. Toxicol.*, 3, 31.

Carpenter, A.W., de Lannoy, C.-F., Wiesner, M.R. (2015). Cellulose nanomaterials in water treatment technologies. *Environ. Sci. Technol*, 49(9), 5277–5287.

Chang, K.H., Chen, Y.L., Dai, S.Y. (2020). A combined tie-fastening method for the reusable surgical gown with two neck tie belts to improve wearing comfort. *Nurs. Rep.*, 10(2), 1–7.

Cho, K. (2006). Mint: Redesigning hospital gowns to enhance end users' satisfaction. *Family and Consumer Sciences Research Journal*, 4, 332–349.

Cook, T.M. (2020). Personal protective equipment during the Coronavirus Disease (COVID) 2019 pandemic—A narrative review. *Anaesthesia*, 75(7), 920–927.

Das, S., Sarkar, S., Das, A., Das, S., Chakraborty, P., Sarkar, J. (2021). A comprehensive review of various categories of face masks resistant to Covid-19. *Clinical Epidemiology*, 12, 100835.

De Maio, F., Palmieri, V., Babini, G., Augello, A., Palucci, I., Perini, G., Salustri, A., Spilman, P., De Spirito, M., Sanguinetti, M., Delogu, G., Rizzi, L.G., Cesareo, G., Soon-Shiong, P., Sali, M., Papi, M. (2021). Graphene nanoplatelet and graphene oxide functionalization of face mask materials inhibits infectivity of trapped SARS-CoV-2. *iScience*, 24(7), 102788.

Devaki, E., Indumathi, T.R., Sangeetha, K. (2019). Natural antibacterial finished wet wipes. *International Journal for Research in Applied Science & Engineering Technology*, 45–98.

Edwards, N.W.M., Best, E.L., Connell, S.D., Goswami, P., Carr, C.M., Wilcox, M.H., Russell, S.J. (2017). Role of surface energy and nano-roughness in the removal efficiency of bacterial contamination by nonwoven wipes from frequently touched surfaces. *Sci. Technol. Adv. Mater.*, 18(1), 197–209.

Eryuruk, S.H., Karaguzel Kayaoglu, B., Kalaoglu, F. (2017). Mint: A study on ultrasonic welding of nonwovens used for surgical gowns. *International Journal of Clothing Science and Technology*, 4, 539–552.

Ferraro, G., Failler, P. (2020). Governing plastic pollution in the oceans: Institutional challenges and areas for action. *Environ. Sci. Policy*, 112, 453–460.

Glukhikh, V.V., Buryndin, P., Artyemov, A.V., Savinovskih, A.V., Krivonogov, P.S., Krivonogova, A.S. (2020). Plastics: Physical-and-mechanical properties and biodegradable potential. *Foods Raw Mater*, 8, 149–154.

Haider, A., Haider, S., & Kang, I.-K. (2015). A comprehensive review summarizing the effect of electrospinning parameters and potential applications of nanofibers in biomedical and biotechnology. *Arabian Journal of Chemistry*, 11, 1165–1188.

Ho, S. (2020). Vietnamese Company Creates World's First Biodegradable Coffee Mask. Greenqueen. https://www.greenqueen.com.hk/vietnamese-company-creates-world-first-biodegradable-coffee-face-mask/

Kumi-Larbi A. Jnr., Yunana, D., Kamsouloum, P., Webster, M., Wilson, D.C., Cheeseman, C. (2018). Recycling waste plastics in developing countries: Use of low-density polyethylene water sachets to form plastic bonded sand blocks. *Waste Management*, 80, 112–118.

Junter, G.-A., Lebrun, L. (2017). Cellulose-based virus-retentive filters: A review. *Rev. Environ. Sci. Bio/Technol*, 16(3), 455–489.

Kayar, M. (2014). Mint: Analysis of ultrasonic seam tensile properties of thermal bonded nonwoven fabric. *Journal of Engineered Fibers and Fabrics*, 3, 8–18.

Khalid, F.S., Irwan, J.M., Ibrahim, M.W., Othman, N., Shahidan, S. (2018). Performance of plastic wastes in fiber-reinforced concrete beams. *Construction and Building Materials*, 183, 451–464.

Kilmartin-Lynch, S., Roychand, R., Saberian, M., Li, J., Zhang, G. (2022). Application of COVID-19 single-use shredded nitrile gloves in structural concrete: Case study from Australia. *Science of the Total Environment*, 812, 151423.

Knaul, J.Z., Hudson, S.M., Creber, K.A.M. (1999). Improved mechanical properties of chitosan fibers. *J. Appl. Polym. Sci.*, 72(13), 1721–1732.

Konda, A., Prakash. G.A., Moss, M., Schmoldt, G.D., Grant, S.G. (2020). Aerosol filtration efficiency of common fabrics used in respiratory cloth masks. *ACS Nano.*, 14, 6339–6347.

Kutralam-Muniasamy, G., Pérez-Guevara, F., Shruti, V.C. (2022). A critical synthesis of current peer-reviewed literature on the environmental and human health impacts of COVID-19 PPE litter: New findings and next steps. *J. Hazard. Mater*, 422, 126945.

Lannutti, J., Reneker, D., Ma, T., Tomasko, D., Farson, D. (2007). Electrospinning for tissue engineering scaffolds. *Materials Science and Engineering: C*, 27(3), 504–509.

Layt, S. (2020). *Queensland Researchers Hit Sweet Spot with New Mask Material*. The Age. https://www.brisbanetimes.com.au/national/queensland/queensland-researchers-hit-sweet-spot-with-new-mask-material-20200414-p54jr2.html

Lindsley, W.G., Noti, J.D., Blachere, F.M., Szalajda, J.V., Beezhold, D.H. (2014). Efficacy of face shields against cough aerosol droplets from a cough simulator. *J. Occup. Environ. Hyg.*, 11(80), 509–518.

Lipp, A. (2003). The effectiveness of surgical face masks: What the literature shows. *Nursing Times*, 99(39), 22–24.

Liu, K., Kamalha, E., Wang, J., Agrawal, T.K. (2016). Mint: Optimization design of cycling clothes' patterns based on digital clothing pressures. *Fibers and Polymers*, 9, 1522–1529.

Liu, X., Lin, T., Gao, Y., Xu, Z., Huang, C., Yao, G., Jiang, L., Tang, Y., Wang, X. (2012). Antimicrobial electrospun nanofibers of cellulose acetate and polyester urethane composite for wound dressing. *J. Biomed. Mater. Res., Part B*, 100B(6), 1556–1565.

Luo, Z., Li, Z., Xie, Z., Sokolova, I.M., Song, L., Peijnenburg, W.J.G.M., Hu, M., Wang, Y. (2020). Rethinking nano-TiO_2 safety: Overview of toxic effects in humans and aquatic animals. *Small*, 2002019.

Ma, J., Chen, F., Xu, H., Jiang, H., Liu, J., Li, P., Chen, C.C., Pan, K. (2021). Facemasks as a source of nanoplastics and microplastics in the environment: Quantification, characterization, and potential for bioaccumulation. *Environ. Pollut.*, 288, 117748.

Mather, R.R., Wardman, R.H. (2011). Cellulosic fibers. In *The Chemistry of Textile Fibres* (p. 26). London: The Royal Society of Chemistry.

Omollo, E., Zhang, C., Mwasiagi, J.I., Ncube, S. (2016). Electrospinning cellulose acetate nanofibers and a study of their possible use in high-efficiency filtration. *J. Ind. Text.*, 45(5), 716–729.

Posch, A., Chen, Z., Wheeler, C., Dunn, M.J., Raulf-Heimsoth, M., Baur, X. (1997). Characterization and identification of latex allergens by two-dimensional electrophoresis and protein microsequencing. *The Journal of Allergy and Clinical Immunology*, 99, 385–395.

Prasad, G.K., Singh, B., Vijayraghavan, R. (2008). Respiratory protection against chemical and biological warfare agents. *Def. Sci. J.*, 58(5), 686–697.

Razal, J.M., et al. (2009). Wet-spun biodegradable fibers on conducting platforms: Novel architectures for muscle regeneration. *Adv. Funct. Mater*, 19(21), 3381–3388.

Rogina-Car, B., Budimir, A., Katovic, D. (2017). Mint: Microbial barrier properties of healthcare professional uniforms. *Textile Research Journal*, 15, 1–9.

Samper, M.D., Bertomeu, D., Arrieta, M.P., Ferri, J.M., López-Martínez, J. (2018). Interference of biodegradable plastics in the polypropylene recycling process. *Materials*, 11, 1886.

Singh, B., Singh, V.V., Boopathi, M., Shah, D. (2016). Pressure swing adsorption based air filtration/purification systems for NBC collective protection. *Def. Life Sci. J.*, 01, 127–134.

Sionkowska, A. (2011). Current research on the blends of natural and synthetic polymers as new biomaterials: Review. *Prog. Polym. Sci.*, 36(9), 1254–1276.

Siracusa, V., Blanco, I. (2020). Bio-polyethylene (Bio-PE), bio-polypropylene (Bio-PP) and bio-poly(ethylene terephthalate) (Bio-PET): Recent developments in bio-based polymers analogous to petroleum-derived ones for packaging and engineering applications. *Polymers*, 12, 1641.

Song, G., Cao, W., Cloud, R.M. (2011). Medical textiles and thermal comfort. In V.T. Bartels (Ed.) *Handbook of Medical Textiles* (pp. 198–218). Woodhead Publishing series in textiles, Cambridge.

Song, X., Vossebein, L., Zille, A. (2019). Efficacy of disinfectant-impregnated wipes used for surface disinfection in hospitals: A review. *Antimicrobial Resistance & Infection Control*, 8(1), 139.

Staff, R. (2020). From field to compost: French firm develops hemp face masks. *Reuters*, Available from www.reuters.com.

Sun, G. (2011). Disposable and reusable medical textiles. *Textiles for Hygiene and Infection Control*, 125–135.

Sussman, G.L., Beezhold, D.H., Kurup, V.P. (2002). Allergens and natural rubber proteins. *Journal of Allergy and Clinical Immunology*, 110, 33–39.

Tcharkhtchi, A., Abbasnezhad N., Seydani, M.Z., Zirak, N., Farzaneh, S., Shirinbayan, M. (2020). An overview of filtration efficiency through the masks: Mechanisms of the aerosols penetration. *Bioact. Mater.*, 6, 106–122.

Tlili, M.A., Belgacem, A., Sridi, H., Akouri, M., Aouicha, W., Soussi, S., Dabbebi, F., Ben Dhiab, M. (2018). Evaluation of surgical glove integrity and factors associated with glove defect. *Am. J. Infect. Control*, 46(1), 30–33.

Valdiglesias, V., Laffon, B. (2020). The impact of nanotechnology in the current universal COVID-19 crisis: Let's not forget nanosafety! *Nanotoxicology*, 14, 1013–1016.

Vanapalli, K.R., Sharma, H.B., Ranjan, V.P., Samal, B., Bhattacharya, J., Dubey, B.K., Goel, S. (2021). Challenges and strategies for effective plastic waste management during and post COVID-19 pandemic. *Sci. Total Environ.*, 750, 141514.

Vozzola, E., Overcash, M., Griffing E. (2020). Mint: An environmental analysis of reusable and disposable surgical gowns. *AORN Journal*, 3, 315–325.

Wang, Z., An, C., Chen, X., Lee, K., Zhang, B., Feng, Q. (2021). Disposable masks release microplastics to the aqueous environment with exacerbation by natural weathering. *J. Hazard. Mater.*, 417, 126036.

Webb, H.K., Arnott, J., Crawford, R.J., Ivanova, E.P. (2013). Plastic degradation and its environmental implications with special reference to poly(ethylene terephthalate). *Polymers*, 5.

Williams-Wynn, M.D., Naidoo, P. (2020). A review of the treatment options for marine plastic waste in South Africa. *Mar. Pollut. Bull.*, 161, 111785.

Wu, P.F., Lia, J.P., Lua, X.C., Tang, Y.Y., Cai, Z.W. (2022). Release of tens of thousands of microfibers from discarded face masks under simulated environmental conditions. *Sci. Total Environ.*, 806, 150458.

Yang, Y., Liu, W., Zhang, Z., Grossart, H.-P., Gadd, G.M. (2020). Microplastics provide new microbial niches in aquatic environments. *Appl. Microbiol. Biotechnol.*, 104, 6501–6511.

Yip, E., Cacioli, P. (2002). The manufacture of gloves from natural rubber latex. *Journal of Allergy and Clinical Immunology*, 110(2), S3–S14.

7 Compression Bandage and Wound Care Biomaterial With Nanotechnology

Vaibhav Verma, Vivek Dave,
Prashansa Sharma, and Devsuni Singh

7.1 INTRODUCTION

Wound assessment has been a challenge for medical society since ancient times; as we all know, numerous cases exhibit that wounds are frequently associated with higher morbidity and mortality. Although any disturbance or defect in anatomic structure or function is termed a "wound" and is sustained by serious organ breakdown, such as the breakdown of the skin, this rupture has the potential to expand to further organs and tissues, such as muscles and subcutaneous tissue, nerves, tendons, arteries, and bone. It might be claimed that the skin, the biggest organ in the human body, is most vulnerable to harm since it is readily burned or hurt by surgery or trauma. Wounds are predominantly categorized as acute or chronic wounds. Acute injuries recover normally via the stages of wound healing and show clearly defined evidence of healing within four weeks. The extent of the wound's damage, including its size, depth, and degree, has an impact on how quickly it heals, but chronic wounds don't recover normally through the levels of healing, and healing is not apparent within four weeks, which means healing from chronic wounds takes longer than it does from acute wounds (Okur et al., 2020; Shi et al., 2020).

A procedure that is very complex in multicellular organisms is wound healing. The hemostasis phase, inflammation phase, and plex in multicellular organisms are wound healing. The hemostasis phase, inflammation phase, proliferation phase, and remodeling phase are some of the stages that are involved in it (Gosain & DiPietro, 2004). The proper sequence, timing, and level of intensity must be followed by these phases and the related bio-physiological processes as shown in Table 7.1. Although a wound's healing activity might be slowed in one or more phases by a variety of causes, this results in insufficient tissue repair (Guo & DiPietro, 2010).

Medical dressings are essential equipment for the healthcare sector. Dressings may be applied to the wound's surface to encourage healing, depending on the kinds and stages of the wounds. Although gauze, sterile absorbent cotton, and bandages are often used in clinical practice and are cost-effective, their benefits for wound

DOI: 10.1201/9781003331612-9

healing and infection control are limited. Dressings and wound adherence will cause secondary harm when the dressing and the wound are ultimately separated. Contemporary dressings offer several benefits over conventional dressings, and their creation and development are focused on the curing principle of the wet environment (Skorkowska-Telichowska et al., 2013). Contemporary dressings also encourage cell proliferation, division, and epithelial migration to prevent damage to fresh connective tissue caused by injury. They may be particularly important in minimizing wound exposure to external microorganisms and successfully preventing cross-contamination (Murakami et al., 2010). We discuss the mechanics of wound healing, conventional and contemporary wound dressings, types and developments, and the benefits and applications of nano-based wound dressings throughout this chapter.

7.2   WOUND CLASSIFICATION

The manner in which a skin injury takes place has a significant impact on how the wound will heal. The various criteria under which wounds are classified are shown in Figure 7.1.

7.2.1   INJURY

7.2.1.1   Incised

Little soft tissue damage results from incised wounds; therefore, the blood flow is not significantly affected. If sutured, these wounds will usually heal with the original intent.

7.2.1.2   Shearing or Degloving

Shearing or degloving injuries to the skin border frequently result in modest damage to the skin's upper layer but considerable devascularization of the soft tissue and skin. These injuries may have resulted from a serious accident, such as when a truck tire crossed a person's leg or crushed their leg. Failure to detect this kind of injury

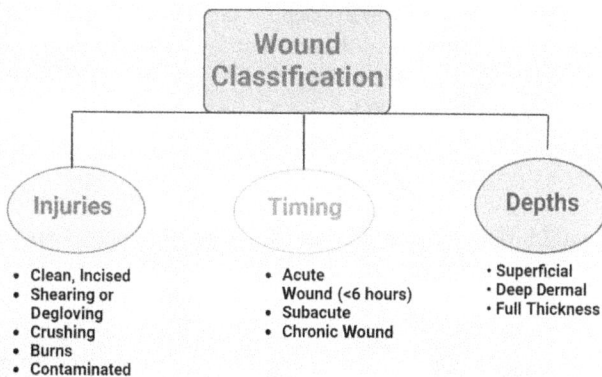

FIGURE 7.1   Classification of wounds

will result in substantial necrosis of the skin and subcutaneous tissue, with the possibility of an infection and slow wound healing. The skin often appears uneven in color, and capillary filling is difficult to see. An efficient approach is to cut or debride the skin to a safe bleeding edge. Before suturing, thorough debridement and disinfection are required.

7.2.1.3 Crushing
Crushing injuries will also result in quick cell death and damage to the underneath blood supply. Excision or wound debridement will be required for tissue that has been taken to a severe crushing force. Nerve and blood vessel avulsion is frequently associated with these types of injuries, notably in the limb, resulting in a poor prognosis for wound healing and revascularizations. Because the tissue in a fracture injury is fragile, a "second-look" procedure should be performed up to 24 to 48 hours after the interim surgical intervention. In this manner, the surgeon is able to ensure that no non-viable tissue remains. The threat of infection rises if the wound is sealed with non-viable tissue. Furthermore, an increase in the population of macrophages (a type of white blood cell) as a result of infection will result in massive scarring.

7.2.1.4 Burn
Burn wounds are categorized based on their size, the body covering an area, and the deepness of skin damage. The wound surface area is critical because fluid losses via the injured epidermis might be significant. In order to restore considerable body tissue fluid loss after burns, which occupy more than 10% of the body's covering area in children and 15% in adults, respectively, proper intravenous fluid resuscitation was required. The depth of the burn damage is particularly crucial since it influences wound healing, both in perspective of how long the lesion takes to heal and future scar development.

7.2.1.5 Contaminated
Wounds can also be classified based on their sterility or bacterial infection. In general, burn injuries and incision wounds are sterile for around six hours after damage but will become colonized by skin bacteria unless additional steps are taken to preserve the wound. The wound must be cleaned with sterile normal saline or an antiseptic before applying a sterile dressing.

Subtypes of Contaminated Wounds:

7.2.1.5.1 Clean Wound
They are typically closed, uninfected, and irritable; if these wounds need to be drained, a closed draining treatment is necessary. Furthermore, these wounds have little effect on the respiratory, digestive, vaginal, or urine systems.

7.2.1.5.2 Contaminated Clean
When an internal organ is repaired or removed from a clean, contaminated wound, no signs of infection are present at that time. Examples of this kind of wound include vaginal, lung, and appendix surgeries. The infection risk is typically less than 10%.

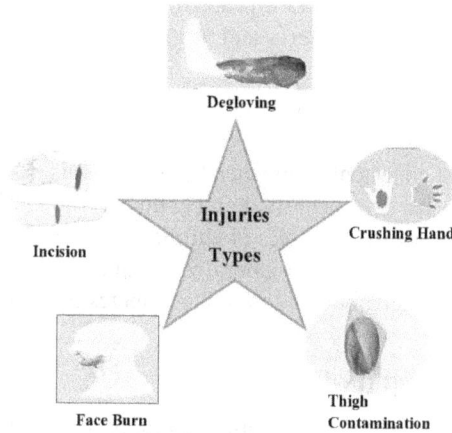

FIGURE 7.2   Schematic diagram—types of injuries

7.2.1.5.3   Severe Contaminated

Open, recent accidental wounds as well as wounds resulting from the repair or removal of an internal organ are examples of severely contaminated wounds. The organ may leak blood or other liquids into the wound. Infection risk typically ranges from 13% to 20%. The risk of infection following surgery on the digestive (gastrointestinal) tract may be very high.

7.2.1.5.4   Dirty Contaminated

An infection is already present in dirty, contaminated wounds at the time of surgery. In these circumstances, the chance of infection is typically around 40%. These wounds normally result from trauma that has not been properly treated. Wounds exhibit weak tissue, and they typically arise from bacteria in the surgical field or ruptured viscera (Onyekwelu et al., 2017; Timothy & Herman, 2022).

7.2.2   TIMING

7.2.2.1   Acute Wounds

Acute wounds are defined as ones that are not older than six hours and hence possibly sterile. Acute wounds are caused by the exterior deterioration of the entire skin and involve surgical wounds, bites, burns, small cuts, and abrasions. However, the chosen healing therapy will be adjusted according to the kind, location, and depth of the wound. To allow for spontaneous and rapid healing, the initial closure of a washed surgical wound requires the least amount of intervention.

7.2.2.2   Subacute

A subacute injury is one that happened longer than six hours ago but lasted less than or up to five days. During this period, simple wound colonization may occur unless the wound is cleaned routinely and a protective dressing is used. Five days later, all wounds are colonized by bacteria and are thus classified as chronic in nature. Chronic wounds require debridement.

7.2.2.3 Chronic Wounds

Chronic wounds most commonly happened by endogenous processes as a result of a predisposing disease that affects dermal and epithelial tissue integrity. Stress sores, ulceration, and leg ulcers are examples of chronic wounds that may form as a result of inadequate arterial blood flow (peripheral vascular disease), poor venous drainage (venous hypertension), metabolic diseases like diabetes mellitus, or both.

7.2.3 Wound Healing (In-Depth)

Wound healing is a repair and regeneration operation that includes wound contraction, collagen production, and epithelialization. Diabetes, dietary deficiencies, and metabolic imbalances can all hinder wound healing, resulting in chronic, non-curable wounds. The capacity of the skin to mend itself is also affected by the degree of the injury, which might be superficial, deep dermal, or full thickness.

7.2.3.1 Superficial Wounds

Wounds that only affect the epidermis and papillary dermis are referred to as superficial wounds. They heal by re-epithelializing the remaining pilosebaceous units, such as the sweat glands, hair follicles, and sebaceous glands. There is no substantial scarring or wound contraction. If an ideal wound environment is formed and infection is avoided, this depth of wound will recover in 10 days.

7.2.3.2 Deep Dermal Wounds

A combination of wound contraction, scar emergence, and re-epithelialization from pilosebaceous "units" can be used to treat incomplete or deep skin wounds. Normally, these wounds heal in 10 to 21 days.

7.2.3.2 Full-Thickness Wounds

Full-thickness wounds can heal in two ways: either primary or secondary healing.

7.2.3.2.1 Primary Wound Healing

Primary healing occurs when surgical injuries are cleansed, incised, and closed in six hours or less using sutures, staples, adhesives, or steristrips. Within the tissue, the injury triggers a series of regulated reactions. Blood coagulation begins within 24 hours, followed by a preliminary stage of inflammation with granulocyte activation. Granulocytes take out bacteria and foreign material from the injury, minimizing the risk of infection. Macrophages take control as the dominant cell type 48–72 hours after injury. These are phagocytic and generate growth elements that stimulate fibroblasts to build an extracellular lattice, smooth muscle cell expansion, and endothelial cell proliferation, which all result in angiogenesis. Fibroblasts are the dominant cell type after seven days of damage. They can produce collagen for 21 days. The collagen is then remodeled. Re-epithelialization begins 48 hours after damage to repair the skin gap and seal the injury.

7.2.3.2.2   Secondary Wound Healing

It occurs when the wound is not medically closed but is permissible to mend naturally via the narrowing and recovery of the epithelium. Myofibroblasts (which are generated from fibroblasts) emerge and multiply on the third day following injury. These cells have an actin microfilament structure that appears to aid in wound contraction. Re-epithelialization is feasible if dermal elements are present; however, wounds without dermal components heal totally through constriction and tissue regeneration of the wound from the wound boundary (Percival, 2002). The different types of injuries are illustrated in Figure 7.2.

7.3   PHASES OF WOUND HEALING

7.3.1   Hemostasis

Hemostasis is the natural response of a vessel to disruption, which includes the formation of a clot that stops bleeding. In a few minutes, the reduced blood flow caused by arteriolar constriction causes tissue hypoxia and acidosis. Histamine is released from mast cells at the same moment. This can also increase vasodilation and blood vessel permeability, allowing inflamed cells to penetrate the wound's extracellular space (ECS) (Singh et al., 2017). Coagulation is caused by the clumping of thrombocytes and platelets in a fibrin cascade, which is dependent on the activity of particular stimuli via the excitation and consolidation of these cells. At the same time, establishing new homeostasis and establishing a barrier against microbe colonization, the network of fibrin coordinates with the temporary matrix required for cell migration, preserving the skin's protective barrier function to maintain skin integrity (Shaw & Martin, 2009).

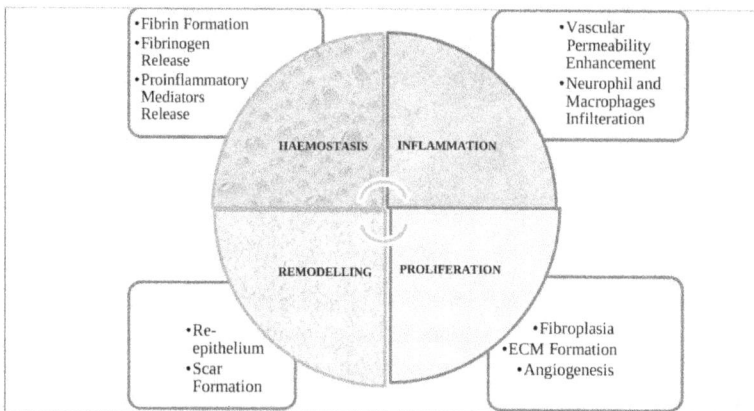

FIGURE 7.3   Wound healing phases

7.3.2 Inflammation

The inflammatory response is activated shortly after circulating neutrophils from ruptured blood vessels are passively exposed to wounds. The work of active neutrophils and later macrophages from the surrounding arteries maintains the inflammatory response, which is regulated by growth factor indicators from regional cells and serum, as well as invading autoantigens such as lipopolysaccharides of invading bacteria. Near the site of the lesion, neutrophils are recognized to produce pro-inflammatory cytokines and active bactericidal as well as bacteriostatic agents such as cationic proteins, peptidases, and reactive oxygen species (ROS). The recruitment of active neutrophils in response to support system activation, platelet agglomeration, and bacterial deterioration products maintains the inflammatory reaction. Then, neutrophils are primarily stimulated immune cells employed by the blood that help to remove the tissue while also contributing to the death of the invading organisms (Eming et al., 2007). Endothelial cells in the blood capillary walls are stimulated by pro-inflammatory cytokines such as tumor necrosis factor alpha (TNF- α) and interferon gamma (IFN- γ) at the lesion site and transmigrate a significant amount of neutrophils only a few hours after the lesion forms. Neutrophils are either expelled from the wound's surface, undergo apoptosis, or are phagocytosed by macrophages (Gurtner et al., 2008).

7.3.3 Proliferation

The proliferative phase lasts four to 21 days and includes endothelial progenitor cells, extracellular matrix (ECM) production, and epithelization. Because platelet-derived growth factor (PDGF) is a recognized supporter and booster of proteoglycan and collagen production, ECM development begins with platelet degranulation (Elnar & Ailey, 2009). Throughout the proliferative phase, the wound fault is covered up by connective tissue that is extremely vascular, which is frequently referred to as "granulation tissue" (Beldon, 2010). When the hemostatic plug forms as a result of platelet release of transforming growth factor (TGF- β), platelet-derived growth factor (PDGF), and fibroblast growth factor (FGF), angiogenesis begins. In reaction to hypoxia, VEGF and other cytokines are produced, which subsequently stimulate endothelial cells to induce neovascularization and the repair of injured blood vessels (Childs & Murthy, 2017).

7.3.4 Remodeling

Remodeling is the final stage of recovery, which starts two to three weeks after the lesion appears and remains for a year or more (Sorg et al., 2017). Remodeling takes place due to the creation of a fibrin clot in the early III phase and during the proliferative phase of blood vessels. As a result, it is assimilated via a scar made of type I collagen, which is collagenous and has very new blood vessels (Li et al., 2007). The key elements of the wound healing

TABLE 7.1

Cellular and biophysiological events in the wound healing process

PHASE	DAYS	KEY AIM	MAIN CELL TYPE	CELLULAR AND BIOPHYSIOLOGICAL EVENTS
HAEMOSTASIS	Immediate	To stop bleeding	Platelets	• Vascular tightening • Platelets activation • Loss of granules (cellular process, also termed as degranulation) • Fibrin production (thrombus)
INFLAMMATION	1–3	To prevent wound infection and initiate the repair process	Leucocytes (neutrophils monocytes, macrophages)	• Neutrophil infiltration and monocyte infiltration • Differentiation to macrophages lymphocyte infiltration
PROLIFERATION	Day 3 to 2 weeks	To provide mechanical supports, control cell proliferation, and provide a scaffold for tissue renewal	Kerathocytes, fibroblasts, endothelial cells	• Reepithelization • Angiogenesis • Collagen synthesis • ECM formation
REMODELING	Week 1 to several weeks	To provide strength to the wound	Fibroblasts	• Collagen remodeling • Vascular maturation regression

procedure are the growth part, which are polypeptides produced by many triggered cells at the wound area that drive cellular multiplication as well as draw additional cells to the wound (Welch et al., 1990). Thus, in remodeling, granulation tissue becomes a scar, and the tensile strength of the tissue increases (Guo & DiPietro, 2010; Okur et al., 2020). The phases throughout wound healing are depicted in Figure 7.3, along with a detailed description of cellular and biophysiological events in Table 7.1.

7.4 FACTORS IMPORTANT IN THE WOUND HEALING PROCESS

Many wounds have been found to heal quickly, whereas others are likely to stay chronic and stuck in the inflammatory period. There are several elements involved in such a settlement. To begin with, excessive amounts of inflammatory chemicals caused harm to growth elements and the extracellular matrix, both of which are required for healing. The probability of a wound quickly colonizing with bacteria or fungus is a serious issue throughout the wound-healing operation. This is due to a decrease in wound infection, the inhibition of growth hormones, and the destruction of the necessary fibrin for healing. Furthermore, bacteria cause an inflammatory response; therefore, chronic wounds frequently have high amounts of bacteria. Clearly, limiting bacterial growth will help the healing process. Furthermore, biofilm, a complicated structural form that can attach to a surface, is implicated in the formation and continuation of the long-term wound habitat. Hypoxia, among other things, slows wound healing via inhibiting fibroblast generation and collagen formation and allowing definite negative organisms, such as bacteria, to thrive. Hypoxia appears to be caused by prevalent chronic illness and peripheral vascular disease has been associated with multiple risk factors, including smoking, diabetes, prior coronary artery disease, and a sedentary lifestyle. As a result, careful management of these disorders can aid in wound healing. Additionally, smoking inhibits wound healing by interfering with chemotaxis, migratory function, and aerobic bacterial processes during the period of inflammation. Many medicines that suppress the inflammatory response can also interfere with the healing operation. For example, oral steroids were discovered to reduce cytokine abundance, resulting in reduced collagen deposition. Diabetes, the most common metabolic illness, causes delays in wound healing procedures. Furthermore, since they have a narrow epidermal barrier and weaker inflammatory, transient, and proliferative responses, senior individuals are more prone to acquire chronic wounds, and they are also more likely to develop the ongoing illness. Finally, an inadequate diet with minimal protein levels might cause wound healing to be delayed (Okur et al., 2020). Some factors that affect wound healing operations are represented in Figure 7.4.

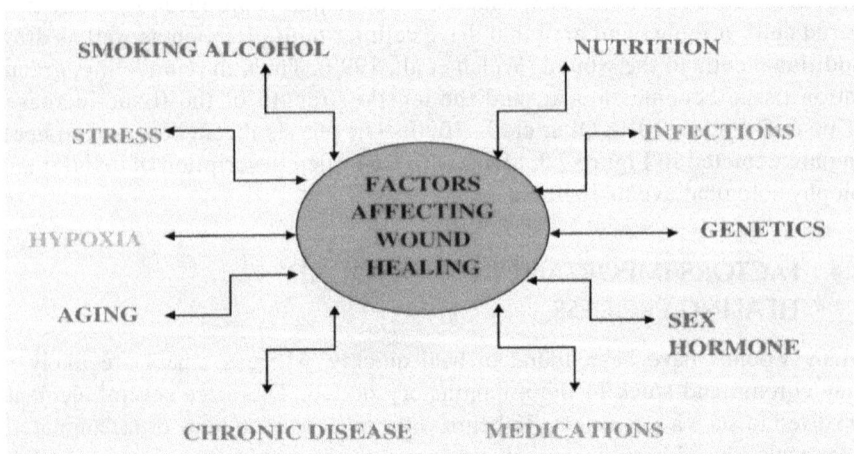

FIGURE 7.4 Factors that influence wound healing

7.5 MEDICAL DRESSINGS, BANDAGES, AND STOCKINGS

7.5.1 DRESSINGS

The phrases "dressing" and "bandage" are sometimes used interchangeably. In reality, the term "dressing" refers to the main layer in touch with the wound. Dressings are used to cover wounds, keep them clean, and control bleeding. We frequently utilize self-adhesive bandages or gauze dressings when administering first aid.

- Adhesive dressings are mostly used on minor wounds. They are available in a variety of sizes, including particular varieties for use on the fingers.
- Massive wounds are covered with gauze bandages, which are made of thick cotton. They are held in place by wrapping a gauze strip around them or using tape to keep them in place (a bandage).
- To stop the growth of germs, dressings must be sterilized and permeable. Unless a lesion needs frequent cleaning, dressings should be kept in place until the wound heals. The various types of dressings are depicted in Figure 7.5.

7.5.2 BANDAGES

A bandage is a material component that is applied to a wound to provide protection, keep dressings in place, provide pressure to stop bleeding, support splints or other medical equipment, or provide assistance to the body on its own. It can also be used to bind a portion of the body. The different varieties of bandages are shown in Figure 7.6.

7.5.2.1 Role
- Covering the wound
- Applying pressure to stop the bleeding
- Managing a strain or sprain

Note: Each of these tasks requires a unique bandage (Todd, 2011).

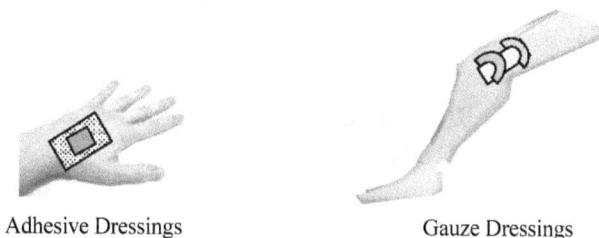

Adhesive Dressings   Gauze Dressings

FIGURE 7.5   Different types of dressings

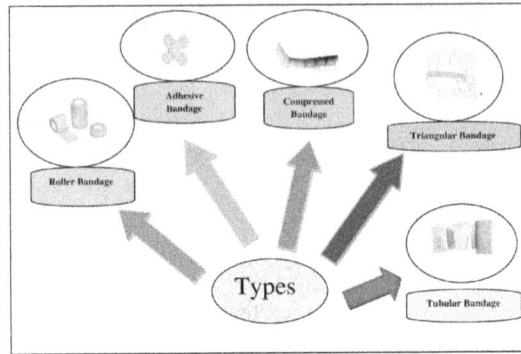

FIGURE 7.6 Bandage varieties

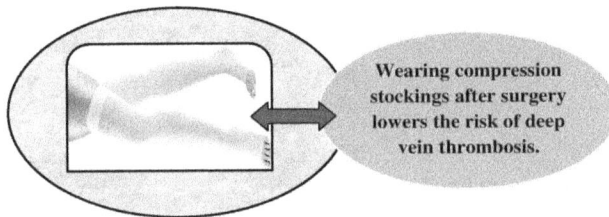

FIGURE 7.7 Stockings

7.5.3 Stockings

Medical stockings (usually compression) are a common, non-invasive therapeutic option for all venous and lymphatic illnesses. The image of the stockings is displayed in Figure 7.7. Deep-vein thrombosis, in which a blood clot develops in one of the deep veins, commonly in the leg, is more common in surgical patients. The clot fragments and travels to the lungs, potentially fatally causing pulmonary embolism. The NICE (full name: National Institute for Health and Care Excellence) strongly recommends and refers to prophylactic pharmacological (such as low molecular weight heparin) and/or mechanical (such as graded compression stockings) treatment.

Patients have reported difficulty utilizing both knees and thigh-length compression stockings. Incorrectly worn or poorly fitted stockings can cause skin injury or roll down, restricting blood flow; hence, patient adherence is critical for effective DVT prevention (Benigni et al., 2003).

7.6 COMPRESSION BANDAGES, STOCKINGS AND CLASSIFICATION

7.6.1 Compression Bandages

Compression bandages are perhaps the most essential concept for the treatment and prevention of venous disorders during compression therapy. Compression bandages

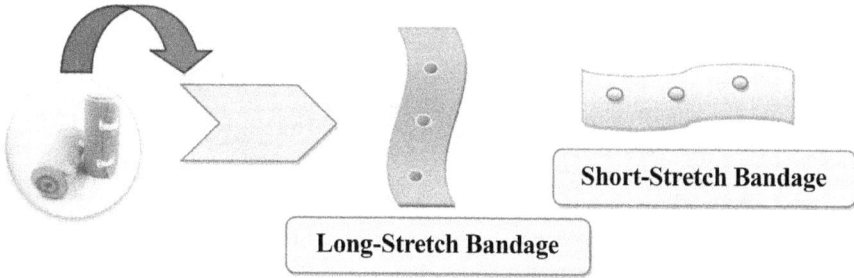

FIGURE 7.8 Types of compression bandages

are made of fibrous materials that are viscoelastic in nature, which causes the internal pressure to develop in the bandage when wrapped. The different types of compression bandages are displayed in Figure 7.8.

Compression bandaging is recommended for people who have any of the following conditions:

- Swollen limbs which are too big to fit into compression garments
- Leg form distortion and reinforced skin folds
- Tissue and skin alterations
- Ulceration
- Lymphorrhoea

7.6.2 CLASSIFICATION OF COMPRESSION BANDAGES

Compression bandages are primarily divided into two types.

- Long-stretch (elastic) bandages
- Bandages with a short stretch (elastic)

7.6.2.1 Long-Stretch Bandages

Long-stretch bandages (also called extensible or elastic bandages) are made of knitted or woven fibers that contain polyamide or polyurethane synthetic threads. These bandages' flexibility is offered via elastic thread, which may be stretched up to 120%.

They expand as the limb's volume increases, as during muscle activity, and return with a lower volume instead of losing pressure, likely to result in consistent pressure independent of activity. Their high resting pressure efficiently squeezes superficial veins upon surgery, sclerotherapy, and orthrombophlebitis (Todd, 2011).

The long-stretch, textured bandage is simple to use and adapts nicely to body shapes. The compressive strength of this bandage may be readily altered thanks to its lengthy stretch capabilities. The very pliable and soft bandage can be used for compression, support, limb immobilization, and dressing retention.

TABLE 7.2

Elastic compression bandage classification, function, and uses

CATEGORY	TYPE OF BANDAGE	BANDAGE FUNCTION	USES INDICATION
1	Lightweight conforming	Exert very little sub-bandage pressure	Used to keep dressings in position
2	Light support	Exert normal sub-bandage pressure	Used to treat mixed-etiology ulcers or to prevent edema
3A	Light compression	Apply pressure on the ankle in the 14–17 mmHg range	Superficial or premature varices Varicosities that developed during pregnancy
3B	Moderate compression	Apply pressure on the ankle in the range of 18–24 mmHg	Varices of moderate severity Ulcer prevention and treatment Mild edema management
3C	High compression	Apply pressure on the ankle in the range of 25–35 mmHg	Significant varices Venous insufficiency after thrombosis Leg ulcer management Management of severe edema
3D	Extra high compression	Apply pressure on the ankle up to 60 mmHg	Assistance for the prevention of venous leg ulcers, the treatment of DVT, and varicose veins

The bandage shouldn't be worn overnight or for lengthy stretches of time while resting because of the high resting pressure level. The classification of elastic bandages with descriptive knowledge is illustrated in Table 7.2.

7.6.2.2 Short-Stretch Bandages

Short-stretch bandages (also referred to as non-elastic bandages) are frequently comprised of 100% cotton fibers or a cotton-polyamide mixture. The slightest stretch in the 100% cotton bandages is attained via the way the fibers are woven; this interlocking pattern also makes it easier for air to get through. These bandages may be stretched to 100% of their original length, creating a solid case around the limb. Muscular activity yields little, resulting in a low clinical-curative working pressure and a lowered resting pressure, enhancing individual comfort when lying down, and so promoting compliance. To deliver compression in the therapy of chronic edema or lymph-edema, expert lymph-edema practitioners prefer the short-stretch bandaging system (Todd M., 2011; Arthur & Lewis, 2000).

Further, compression bandages are classified into three types based on their adhesive properties:

- Non-adhesive bandages
- Cohesive bandages
- Adhesive bandages

7.6.2.2.1 How to Use a Compression Bandage
- Only use elastic bandages for the first 24 to 48 hours following an accident
- Avoid wrapping or covering too tightly
- Combine rest and elevation with compression
- Do not use ice and compression at the same time

7.6.2.2.2 Application of Compressed Bandages
- Venous insufficiency treatment
- Venous leg ulcer treatment
- Post-thrombotic syndrome treatment
- Treatment for dependent oedema

7.6.3 COMPRESSION STOCKINGS

Compression stockings are a common, non-invasive therapeutic option for all venous and lymphatic illnesses. A varicose vein is a prominent vein situated just beneath the skin's surface. Compression stockings may aid in reducing the appearance and uncomfortable symptoms of varicose veins. Compression stockings have long been used to promote circulation. During long marches, people would wrap their legs in leather bands to enhance circulation.

Modern compression socks are more advanced, supplying steady pressure to the legs and encouraging blood to return to the heart. Typically, stockings provide more pressure on the area around the ankles and feet, causing an excess squeeze that improves blood flow. In studies, compression stockings have been shown to relieve the symptoms of varicose veins, but there is little proof that they would completely eradicate them. Different styles of stockings exert varying degrees of pressure (Shi et al., 2020). The application of compression stockings is displayed in Figure 7.9.

7.6.3.1 Classification of Compression Stockings
Stockings are categorized based on the amount of compression they provide to the limb. Significantly, stockings provide less pressure than bandages and are less

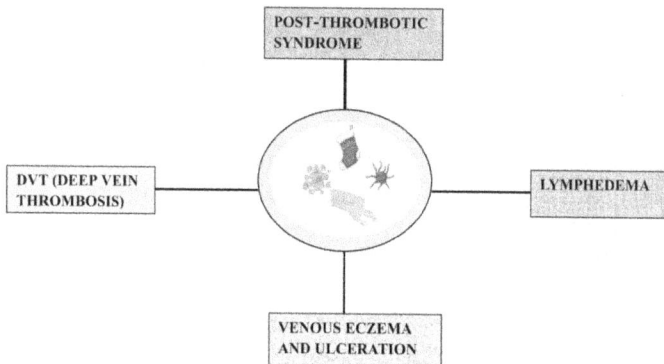

FIGURE 7.9 Application of compressed stockings

TABLE 7.3

Stocking classification, function, and indication

CLASS	STOCKING TYPES	STOCKINGS FUNCTION	USES INDICATION
I	Light support stockings	Put pressure of 14 to 17 mmHg on the ankle	Varicose veins treatment
2	Medium support stockings	Pressurize the ankle with 18 to 24 mmHg of pressure	To prevent venous leg ulcers and to repair more severe varicosities
3	Strong support stockings	Pressurize the ankle with 25 to 35 mmHg of pressure	Avoid venous leg ulcers and cure serious chronic hypertension and varicose veins

susceptible to operator variation. Table 7.3 shows the classification of stockings along with a brief description of their function and uses.

7.6.3.2 The Benefits of Compressed Stocks

Compression socks and stockings are specifically designed to help with compression treatment. They apply gentle pressure to your legs and ankles in order to increase blood flow from your legs to your heart.

Benefits are:

- Avoid having blood collect in your leg veins
- Minimize leg edema and orthostatic hypotension (lightheadedness or unsteadiness when standing)
- Help to avoid venous ulcers
- Avoid developing deep vein thrombosis in your legs
- Assist in reducing the discomfort caused by varicose veins
- Roll back or reverse venous hypertension
- Enhance lymphatic drainage

7.6.3.3 Compression Stockings Wearing Technique

After bandaging any sores, put on your stockings before getting out of bed in the morning. It is because, in the early morning, your legs have the minimum swelling.

Steps:

- Roll the stocking down to the heel while holding the top.
- As deeply as you can, tuck your foot inside the sock. Insert your heel into the stocking's heel.
- Draw up the stocking. Over your leg, unroll the stocking.
- After you've secured the stocking's top, straighten out any creases.
- Keep the stockings from bunching up or wrinkling.
- Stockings that are knee-length should terminate two fingers below the knee bend.

(Alavi & Kirsner, 2017; Holsche & Haut, 2023; Markovic & Shortell, 2023)

7.6.3.4   Application of Compressed Stockings

7.7   BIOMATERIALS FOR WOUND MANAGEMENT

7.7.1   BIOMATERIAL

A biomaterial is a non-drug that can be used in systems to enhance or take the place of physiological tissues or organs in their function. These substances may stay in contact with physiological fluids and tissues over extended periods of time without producing any negative effects or minimal side effects (Nicolai & Rakhorst, 2008; Heness & Ben-Nissan, 2004). Biomaterials are classified as either synthetic or natural biopolymers, as shown in Figure 7.9.

7.7.1.1   Wound Dressings Made From Naturally Occurring and Synthesized Biopolymers

Natural polymers are often preferred over synthetic polymers for wound treatment since they are less expensive, non-poisonous to the human body, and environmentally safe. Polysaccharides are naturally occurring polymers that are frequently employed as materials for wound dressing. Among the materials most commonly employed along with collagen, hyaluronic acid, and alginate, polymers including cellulose, chitosan, pullulan, starch, and glucan are utilized as wound dressings.

7.7.1.1.1   Chitosan-Based Wound Treatments

Chitosan (CS) is considered a natural polymer that is commonly used in biomedical applications attributed to its antibacterial activity and ability to stimulate healing (Siafaka et al., 2016b). In wound care, it also facilitates drainage, minimizes the accumulation of toxins, and acts as a bed for autograft. Moreover, chitosan stimulates gas exchange, which is necessary for wound healing (Siafaka et al., 2015b). Literature is filled with chitosan-based drug delivery methods for wound care. The resultant polymer may provide a therapy option for both chronic and acute wounds, including hydrogels and nanoparticles containing chitosan. Because of the chemical characteristics of chitosan, gels may develop in acidic solutions (Filippousi et al., 2015). The hydrogels exhibit robust characteristics and can absorb a substantial amount of water, concurrently forming a three-dimensional network or 3D structure. When in contact with chitosan-based wound dressings, they demonstrate excellent properties for enhancing wound healing. Because they are biocompatible and exhibit action against pathogenic bacteria, chitosan-based hydrogels have been extensively employed in wound healing (Ferreira et al., 2019). Research scholars designed and analyzed a chitosan gel system containing chlorhexidine (2% and 4%). This hydrogel system's therapeutic and bactericidal-bacteriostatic capabilities were investigated, with 100% suppression of bacterial spread when strain *S. aureus* was used. After 14 days of treatment using chitosan hydrogel containing 2% chlorhexidine, histologic assessment confirmed healing; healing was faster in groups that received 4% chlorhexidine, and any additional lesions were closed by the 14th day. The findings show that a favorable substance with antibacterial capabilities was produced and utilized as a therapeutic agent (Martínez-Ibarra et al., 2018).

The primary drawbacks of chitosan-based hydrogels are their weak mechanical characteristics and unsatisfactory anti-bacterial activity. As a result, numerous research groups are focused on combining chitosan with some other polymers to enhance its hydrophilic nature, boost antibacterial action, and improve mechanical qualities (Yao et al., 2019). Although quaternized chitosan nanocomposite films were recently combined with AgNPs to generate excellent wound dressings. The quaternized chitosan (CS) film with AgNPs was shown to have strong bactericidal as well as bacteriostatic activity on both gram-positive and gram-negative bacteria strains. More notably, all of the films demonstrated biocompatibility with HFF (human foreskin fibroblast) cells, showing that the nanocomposite films made of quaternized chitosan may be employed as wound-covering materials effectively (Okur et al., 2020).

7.7.1.1.2 Other Natural Polymeric Wound Dressings

Aside from chitosan, researchers are looking at other natural polymers that might be used to make wound dressings, although it can be stated that the majority of the investigations include the usage of natural polymer combinations. The most prevalent natural polymer derived from sustainable energy sources is cellulose. Bacterial cellulose is a biopolymer manufactured by bacteria that has various benefits, including purity, high porosity, and excellent biocompatibility (Portela et al., 2019). Moreover, bacterial cellulose (BC) may be easily changed to acquire antibacterial action as well as potential local drug delivery properties. Alginate is a commonly accessible anionic biopolymer derived from brown seaweed with good biocompatibility, and wound dressings containing alginate (AG) provide a wet atmosphere and prevent bacterial contagion, both of which are significant elements in wound healing (Aderibigbe & Buyana, 2018). Collagen, which is generated by fibroblasts, is an extremely abundant protein element in the human body, triggering cellular migration and contributing to the formation of new tissues. Biomaterials formed from collagen activate and attract particular cells, such as scavenger and fibroblast cells, influencing wound healing (Fleck & Simman, 2010). HA stands for hyaluronic acid, a glycosaminoglycan that is abundant in various soft connective tissues, including the skin. In reality, hyaluronic acid is essential for tissue integrity as well as cell stickiness and division throughout inflammation, wound healing, and embryonic development (Longinotti, 2014). Because of the positive results associated with biocompatibility and biodegradability, a variety of wound dressings incorporating HA for human medical use have been developed (Yu et al., 2021).

7.7.1.2 Wound Dressings Composed of Synthetic Polymers

Synthetic polymers like PCL (Polycaprolactone), PLA (Polylactic Acid), PLGA (Polylactic Co-Glycolic Acid), and PVA (Polyvinyl Alcohol) are broadly employed as biomaterials due to their outstanding biocompatibility and biodegradability, as well as active groups (-OH) that can be covalently linked or conjugated with the several receptors to promote cellular absorption and circulation time to the RES (reticuloendothelial system) (Mir et al., 2018). The polymers listed earlier are available as wound dressings for acute or severe persistent wounds in the manner of micro- or nanoparticles, electrospun fibrous structures, sponges, and so on. Antibiotic elements, growth enhancers, or natural components such as honey, cinnamaldehyde, and so on are commonly found in polymeric formulations (Siafaka et al., 2016a).

7.7.1.2.1   Polycaprolactone (PCL)-Based Systems

PCL (Polycaprolactone) is an aliphatic polyester that is widely employed in medicinal usage owing to its excellent biocompatibility, eco-friendliness, and mechanical features. However, the bulk of aliphatic polyesters exhibited a strong lack of affinity towards water and crystallinity (degree of molecule arrangement), limiting their use as wound dressing materials (Filippousi et al., 2016). As a result, in most situations, PCL is combined with hydrophilic substances to address the issues raised by its hydrophobicity. Many studies have been conducted on the use of PCL as a wound dressing material. As previously stated, PCL is hydrophobic but biocompatible (Siafaka et al., 2015a), which is why many studies are being conducted on PCL electrospun fibers or micro- or nanoparticles containing active substances such as growth factors or antibiotics, or PCL blends with hydrophilic polymers such as chitosan, PEG, and others (Egri & Erdemir, 2019).

7.7.1.2.2   Polyvinyl Alcohol (PVA)-Based System

PVA (polyvinyl alcohol) is a neutral, unbiased hydrogel with excellent biocompatibility, hydrophilicity, and biomechanical characteristics. PVA is a potential wound dressing material since it can easily create hydrogels and is frequently employed in controlled-release applications. During the literature search, PVA electrospun fibers were discovered, as predicted (Tavakoli & Tang, 2017). Furthermore, this is the most simple and inspiring way of producing structures that replicate the extracellular matrix. PVA hydrogels and NPs, in addition to nanofibrous systems, are commonly encountered in research (Ardekani et al., 2019; Kim et al., 2020).

7.7.1.2.3   System Based on Polylactic Acid (PLA) and Polylactic-Co-Glycolic Acid (PLGA)

Some other aliphatic polyesters discovered in past research and employed to develop quality wound dressings, besides PCL (polycaprolactone), is PLA (polylactic acid) and PLGA (polylactic-co-glycolic acid). Because of its cytocompatibility and biodegradability, PLA is a crucial biomaterial employed in various biomedical implementations, such as medication delivery methods, gene therapy, surgical stitches, biomedical engineering, genetic engineering, and tissue regeneration. PLA (polylactic acid) and PGA (polyglycolic acid) are combined to form the copolymer PLGA (polylactic-co-glycolic acid) (Perumal et al., 2017). This copolymer has high biocompatibility, mechanical strength, and other beneficial properties. Furthermore, PLGA has tunable degradation and mechanical qualities, depending on the application (Siafaka et al., 2016a). Furthermore, when PLGA is employed as a dressing material, the breakdown rate is synced with the epithelialization rate, accelerating the healing task (Ahmed & Ikram, 2016). The description of biomaterial types with an example along with a graphical depiction of biomaterial application in dressings (especially the mechanism of drug incorporation through biomaterial in dressings that are then applied to a wound for healing purposes) is shown in Figure 7.10.

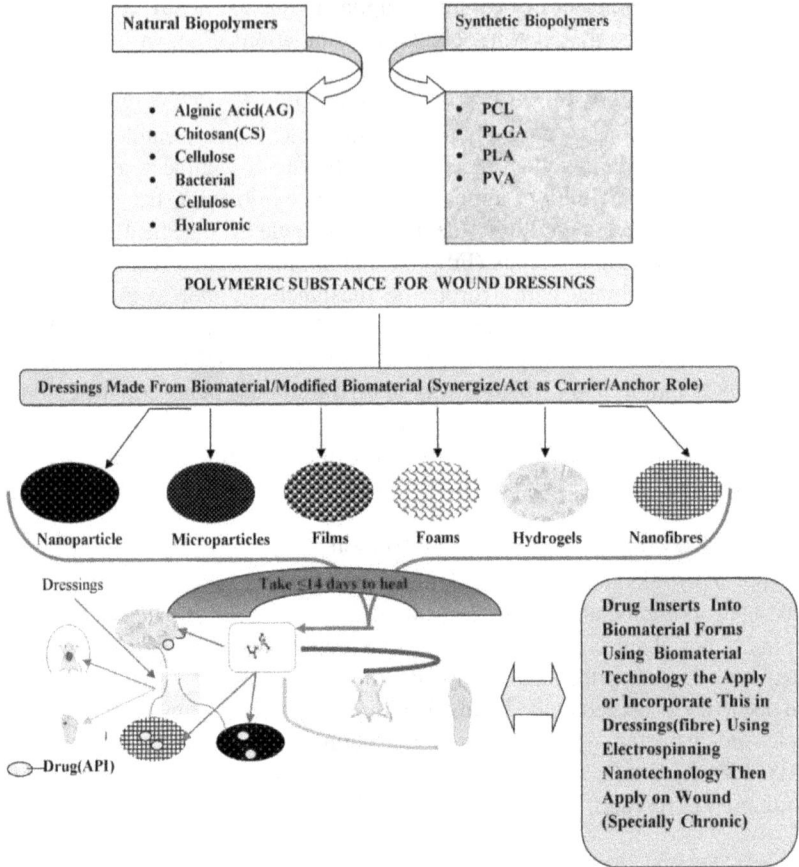

FIGURE 7.10   Wound dressings made from naturally occurring and synthesized biopolymers

7.8   NANOTECHNOLOGY IN WOUND HEALING

7.8.1   NANOTECHNOLOGY—DEFINITION

Nanotechnology is the study of the production, architecture, and dynamics of atomic and molecular nanometric particles (with a maximal diameter of 100 nm), after which nanoproducts are formed. When a particle is downscaled to the nanometric range, its surface rises rampantly while its volume shrinks, resulting in certain physicochemical properties that account for several medicinal uses. CD (circular dichroism), IR (infrared spectroscopy), and MS (mass spectroscopy) help in the examination of the structure, configuration, and outer edge properties of nanoparticles. DLS (dynamic light scattering), FCS (fluorescence correlation spectroscopy), and RS (Raman scattering) deliver knowledge on the hydro mechanical nanoparticle size distribution. Furthermore, in order to investigate the dynamics properties (such as mobility and adhesion) of nanomaterials, electron microscopy, in general, and TEM (transmission

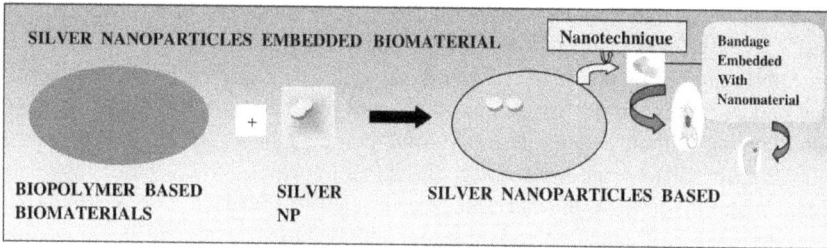

FIGURE 7.11   Silver NP-based textile in wound healing

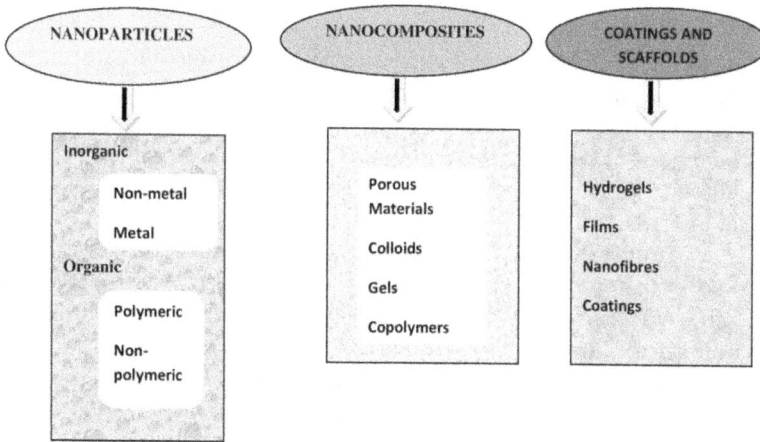

FIGURE 7.12   Different varieties of nanomaterials

electron microscopy), in particular, have been identified as valuable analytical tools. The morphology of nanomaterials can be explored with TEM, although SEM only generates a surface picture of the nanomaterial and is thus used to research dimensions and general forms (Mihai et al., 2019). The silver NP-based textile in wound healing is shown in Figure 7.11.

7.8.2   Nanomaterial Categories Used in Wound Care

7.8.2.1   Nanoparticles

Nanoparticles are tiny particles that range in size from 1 to 100 nanometers. The different varieties of nanomaterial are shown in Figure 7.12.

7.8.2.1.1   Silver Nanoparticles

Silver nanoparticles (AgNPs), among the different metallic nanoparticles employed in biomedical applications, are one of the most important and fascinating nanomaterials.

The drawbacks of traditional silver compounds can be addressed using silver nanoparticles (AgNPs) (Zhang et al., 2016). Since they have a higher surface-to-volume proportion, AgNPs are highly effective at lower doses and have lower toxicity. Unadulterated silver nanoparticles trigger the liberation of anti-inflammatory cytokines to hasten wound healing without leaving scars (Hamdan et al., 2017). AgNPs increase wound contractility by differentiating myofibroblasts from normal fibroblasts, thereby expediting the healing process. Furthermore, AgNPs elevate epidermal re-epithelialization via keratinocyte multiplication and relocation (Vijayakumar et al., 2019). On the other hand, research has found that too high concentrations of AgNPs reduce keratinocyte viability, metabolism, migration, and differentiation by triggering caspase 3 and 7 (programmable cell death caused by proteases) and prompting dependent DNA damage (Szmyd et al., 2013). The application of silver nanoparticles is shown in figure 7.13.

7.8.2.1.2 Gold Nanoparticles

Gold nanoparticles (AuNPs) are a good alternative for wound treatment because of their chemical firmness (in other words, stability) and affinity to absorb near-infrared light while being relatively easy to synthesize (Niska et al., 2018). Furthermore, by fine-tuning with the surface plasmon resonance, AuNP gels acquire thermo-responsiveness, as explained by Arafa and El-Kased (2018), who displayed antibacterial and healing activities in vitro and in vivo, supported by microscopic examination of disease tissue. A bacterial cell wall is directly targeted by silver nanoparticles, or they can attach to bacterial DNA, preventing the double-helix from uncoiling throughout replication or transcription, giving rise to bacterial killing and inhibiting activity. As a result, multi-drug-resistant bacteria such as *S. aureus* (Staphylococcus) and *P. aeruginosa* (Pseudomonas) can be inhibited. Furthermore, silver nanoparticles inhibit the generation of reactive

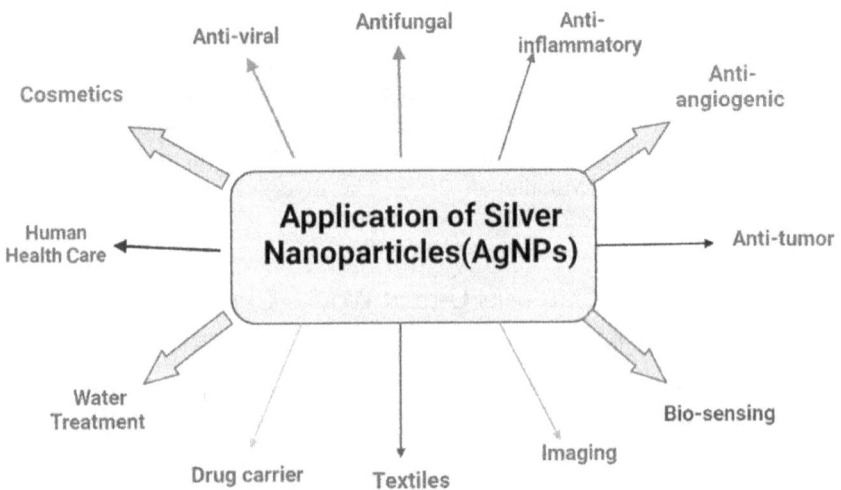

FIGURE 7.13   Silver nanoparticles (AgNPs) applications

oxygen species, functioning as antioxidants and assisting in healing operations. As per research, minimal concentrations of silver nanoparticles promote keratinocyte proliferation and differentiation, while greater quantities cause cytotoxicity (Lu, 2016). In the investigation, it was also found that the effect of bFGF (basic fibroblast growth factor) combined with AuNPs in Vaseline mixtures on wound healing for 14 days was based on the finding that bFGF (basic fibroblast growth factor) and VEGF (i.e., vascular endothelium growth factor) are released when bioactive glass triggers a local cell response. The chemically induced angiogenesis and fibroblast proliferation encouraged fast wound closure rather than cell toxicity (Marza & Magyari, 2019). AuNPs can also be effective in burn treatment, promoting healing and inhibiting microbial colonization while also being transdermal dynamic, as proven by recent ex vivo permeation research.

7.8.2.1.3   Zinc Oxide Nanoparticles

Zinc oxide nanoparticles (ZnONPs) function as a credible and effective bacterial inhibitor by producing holes in bacterial cell membranes. Additionally, when combined with hydrogel-based wound dressings (Hamdan et al., 2017), the entire contact period increases, increasing keratinocyte migration and thereby boosting re-epithelialization (Vijayakumar et al., 2019). Furthermore, a microporous chitosan hydrogel or ZnONPs dressing demonstrated huge abilities for collecting wound exudates and allowing the development of hemostatic blood clots, as well as antibacterial capabilities with low cytotoxicity.

It is found in research that dressings integrated with ZnONPs in a biodegradable matrix consisting of collagen and orange essential oil give a better option to heal burns while also minimizing the occurrence of related infections (Balaure et al., 2018). In in vitro and in vivo evaluation, it was observed that ZnONP-based wound dressing quickened wound closure and inhibited bacterial enhancement while also exhibiting great biocompatibility and low cytotoxicity (Balaure et al., 2018; Shao et al., 2018).

7.8.2.2   Nanocomposites or Nanoparticles From Nanocomposites

Materials with solid structures are known as nanocomposites, which often take the shape of an inorganic polymer matrix set in an organic phase or an organic polymer matrix set in an inorganic phase and have a space between the phases that is minimally constructed of a dimension comprising nanoscale size. Nanocomposite materials can display distinct qualities, including properties in terms of biomechanical, biochemical, electrochemical, optic, and catalytic. Nanocomposite membranes offer these conditions for the penetration of the required elements while functioning as a protective curtain against other undesirable elements. Modifying the underlying polymeric matrix and the mineral nanofillers can significantly increase the characteristics of the interaction between organic polymers and nanoparticles, which is crucial. As an organic base matrix, glass or rubber polymers can be used in the membrane construction of nanocomposite-based membranes. Mineral nanofilters can be constructed using an array of nanoparticles. Mineral materials such as carbon, zeolites, metal oxides, pure metals, and others may all be referenced as examples. In particular, zeolite 4A, silicate, and ZSM-5 (Zeolite Socony Mobil-5) from zeolites, as well as nanosilver made from pure metals, carbon nanotubes, and C60 fullerenes made from carbon materials, might be highlighted.

Nanocomposite membranes, especially in innovative and cutting-edge applications, are crucial to membrane-based procedures. Compared to other types of conventional membranes, nanocomposite membranes offer a lot more benefits, such as:

- Compared to conventional membranes, nanocomposite membranes have greater penetration.
- Systems employing nanocomposite membranes need less pressure than typical membrane processes.
- The structural design of nanocomposite membrane systems is dense.
- Compared to other membrane activities, systems using nanocomposite membranes consume less energy.
- Systems utilizing nanocomposite membranes need less membrane surface area than other membrane procedures.
- Systems using nanocomposite membranes have less environmental impact than existing membrane processing methods in industrial settings.

(Rahimi & Mosleh, 2022)

7.8.2.3   Nanocarriers for Management

Nanomaterials can also operate as carriers for medicinal medicines, regulating their release. Nitric oxide is involved in the inflammatory mechanism, cellular growth, blood vessel formation, extracellular matrix accumulation, and remodeling processes. Furthermore, nitric oxide has broad-spectrum antibacterial effects while simultaneously interfering with the development of biofilms. As an outcome, several studies have attempted to develop a delivery method with a regulated release, high loading capacity, and minimal cytotoxicity. In order to facilitate longer nitric oxide liberation and antibacterial activity against methicillin-resistant *s. aureus* and *p. aeruginosa* as well as fast wound healing in vivo, nitric oxide-releasing PLGA-PEI nanoparticles were constructed (Nurhasni et al., 2015).

7.8.2.4   Coatings and Scaffolds

7.8.2.4.1   *Coatings*

The polymer coating is a process that modifies surface properties to meet the requirements of various practical applications. It is a paint or coating designed to utilize polymers with superior qualities to those found in use today. In many different applications, including stickiness, tolerance, cracks and abrasion, rusting, water sorption, and biological functionalization, polymer coatings have been employed. Because polymer coatings provide versatility in terms of the chemical groups that may be bonded to surfaces, which is advantageous for interactions between biomaterials and tissues, they are thought to be very valuable in bio-medical applications. Additionally, they share many mechanical and elastic characteristics with biological tissues. Different techniques have been developed and put into use for the manufacture of polymer coatings for various purposes (Nathanael & Oh, 2020).

7.8.2.4.2   Scaffolds

Scaffolds are the finest materials for promoting cellular functions, repair, and tissue longevity. They have a specific role in angiogenesis and, more importantly, restoration by enabling the flow of different materials essential for cell survival, growth, and division (Chaudhari et al., 2016). Figure 7.14 depicts the various types of scaffolds, their advantages, and future prospects.

A variety of techniques are used to assemble polymers into coatings and films as well as to create three-dimensional nanostructured scaffolds, as shown in Figure 7.15. The most common method used in 3D scaffold creation is electrospinning, which makes porous polymeric nanofibers that are suitable for use as hybrid scaffolds for fibroblast adhesion and growth in wounds. Figure 7.15 shows various methods used in coatings and scaffolds (Nathanael & Oh, 2020; Lu et al., 2013).

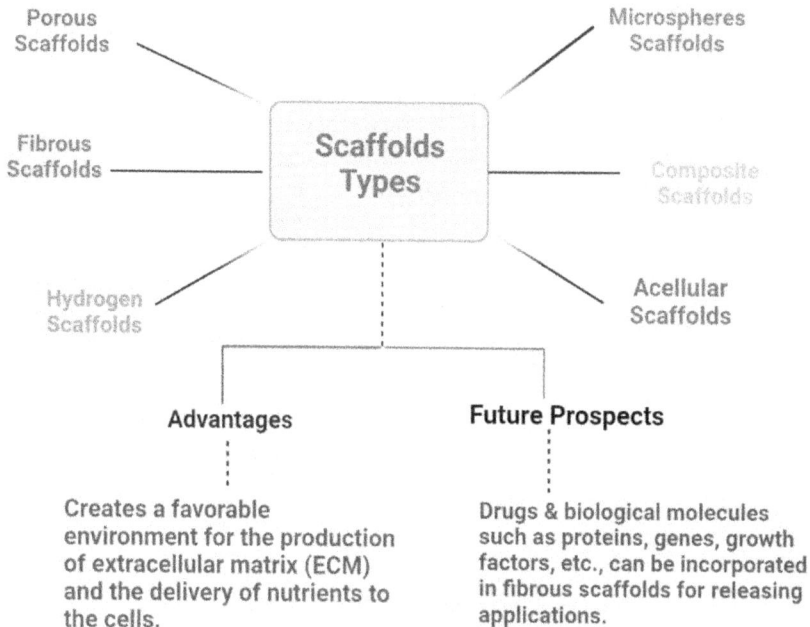

FIGURE 7.14   Scaffold types, advantages, and future approach

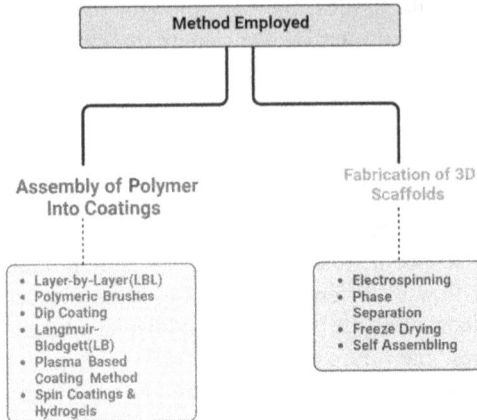

FIGURE 7.15   Method employed in coatings and scaffolds

7.9   SUMMARY AND FUTURE VISION

Wound management is a critical medical field because an infected wound may result in serious complications. This chapter showed contemporary information related to wound care and monitoring in order to aid researchers, practitioners, and anyone else interested in the wound field in grasping the complicated mechanism of wound healing. Among the existing materials employed in drug delivery systems, this chapter mentioned the utilization of biomaterials made from natural polymers such as chitosan, hyaluronic acid, and others, as well as synthetic polymers such as PCL, PVA, and PLGA. We also discussed modern wound healing dressings extensively and proved the benefits and applications of biomaterials and nanomaterials-based compression, bandages, stockings, and dressings in wound healing. Overall, we learned from the discussed knowledge that customized wound bandages made from nanomaterials have enormous potential for personalized wound care. Biomolecules, growth factors, and antibiotics coupled with polymeric nanomaterials of natural origin possess the ability to go beyond the limitations of modern wound healing stuff, resulting in scaffolds with improved mechanical resistance.

Future attempts should pay attention to enhancing site particularity and targeted efficacy for more sophisticated wound treatments, preferably based on the utilization of nanomaterials. As a result, scientists should work to create biocompatible and biodegradable nanomaterials that can be utilized to correct all levels of wound healing.

REFERENCES

Aderibigbe, B.A., Buyana, B. (2018). Alginate in wound dressings. *Pharmaceutics*, 10(2), 42.
Ahmed, S., Ikram, S. (2016). Chitosan based scaffolds and their applications in wound healing. *Achievements in the Life Sciences*, 10, 27–37.
Alavi, A., Kirsner, R.S. (2017). Dressings. In J. Bolognia, J. Schaffer, L. Cerroni (Eds.), *Dermatology* (4th ed.). Philadelphia, New York: Elsevier.

Arafa, M.G., El-Kased, R.F. (2018). Thermoresponsive gels containing gold nanoparticles as smart antibacterial and wound healing agents. *Sci. Rep.*, 8.

Ardekani, N.T., Khorram, M., Zomorodian, K., Yazdanpanah, S., Veisi, H., Veisi, H. (2019). Evaluation of electrospun poly (vinyl alcohol)-based nanofiber mats incorporated with Zataria multiflora essential oil as potential wound dressing. *Int. J. Biol. Macromol.*, 125, 743–750.

Arthur, J., Lewis, P. (2000). When is reduced compression bandaging safe and effective. *J. Wound Care*, 9(10), 469–471.

Balaure, P.C., Holban, A.M., Grumezescu, A.M., Mogosanu, G.D., Balseanu, T.A., Stan, M.S., Dinischiotu, A., Volceanov, A., Mogoanta, L. (2018). In vitro and in vivo studies of novel fabricated bioactive dressings based on collagen and zinc oxide 3D scaffolds. *Int. J. Pharm.*, 557, 199–207.

Beldon, P. (2010). Basic science of wound healing. *Surgery*, 28, 409–412.

Benigni, J.L., Sadoun, S., Allaert, F. (2003). Efficacy of class 1 elastic compression stockings in the early stages of chronic venous disease. *Int. Angiolg.*, 24(3), 224–238.

Chaudhari, A.A., Vig, K., Baganizi, D.R., et al. (2016). Future prospects for scaffolding methods and biomaterials in skin tissue engineering: A review. *International Journal of Molecular Sciences*, 17, 1–31.

Childs, D.R., Murthy A.S. (2017). Overview of wound healing and management. *Surg. Clin. North Am.*, 97, 189–207.

Egri, O., Erdemir, N. (2019). Production of hypericum perforatum oil-loaded membranes for wound dressing material and in vitro tests. *Artif Cells Nanomedicine Biotechnol*, 47(1), 1404–1415.

Elnar, T.V., Ailey, T.B. (2009). The wound healing process: An overview of the cellular and molecular mechanisms. *J. Int. Med. Res.*, 37(15), 28–42.

Eming, S.A., Krieg, T., Davidson, J.M. (2007). Inflammation in wound repair: Molecular and cellular mechanisms. *J. Invest. Dermatol.*, 127, 514–525.

Ferreira, M.O.G., de Lima, I.S., Morais, A.Í.S., Silva, S.O., de Carvalho, R.B.F., Ribeiro, A.B., et al. (2019). Chitosan associated with chlorhexidine in gel form: Synthesis, characterization and healing wounds applications. *J. Drug Deliv. Sci. Technol.*, 49, 375–382.

Filippousi, M., Siafaka, P.I., Amanatiadou, E.P., Nanaki, S.G., Nerantzaki, M., Bikiaris, D.N., et al. (2015). Modified chitosan coated mesoporous strontium hydroxyapatite nanorods as drug carriers. *J. Mater. Chem. B.*, 3, 5991–6000.

Filippousi, M., Turner, S., Leus, K., Siafaka, P.I., Tseligka, E.D., Vandichel, M., et al. (2016). Biocompatible Zr-based nanoscale MOFs coated with modified poly (ε-caprolactone) as anticancer drug carriers. *Int. J. Pharm.*, 509, 208–218.

Fleck, C.A., Simman, R. (2010). Modern collagen wound dressings: Function and purpose. *J. Am. Col. Certif. Wound Spec.*, 2, 50–54.

Gosain, A., DiPietro, L.A. (2004). Aging and wound healing. *World J. Surg.*, 28, 321–326.

Guo, S., DiPietro, L.A. (2010). Factors affecting wound healing. *Journal of Dental Research*, 220–227.

Gurtner, G.C., Werner, S., Barrandon, Y., Longaker M.T. (2008). Wound repair and regeneration. *Nature*, 453, 314–321.

Hamdan, S., Pastar, I., Drakulich, S., Dikici, E., Tomic-Canic, M., Deo, S., Daunert, S. (2017). Nanotechnology-driven therapeutic interventions in wound healing: Potential uses and applications. *ACS Cent. Sci.*, 3, 163–175.

Heness, G., Ben-Nissan, B. (2004). Innovative bioceramics. *Mater. Forum*, 27, 104–114.

Holsche, C.M., Haut, E.R. (2023). Venous thromboembolic disease: Mechanical and pharmacologic prophylaxis. In A.N. Sidawy, B.A. Perler (Eds.), *Rutherford's Vascular Surgery and Endovascular Therapy* (10th ed.). Philadelphia, New York: Elsevier.

Kim, M.S., Oh, G.W., Jang, Y.M., Ko, S.C, Park, W.S., Choi, I.W., et al. (2020). Antimicrobial hydrogels based on PVA and diphlorethohydroxycarmalol (DPHC) derived from brown alga Ishige okamurae: An in vitro and in vivo study for wound dressing application. *Mater. Sci. Eng. C*, 107, 1–12.

Li, J., Chen, J., Kirsner, R. (2007). Pathophysiology of acute wound healing. *Clin. Dermatol.*, 25, 9–18.

Longinotti, C. (2014). The use of hyaluronic acid based dressings to treat burns: A review. *Burn Trauma*, 2(4), 162–168.

Lu, L. (2016). Essential components clinical applications & health benefits. *Chinese Herbs & Herbal Medicine*, 9–10.

Lu, T., Li, Y., Chen, T. (2013). Technique for fabrication and construction of three-dimensional scaffolds for tissue engineering. *International Journal of Nanomedicine*, 8, 337–350.

Markovic, J.N., Shortell, C.K. (2023). Treatment of chronic venous disorders. In A.N. Sidaway, B.A. Perler (Eds.), *Rutherford's Vascular Surgery and Endovascular Therapy* (10th ed.). Philadelphia, New York: Elsevier.

Martínez-Ibarra, D.M., Sánchez-Machado, D.I., López-Cervantes, J., Campas-Baypoli, O.N., Sanches-Silva, A., Madera-Santana, T.J. (2018). Hydrogel wound dressings based on chitosan and xyloglucan: Development and characterization. *J. Appl. Polym. Sci.*, 136, 47342.

Marza, S., Magyari, K. (2019). Skin wound regeneration with bioactive glass-gold nanoparticles ointment. *Biomed. Mater.*, 14.

Mihai, M.M., Dima, M.B., Dima, B., Holban, A.M. (2019). Nanomaterials for wound healing and infection control. *Materials*, 12, 1–16.

Mir, M., Ali, M.N., Barakullah, A., Gulzar, A., Arshad, M., Fatima, S., et al. (2018). Synthetic polymeric biomaterials for wound healing: A review. *Prog. Biomater.*, 7, 1–21.

Murakami, K., Aoki, H., Nakamura, S., Nakamura, S., Takikawa, M., Hanzawa, M., et al. (2010). Hydrogel blends of chitin/chitosan, fucoidan and alginate as healing-impaired wound dressings. *Biomaterials*, 31, 83–90.

Nathanael, A.J., Oh, T.H. (2020). Biopolymer coatings for biomedical application. *Polymers*, 12, 1–26.

Nicolai, J., Rakhorst, G. (2008). Introduction. In G. Rakhorst, R. Ploeg (Eds.), *Biomaterials in Modern Medicine: The Groningen Perspective*. New Jersey, USA, NY: World Scientific Publishing Co.

Niska, K., Zielinska, E., Radomski, M.W., Inkielewicz-Stepniak, I. (2018). Metal nanoparticles in dermatology and cosmetology: Interactions with human skin cells. *Chem. Biol. Interact*, 295, 38–51.

Nurhasni, H., Cao, J., Choi, M., Kim, I., Lee, B.L., Jung, Y., Yoo, J.-W. (2015). Nitric oxide-releasing poly (lactic-co-glycolic acid)-polyethylenimine nanoparticles for prolonged nitric oxide release, antibacterial efficacy, and in vivo wound healing activity. *Int. J. Nanomed.*, 10, 3065–3080.

Okur, M.E., Karantas, I.D., Zeynep, S., Okur, N.U., Siafaka, P.I. (2020). Recent trends on wound management: New therapeutic choices based on polymeric carriers. *Asian Journal of Pharmaceutical Sciences*, 15, 662–663.

Onyekwelu, I., Yakkanti, R., Protzer, L., Pinkston, C.M., Tucker, C., Seligson, D. (2017). Surgical wound classification and surgical site infections in the orthopaedic patient. *J. Am. Acad. Orthop. Surg. Glob. Res. Rev.*, 1(3), e022.

Percival, N.J. (2002). *Classification of Wounds and their Management*. Surgery (oxford), 20, 114–117. https://doi.org/10.1383/surg.20.5.114.14626

Perumal, G., Pappuru, S., Chakraborty, D., Maya Nandkumar, A.M., Chand, D.K., Doble, M. (2017). Synthesis and characterization of curcumin loaded PLA—Hyperbranched polyglycerol electrospun blend for wound dressing applications. *Mater. Sci. Eng. C.*, 76, 1196–1204.

Portela, R., Leal, C.R., Almeida, P.L., Sobral, R.G. (2019). Bacterial cellulose: A versatile biopolymer for wound dressing applications. *Microb. Biotechnol.*, 12, 586–610.

Rahimi, R.M., Mosleh, S. (2022). Chapter five-membrane-based sorption processes: Intensification of sorption processes. *Active & Passive Mechanism*, 133–189.

Shao, F., Yang, A., Yu, D.M., Wang, J., Gong, X., Tian, H.X. (2018). Bio-synthesis of barleria gibsoni leaf extract mediated zinc oxide nanoparticles and their formulation gel for wound therapy in nursing care of infants and children. *J. Photochem. Photobiol. B*, 189, 267–273.

Shaw, T.J., Martin, P. (2009). Wound repair at a glance. *J. Cell Sci.*, 122, 3209–3213.

Shi, C., Wang, C., Liu, H., Li, Q., Li, R., Zhang, Y., Liu, Y., Shao, Y., Wang, J. (2020). Selection of appropriate wound dressing for various wounds. *Frontiers in Bioengineering and Biotechnology*, 8, 1–12.

Siafaka, P.I., Barmbalexis, P., Bikiaris, D.N. (2016a). Novel electrospun nanofibrous matrices prepared from poly (lactic acid)/poly (butylene adipate) blends for controlled release formulations of an anti-rheumatoid agent. *Eur. J. Pharm. Sci.*, 88, 12–25.

Siafaka, P.I., Barmpalexis, P., Lazaridou, M., Papageorgiou, G.Z., Koutri, E., Karavas, E., et al. (2015a). Controlled release formulations of risperidone antipsychotic drug in novel aliphatic polyester carriers: Data analysis and modelling. *Eur. J. Pharm. Biopharm.*, 94, 473–484.

Siafaka, P.I., Titopoulou, A., Koukaras, E.N., Kostoglou, M., Koutris, E., Karavas, E., et al. (2015b). Chitosan derivatives as effective nanocarriers for ocular release of timolol drug. *Int. J. Pharm.*, 495, 249–264.

Siafaka, P.I., Zisi, A.P., Exindari, M.K., Karantas, I.D., Bikiaris, D.N. (2016b). Porous dressings of modified chitosan with poly (2-hydroxyethyl acrylate) for topical wound delivery of levofloxacin. *Carbohydr. Polym.*, 143, 90–99.

Singh, S., Young, A., McNaught, C.E. (2017). The physiology of wound healing. *Surg (United Kingdom)*, 35, 473–477.

Skorkowska-Telichowska, K., Czemplik, M., Kulma, A., Szopa, J. (2013). The local treatment and available dressings designed for chronic wounds. *J. Am. Acad. Dermatol.*, 68, 117–126.

Sorg, H., Tilkorn, D.J., Hager, S., Hauser, J., Mirastschijski, U. (2017). Skin wound healing: An update on the current knowledge and concepts. *Eur. Surg. Res.*, 58, 81–94.

Szmyd, R., Goralczyk, A.G., Skalniak, L., Cierniak, A., Lipert, B., Filon, F.L., Crosera, M., Borowczyk, J., Laczna, E., Drukala, J., et al. (2013). Effect of silver nanoparticles on human primary keratinocytes. *Biol. Chem.*, 394, 113–123.

Tavakoli, J., Tang, Y. (2017). Honey/PVA hybrid wound dressings with controlled release of antibiotics: Structural, physico-mechanical and in vitro biomedical studies. *Mater. Sci. Eng. C*, 77, 318–325.

Timothy, F., Herman, B.B. (2022). Wound classification: National library of medicine. *StatPearls*.

Todd, M. (2011). Compression bandaging types and skills used in practical application. *Bristish Journal of Nursing*, 20(4), 239–240.

Vijayakumar, V., Samal, S.K., Mohanty, S., Nayak, S.K. (2019). Recent advancements in biopolymer and metal nanoparticle-based materials in diabetic wound healing management. *Int. J. Biol. Macromol.*, 122, 137–148.

Welch, M.P., Odland, G.F., Clark, R.A. (1990). Temporal relationships of F-actin bundle formation, collagen and fibronectin matrix assembly, and fibronectin receptor expression to wound contraction. *J. Cell. Biol.*, 110, 133–145.

Yao, H.Y., Lin, H.R., Sue, G.P., Lin, Y.J. (2019). Chitosan-based hydrogels prepared by UV polymerization for wound dressing. *Polym. Polym. Compos.*, 27, 155–167.

Yu, R., Zhang, H., Ga, B. (2021). Conductive biomaterials as bioactive wound dressing for wound healing and skin tissue engineering. *Nano-Micro Letters*, 5–46.

Zhang, X.F., Liu, Z.G., Shen, W., Gurunathan, S. (2016). Silver nanoparticles synthesis, characterization, properties, applications, and therapeutic approaches. *International Journal of Molecular Sciences*, 17, 1534.

8 Nanotechnology in Hospital Clothing and Odor Control of Medical Textiles

Tasnim N. Shaikh and Bharat H. Patel

8.1 INTRODUCTION

Four main criteria related to human skin, viz., freshness, care, protection, and comfort, are considered while engineering textiles that are going to be used in a hospital environment. These desired parameters can be imported to the base textile material in association with active ingredients. Attributed to such composition, the human skin deliberately gets freshened and revitalized with the simple natural movement of the body. This subsequently offers a much fresher and hygienic environment to the people living in a highly traumatic hospital work culture. A major factor that has stimulated interest in antimicrobial finishes has been the current vogue that promotes a healthier and physically active lifestyle.

Hence, textiles and especially natural resourced fibers are proving good inhabitations for the microorganisms by serving as food for their grooming. The bacteria-laden medium becomes acute with microbe friendly environmental changes: higher humidity, rain, and cold. The presence of such microbes in textile structures is unhygienic and often causes staining, fading of the fabric color, and a bad smell. Accumulation of dust mites on continuous foot paths in floor covering, rugs, etc., damp towels and napkins, and blood- or urine-stained patient bed sheets invite breeding of microbes, insects, and other vermin, even though subjected to a regular cleaning cycle in the hospitals. Protection of the users and service-providers against such multivariate microbes grooming mediums in the hospital environment is indeed a big challenge. Fortunately, there is a continuously growing cognizance of textile consumers about the deleterious impacts on textiles by microorganisms and thereby humanoid hygiene (Home, 2002). Similarly, equally important is that the increased consumption of such antimicrobials sterilized textile materials on making direct contact with the human body should not leave undesirable traces (Patel & Tandel, 2005; Gao & Cranston, 2008).

8.1.1 Basic Requirements in Hospital Clothing

Clothing wearers are exposed to an environment where there is microbial cross-contamination, be it in schools, hospitals, pathological labs, food processing, milk

DOI: 10.1201/9781003331612-10

processing, hotels, airline companies, IT companies, etc. This further exacerbates microbial growth. Microbial growth on textiles, in particular, and textiles in general, leads to issues such as bad odor, itching, yellowing, and the rapid deterioration of such textile products.

Hospitals and pathological labs are the breeding ground for microbes due to blood, body fluids, stools, urine, etc. Medical workers, especially doctors and medical staff, are prone to contaminating their clothing with these microbes. Anti-microbial finished textiles can restrict the grooming and spread of such harmful bacterium found in hospital environment and safeguard doctors and patients alike from the "hospital-generated diseases" also known as Nosocomial infections. Special importance is given to the antibacterial fabric used for personnel hygiene by maintaining surroundings cleaner and fresher in the hospitality sector (Home, 2002; Francois et al., 2006). Some common pathogens found in the hospital environment are summarized in Table 8.1.

8.1.2 Nanotechnology in Medical Textiles

Preliminarily nanotechnology deals in designing, characterizing, production, and application of structures, devices, and systems via controlled nanometer scale shape and size. It holds a commendable quality and economical potential for the medical textile industry, extensively using the different formats of textile materials. This is mainly because conventional technologies failed in implanting permanent added functional characteristics to fiber/yarn/fabric and thereby often such articles lose their functionality in a due course of time. Also, the breathability or hand feel of the fabrics will not be altered while coated with nanoparticles. Anti-bacterial, water repellency, flame retardancy, anti-static, improved dyeability, soil resistance, wrinkle resistance, and UV protection, are a few functional parameters that get introduced or enhanced in textiles using nanotechnology. The thermal, mechanical, and barrier properties of the pure polymer matrix get substantially enhanced by reinforcing a small percentage of strong fillers. Furthermore, it should be noted that these positive shifts are attained via conventional processing techniques only, but without leaving

TABLE 8.1
List of pathogens in hospital environments

Gram +ve/-ve	Name of pathogens
Gram +ve	Staphylococcus Aureus
	Staphylococcus Epidermidis
	Staphylococcus Pyogenes
	Micrococcus luteus
Gram −ve	E. coli
	Acinetobacter baumanni
	Klebsiella sp
	Klebsiella pneumonia

any negative traces on the processability, ageing performance, density, and appearance of the material.

The hybrid structure of inorganic-organic nanocomposite materials, commonly known as a hybrid polymer, is widely used nowadays for the amalgamation of dirt-repellent effect with scratch resistance, superior transparency, antimicrobic activities, or distinct barrier characteristics to material (Mandot et al., 2012). Governing categories of nanomaterials are metals and their oxides at the present moment. Amongst them, gold (Au) and silver (Ag) are drawing the highest attention (Chattopadhyay & Patel, 2014a, 2014b). Whereas, iron oxide (Fe_3O_4, FeO), silica (SiO_2), Zinc oxide (ZnO), alumina (Al_2O_3), and titanium (TiO_2) are recognized metal oxides. A diverse set of properties. such as electrical conductivity, protection, photocatalytic activity, and UV absorption are owned by this group of nanomaterials. In the present scenario, the parameters of UV-blocking functions, self-decontamination, and anti-microbial are getting prime consideration irrespective of the domain of research (Shaikh et al., 2018).

8.2 PREPARATION TECHNIQUES FOR NANOMETAL COMPOSITE TEXTILES

Nanometal composite textiles can be prepared by several methods depending on the class of nanomaterial and also on the class of textiles to be composite. Broadly, it can be classified according to the stage at which the nanoparticles are incorporated into the textile polymer matrix. Application of the nanoparticles to textile materials can be carried out at different processing steps, like:

1) At the point of fiber or filament preparation
2) Undergoing finishing
3) Processing of garment

8.2.1 FILAMENT OR FIBER PREPARATION STAGE

Sols have served as an elementary solution in fiber spinning. The simple glass fibers are spun successfully by adopting this technique; just for an example, Peltola et al. (2001) and Celzard et al. (2002) have cited silica sols spun using dry spinning. The inorganic composite fibers can be produced by spinning directly from appropriate sols, and this formulation is equally true for the fibers resourced from pure SiO_2, oxides of other metals, or their combinations. According to Amalvy (2002) inorganic/organic amalgamation-based or pure inorganic routed composite fibers represent the two different categories of sol-gel-based fibers. The possible morphologies acquired by the nanocomposite particle are illustrated schematically in Figure 8.1.

Polymer-based nanocomposites synthesized from the organic or inorganic sources have perpetually achieved incredible attention in the area of materials science. This is attributed to the collective benefits of the organic polymer and the inorganic material owned by such organic/inorganic nanocomposites. Preparation of polymer/inorganic nanocomposite materials incorporates the use of nanoscale inorganic materials, like oxides or nanoparticles of metal, silicate, and semiconductors.

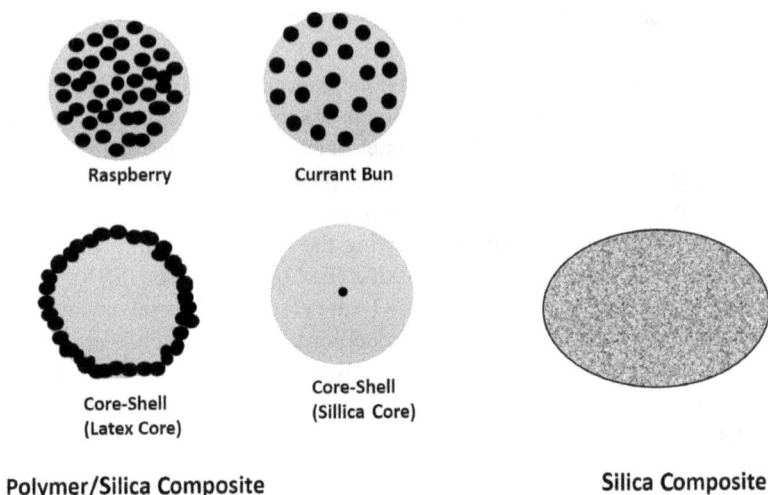

FIGURE 8.1   The common morphologies acquired by the nanocomposite particle

According to Zhang (2008) as well as Ahmadi (2004), the polymer- nanocomposites are fundamentally synthesized via four different routes: "Melt intercalation, Solution method, in situ polymerization and Electrospinning."

8.2.2   FINISHING STAGE

8.2.2.1   Pad-Dry-Cure and Spray Finishing Method

The simple dipping, padding, spray technique and foam finishing have been the foremost textile finishing methods for a long period of time. Nanosols can be applied successfully to the textile materials using either of these classical finishing methods as well as printing techniques. Perhaps, dipping a textile sample into the nano sol can be regarded as the simplest method amongst all.

The process includes immersion of the fabric in the nano sol for a predetermined time interval, followed by take-up and drying under the ambient conditions or thermal curing in an oven or a stenter frame. However, it is not always necessary to dip the textile material completely in the sol. Just for instance, if the product design requires a single-sided repellence characteristic, then nano sol should be applied only on one side. In such a case, rather than dipping followed by padding [Figure 8.2 (A)], the casting [Figures 8.2 (B)] or a spray application [Figures 8.2 (C)] techniques of the nano sol are found more useful.

8.2.2.2   Foam Finishing Method

The chemical finishes in the foam state can also be applied to the fabric. Since the water used in the finish preparation recipe is replaced with air, it radically reduces its consumption and is considered as one of the important water-saving finishing

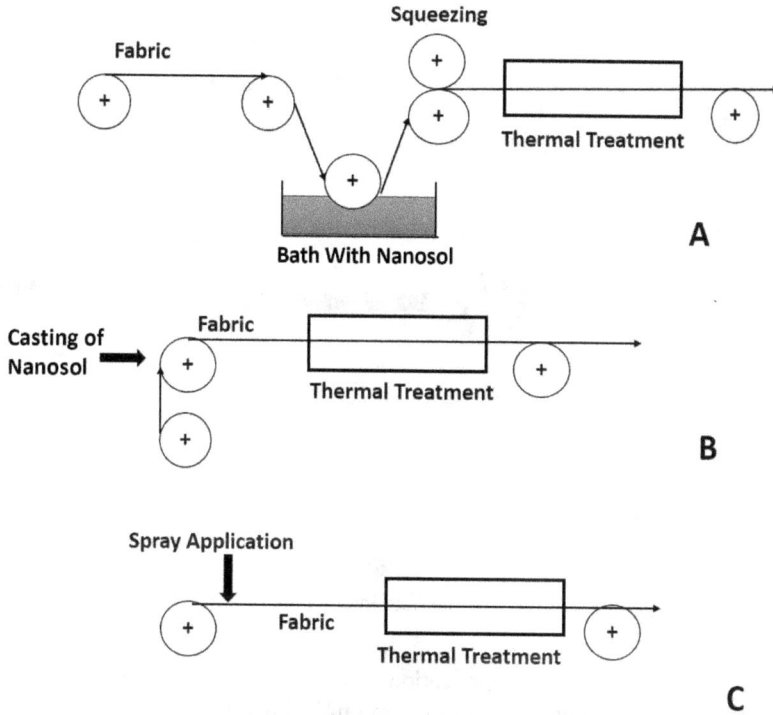

FIGURE 8.2 Diagram for conventional application techniques used in nano sol finishing of textiles A: pad, B: casting, C: spray

(*Source:* https://garph.co.uk/ijarie/jan2013/4.pdf)

techniques. The careful selection of the surfactants used for foaming the formulation can probably lead to an effective reduction of repellent finishes. Production of high volumes of foam is carried out in a foam generator by mixing chemical formulation with air; such foam can be applied to fabrics in several ways.

8.2.2.3   Plasma Technology

Plasma is an ionized gas. The substrate and the gas undergo a mutual interaction on exposing its surface to the plasma. Figure 8.3 reveals the principle of the plasma-substrate interaction mechanism. It commences with the bombarding of electrons, UV radiation from the plasma, ions, neutrals, and radicals on the surface of the substrate, which results in the integration of volatile components and polymer or textile (Patel & Patel, 2006). The electrons in the plasma can break covalent chemical bonding and make physical as well as chemical modification viable for the surfaces of various substrates. The vast diversity of outcomes can be obtained via plasma technology, only by varying combinations and substrates to be treated.

The plasma-activated gasses can be used in film application on textiles substrate. The identical terms for methods used in this course are deposition, coating, or layering and polymerization coating. According to Zou (2008), the plasma treatment

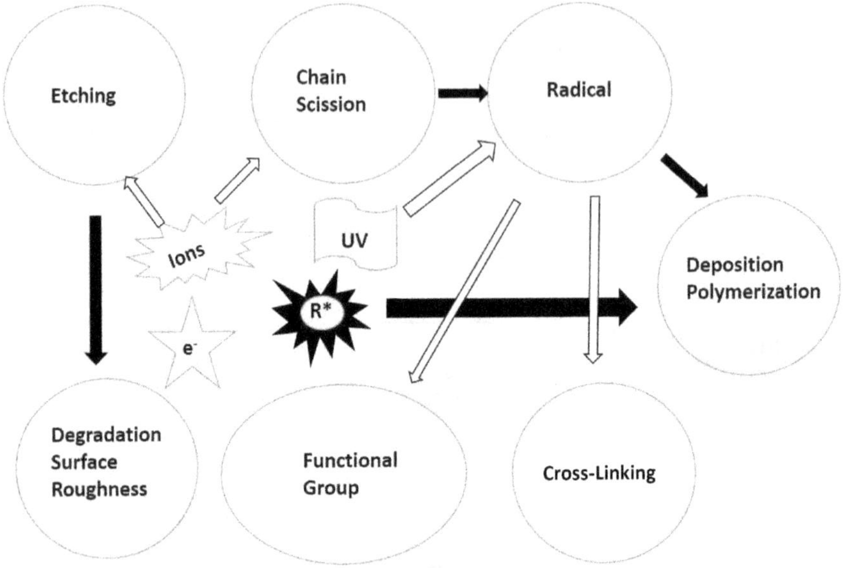

FIGURE 8.3 Mechanism of plasma-substrate interaction

brings key rewards, like lower application temperature, a very short treatment time, and elimination of drying steps after plasma finishing due to the abolition of water or solvents in the course of treatment.

8.2.3 GARMENT PROCESSING STAGE

The exhaustible chemical finishes, like softeners, antimicrobials, ultraviolet (UV) absorbers, etc., are usually applied to the garment after the accomplishment of all other wet processing procedures. These finishes are normally added to the bath of the processing unit for the purpose. Seldomly, an easy-care finish like a non-exhaustible finish, is also anticipated and their special procedures have been established. According to the first technique, the maximum possible water from wet processed garments must be extracted before dipping into the finishing bath. The solution is filled in a trough placed separately or as an integral part of the same garment machine. The garments immersed in the finishing bath for a predefined time interval are subjected to further extraction drying, and curing. In the second technique also after extraction of excess water from wet processed garments, on the processing machine, a precise amount of finish solution has been sprayed on the moving garments. The finish is uniformly dispersed throughout the garment by prolonged spinning of the garments, which can facilitate the migration of the finish. Drying and curing are carried out next in the sequence completing the process. From a commercial point of view, both methods are successful but have their returns and shortcomings. The chemical finish is consumed more with the immersion technique but less with the spray technique. On the contrary, the precise spray procedure unlike the immersion technique needs extra setup on existing garment machines resulting in comparatively higher capital investment.

8.3 CHARACTERIZATION OF NANOMETAL COMPOSITES FOR MEDICINAL TEXTILES

The composition, size of the particles, and interfacial interaction are the major characterization features of any nanocomposite. So, the insight story of the nano-composite structure needs to be investigated to reveal its behavior during end-use applications. Just for example, thermal, mechanical, and other key features of the polymer/silica nanocomposite are evidently affected by the production method adopted, because it defines the kind of interaction that took place between the participating elements. There are recognized characterization techniques for assessing the chemical structure, microstructure, morphology, and physical properties of the nanocomposites. This evaluation is mandatory to completely comprehend structure-property relationships as mentioned before.

Three renowned microscopy techniques, TEM, SEM, and AFM, are used for the morphology study of nanocomposites. Thermal analysis techniques help to study the change in thermal properties of materials with temperature, just like the crystallization behaviors of the nanoparticle-filled composites with cyclic temperature changes can be investigated using Differential Scanning Calorimeter (DSC). Apart from DSC, other popular techniques in this regard are TGA, DTA, and dielectric thermal analysis. The FTIR and solid-state NMR spectra analysis can help in determining the chemical structure of polymer-based nanocomposites. Inorganic fillers are added to polymers mainly for enhancing their mechanical performance, one of the key objectives in the polymer nanocomposite formulation, and that's why measuring for their mechanical properties is the greatest concern. The mechanical properties of nanocomposites should be measured from a different point of view, purely influenced by the need of the application area. Russell et al., in 2002, dictated several criteria, like flexural strength, tensile strength, fracture toughness, hardness, impact strength, etc. considered in this respect.

8.4 NANOENGINEERED TEXTILES AND THEIR COMMERCIAL APPLICATIONS

The possible commercial applications in addition to the medical sector worked out by various researchers in the field are summarized in Table 8.2. Accordingly, a vast application field is covered by these functionality-boosted nanostructures. The utilization formats include all product forms which can be sold directly to the end consumer or the products initially purchased by industrial clients before touching the targeted customers. The textile additives and fabrics materials to be converted into apparel or home furnishing products are common examples of such secondary or intermediate products. Thus, the application domain starts from the classical but to date major stockholder apparel sector and covers almost all specialty segments: medical appliances, civil structures, home furnishing, protective textiles, sports textiles, internal fit and stuffing materials, cosmetics, packaging materials, filter fabrics, and industrial textiles.

8.4.1 MEDICAL TEXTILE

Medtech designates textile materials used in the field of medicine, one of the most important and continuously blooming fields. The textile material used for the purpose

TABLE 8.2
Various application areas of nanomaterial-based products

Automotive industry	Construction	Cosmetics
• Lightweight structure	• Non-thermal conductive	• Sun protection
• Painting (nanofiller)	• Fire retardants	• Lipstick
• Catalysts	• Building materials with surface	• Skin creams
• Sensors	functionality	• Toothpaste
	• Facade coatings	
Chemical industry	**Electronic industry**	**Energy**
• Nanocomposite coating	• Data memory storage devices	• Capacitors
• Paper impregnation	• Glass fibers	• Solar cells
• Magnetic fluids as switchable	• Display devices	• Batteries
adhesives	• Filters (IR-blocking)	• Fuel cells
	• Optical switch	
	• Conductive, antistatic coatings	
	• Laser diodes	
Engineering	**Food and drinks**	**Domestic**
• Tools and machines coating for	• Additives	• Glass cleaner, ceramic,
wear protection	• Packaging materials	floor, windows
• Bearings without lubricant	• Clarification of fruit juice	• Ceramic coatings for irons
	• Storage life sensors	• Odors catalyst
Medicine	**Outdoor-Sports**	**Textile materials**
• Antimicrobic agents	• Antifogging glasses	• Smart textiles
• Vehicle for drug delivery	• Skin ointment	• Functional textiles
• Active agents	• Reinforced tennis balls and	• High-performance textiles
• Contrast medium	rackets	
• Medicinal rapid testing	• Ship and boats with antifouling	
• Implants and prostheses	coatings	
• Cancer therapy agents		

starts from a simple cleaning wipe to an advanced antibacterial fabric used by the surgeon while operating on patients. The product forms include hospital clothing (disposable/non-disposable), bed sheets, bandages, cotton swabs, wraps, gauze-piece, etc. The list is long and typically used in the Out Patient Department (OPD), Operation Theatre (OT), and In-Patient Department (IPD) by the doctors, patients, nurses, and other staff. Healthcare with due hygiene is the most important apprehension for any medical textile manufacturer as well as the user. The manufacturing technology thereby demands constant upgradation in terms of textile material selection, efficacy, and economy of functional finishes induced to them to make a pace with faster-changing genetics of wide species range of bacterium, viruses, etc. Thereby, continuous studies are conducted to explore new but cost-effective means for protecting both clinical staff and patients from getting exposure to microorganisms, body fluid invasions, and viruses in operation room situations. The use of an odor-free antibacterial fabric is always a preference, and fabric possessing a durable in situ, light, and pleasing fragrance reduces the negative impact on the user's mindset, especially in a high-occupant hospital environment.

8.4.1.1 Hospital Clothing

This relates to the outfits worn by the doctors, nurses, ward boys, and other hospital staff as well as patients during normal OPD, IPD, at operation theaters, and casualties. The disposable/non-disposable articles included in this category are baby dresses, maternity wear, nurse uniforms, scrub suits, apron cloth, doctor's coats and lab coats, surgeon's gown-gloves-cap-mask, patient gowns, X-ray protection lead garments, drapes, bed sheets, pillow covers, towels, etc. Apart from these, smart fabrics are developed using nanotechnology for continuous mapping of heart and brain conditions known as wearable textiles. However, the contribution of this hospital clothing segment is very small compared to the apparel sector for the non-disposable category, likewise disposable class of hospital clothing against overall nanocomposite consumption. But still, it is having enormous prospects for researchers to come out with a new functional product.

8.4.1.2 Conductive Wearable Textiles

Textile-structured EEG and ECG wearable electrodes are interactive smart textile devices designed for continuous monitoring of brain and cardiac biopotential signals in long-term mapping. These wearable textile electrodes are developed by integrating conductive nano-polymer composite sensors and can increase or decrease their conductivity as per applied stress. These conductive textiles are found efficient enough to replace skin-irritating gel and hard metallic sensing electrodes used in transmitting electronic signals from human skin to integrated electronic devices (Shaikh et al., 2021).

The popularly used synthetic fibers in medical textiles such as polypropylene (PP) or polyethylene (PE) are made up of low electric conductivity polymers and generally behave as isolators. The additional electromagnetic shielding functionalities can be imparted in these textile fibers by increasing their conductivity. This was done by infusing a very small quantum of a conductive medium into the polymer matrix. The medium can be metal nanoparticles, or carbon nanoparticles in the form of Carbon Black (CB), Carbon Nanotubes (CNT), or blended conductive polymers like polythiophene, polypyrrole, polyaniline, etc., but in a very small proportion (Lubben, 2005). The various techniques adopted by the researchers to date are summarized in Table 8.3.

Wearable electrodes are popular user areas for conductive textiles in hospital environments. As per Lubben (2005) and Patel et al. (2015b), antistatic clothing designed for industrial workers is the major utilization, reported in the clothing segment for conductive nanocomposite textile materials. According to Nanotex (2007), in the case of upholstery and interior trim, conductive fabrics are expected to become a good choice in engineering antistatic furniture textiles. Similarly, the electromagnetic shielding functions integrated into carpets or floor coverings can guard in a much better way underlying electronic devices as stated (Bekaert, 2007). The antistatic dust filters and bulk containers if fitted well with conductive textiles are capable of preventing explosions caused by spark discharges, as cited by Bekaert (2007). Mahltig et al. (2005) have suggested protective clothing applications in the MRI room; according to them, the suits should be entitled to safeguard against undesirable static discharges.

TABLE 8.3

Nanomaterials-based conductive textile composites

Nanoparticle	Textile material	Manufacturing method	Method of incorporation with the textiles
Cu	PA/PP	Physically depositing vapour: sputter coating	Consistent Cu layer with some nm thick
CB (in dispersion: 400–1700 nm)	Polyurethane (PU)	Electrospinning of PU dispersion with CB	CB nanoparticles in PU fibers having nm thickness
CNT	No specific	Coating of finished textile through dipping or spray	Fiber surface with some SWCNT clusters
	PP	Dip coating with polyaniline/CNT dispersion	CNT composite layer within and on PP hollow fiber, polyaniline matrix incorporated with CNT
	–	The wet spinning of dispersive CNT/polyaniline solution	Polyaniline CNT composite fiber

8.4.1.2.1   Commercially Available Products

The most accustomed goods are successfully launched via a digital platform and belong to the described nanoengineered product groups depicted in brief. Nanotex (2007), Eeon technology (2007), and Nanogate (2007) have elaborated on auxiliary products along with their production techniques capable of yielding antistatic and conductive textile characteristics, as well as described additives that ensure an identical level of performance. Eeon technology (2007) recommended polypyrrole and polyaniline to be utilized for the purpose. Lands' End (2007) limelight about nanoengineered clothing belong to consumer product domain, like antistatic jackets, pants, caps, and gloves, etc. Wearable sensors integrated conductive fabric known as "SmartShirts" have been engineered and marketed by Sensatex (2007); they are used for mapping heart rate, body temperature, or respiration.

8.4.1.3   Antibacterial/Hygienic Textiles

The popularity of antibacterial textile products is continuously increasing especially due to their fresh fragrance, skincare, and high-performance characteristics, enough to survive in the rigorous medical textile sector. Antibacterial agents commonly prevent bacterial growth on the surfaces as well as the interior structure of the treated materials, and their small quantities are sufficient enough in the majority of applications. The antibacterial performance can be further enhanced with the nano-size diffusion of the functional element due to increased specific surface area. Various nanomaterials and techniques adopted for engineering antibacterial textiles are summarized in Table 8.4.

TABLE 8.4

Nanomaterials and techniques for antibacterial textiles

Nanoparticle	Textile medium	Manufacture technique	Incorporation into the textile medium
Ag	Cotton, Polyester, Spandex	Coated finished textile via dip: pad: dry: cure method	Partial diffusion into the textile, Textile with some Ag NP on the surface
	PP	Melt spinning, Ag/PP Masterbatch production	PP matrix with PP/Ag nanocomposite
	Silk, PA	Production of Ag/PP Masterbatch, melt spinning	PP matrix with PA/Ag nanocomposite
	PP	Melt compounded Ag/PP	PP matrix with PP/Ag nanocomposite
	Not stated	Acetylene/Ag coated finished fabric: Plasma-polymerized acetylene with co-sputtering of Ag: NP	Some Ag NP on nano porous acetylene coating
TiO2	Cellulosic fibers	Coated finished fabric through sol gel process	TiO2 nanoparticles loaded textile material
	Cotton fibers	Coating of fabric via deposition of plasma enhanced chemical vapor	1 nm TiO2 coating on the fiber
Ag + TiO2	Cotton	Coated finished textile produced by dipping: padding: drying: cure method	Some Ag NP on the textile surface
ZnO	Cotton	Coated finished textile produced by dip: pad: dry: cure system	ZnO NP-coated starch matrix
SiO2 matrix with embedded biocides	No specific	Biocides added to Si nano sol, coated finished textile through sol-gel process	Nanoporous SiO2 coated by way of a cross-linked network

According to Mahltig et al. (2005), biocidal textiles can be divided into three classes as per their basic characteristics:

1) Non-diffusible biocides
2) Photoactive biocides
3) Embedded biocides with their controlled release

Daoud et al. (2005) have stated coating of fabric done with TiO2 as the best explanatory case for the first category of biocides. The photocatalytic process held in the presence of TiO2 can cause the degradation of stains and is useful for the production of self-cleaning textiles. This phenomenon is important for the clothing worn by the surgeons in the operation theater, liable to get blood stains. Parkin and Palgrave (2004) have well described the photocatalytic process for the fabric treated with TiO_2. Accordingly, the valence electrons of TiO_2 on the absorption of light can be lifted into an advanced energy level and generate exciting charge carters, a positive charge electron-hole, and an electron. The organic molecules get oxidized by positively charged holes, whereas the formation of the hyperoxide radicals occurs in an electron reaction with oxygen. These hyperoxide radicals are capable of attacking and oxidizing the cell membranes of microorganisms. Consequently, the antibacterial fabric so engineered also gets enriched with self-cleaning properties.

The second category deals with the immobilization of biocides in the textile matrix itself or the matrix of a coating in the textiles. The negative charge cell membranes on interacting with the positive charge biocide give rise to an antibacterial effect, which damages the microbes, and hinders their grooming and reproduction. The phenomenon was testified by Chattopadhyay & Patel (2009).

The third method for antibacterial fabric preparation via coating deals with diffusing out the biocides from the matrix. Patel et al. (2015a, 2016) have elaborated on their integration phenomenon for metallic antibacterial agents. As per their perceptions, in the use of metallic antibacterial agents, air oxidizes the nanoparticles present in the matrix. The positive ions like triclosan, $Ag+$, and $Cu2+$ formed in the course are then diffused out of the medium and result in deterred bacterial growth.

A biocidal effect has been obtained on the use of Ag, TiO_2, or a combination of both NP, by mainstream researchers. Vigneshwaran et al. (2006) have attained a textile with a projected antibacterial effect on the ZnO nanoparticles integration. Ye et al. (2005) have used Core Chitosan-based NP shell in order to get a desirable antibacterial coating for cotton fabrics. Moreover, Mahltig et al. (2005) have cited a plausible integration of different Ag, Cu like inorganic or chitosan, Triclosan type organic biocides, into a silica coating matrix.

The most common means used for applying reagent TiO_2 on the textile is the sol-gel process, as mentioned in most of the examined research papers: Daoud & Xin (2004a, 2004b); Qi et al. (2006); Bozzi et al. (2005)). The process is well described by Mahltig et al. (2005). Initially, a TiO_2 dispersion containing particles with a size around 50 nm also known as nano sol is prepared. The textile material—fiber, yarn, or finished fabric—needs to be treated and is then immersed into this nano sol. This results in the formation of a solvent-loaded lyogel layer due to particles getting accrual on the textile surface. Thence after the residual solvent in a solid, porous xerogel layer is evaporated by heating the lyogel. Mahltig et al. (2005) have mentioned the antibacterial coatings in which via the sol-gel processes only biocides get embedded with a Si-matrix. Diverse dip-pad-dry-cure techniques were practiced by Yuranova et al. (2006), Vigneshwaran et al. (2006), and Lee et al. (2003) to load the textile materials with antibacterial agents like Ag, Ag/TiO_2, or ZnO coatings. The technique basically involved dipping of the textile material into a nano sol then drying and finally heating to evaporate the solvent. Dubas et al. (2006) have formed an antibacterial coating via a layer-by-layer deposition in which the finished fabric was dipped into an Ag-nano sol and then into a polyelectrolyte solution. Probable techniques apart from the aforementioned comprise the Ag-NP co-sputtering while polymerization of plasma to produce an antibacterial coating as per Hegemann et al. (2007); and by chemical vapor deposition technique cited by Szymanowski et al. (2005) for the deposition of TiO_2 NP. An alternative proposal that is contrary to

NP coating procedure is to incorporate NPs prior to the manufacturing process; for example, Jeong et al. (2005) have anticipated direct melt compounding of the textile polymer with Ag. Yeo et al. (2003) have cited about manufacturing masterbatches for Ag/PP and also subsequent melt spinning belonging to the same class.

8.4.1.3.1   Commercially Available Products

The antibacterial goods have been seen in almost all commercial applications except the products belonging to the automotive sector. No doubt their direct or indirect utilization in the hospital healthcare sector is higher and in a way obligatory. The hospital clothing-related product list is quite long by way of Good Weaver Textile; United Textile Mills; AgActive (2007a); Nano Babies; Song Sing Nanotechnology (2007); Nanoinfinity Nanotech (2007). Accordingly, antibacterial polo shirts, self-cleaning shoe inserts, socks, underclothing, etc. can be procured by various producers. The well-known examples in stuffing and an internal trim class of products are antimicrobial baby bedspreads and bedsheets as revealed by Ag Active, Green Yarn Technology (2007). The biocidal wound dressings are available in the product collection related to the healthcare division, as per Smith & Nephew, while cosmetic utilities like toothbrushes and face cover as per Nanover (2007), Song Sing Nanotechnology, and Nano infinity Nanotech. The protective face masks are also available to care against bacterial and viral infections, Emergency Filtration Products Inc. (2007). Moreover, many companies offered antibacterial augmented fabrics, additives, or technologies for textile treatment, to their trade customers. Thomson Research Associates offer treatment for antibacterial characteristics induced textile useful in making a widespread product, viz., bed sheets, undergarments, kitchen scrubbers, bath towels, sport helmet waddings, or rugs. Both Nanopool (2007) and Nanogate (2007) offer technologies for antibacterial coating, while Murray (2006) has made accessible masterbatches for antibacterial polymer. HeiQ Materials Ltd. (2007) and Polartec have engineered antibacterial fabrics useful in making products for household purposes as well as outdoor clothing.

8.4.1.4   UV-Blocking Medicinal/Cosmetic Clothing for Skin Protection

According to Chaudhari et al. (2019) and Patel et al. (2017), integration of either UV-absorbing finish, pigments, metal particles, or dyes with the fabric can enhance the UV-blocking properties of textiles. All the research papers deliberately emphasize the use of such finishes to accomplish the anticipated effect. Yadav et al. (2006) have reported on the nanoparticulate ZnO- finish application to cotton fabrics employing a dipping: padding: drying: cure method. Vigneshwaran et al. (2006) have described a similar coating method for the synthesis of ZnO-NP carried out with the addition of soluble starch; they realized the prevention of agglomeration along with boosted UV blocking. Daoud and Xin (2004b) have proposed another option for enhancing cotton fabrics with UV-blocking characteristics: the fabrics were coated with a film containing TiO_2 nanoparticles via sol-gel technique by using a process sequence of dipping, padding, dry, and cure. Incorporation of the organic UV absorbers like benzotriazoles into a Si nano sol before application onto the fabric via sol-gel systems can also become one more pathway in addition to the aforementioned procedure. Table 8.5 displays the nanomaterials and various manufacturing methods for UV-blocking textiles.

TABLE 8.5
Nanomaterials and techniques for UV-blocking textiles

Nanoparticle	Textile medium	Manufacturing method	Way of incorporation with the textile medium
ZnO	Cotton	Finished fabric coated via dip: pad: dry: cure method	Data not available
TiO2	Cotton	Finished fabric coated via sol gel process	The fibers having some TiO2-NP
UV absorbers engrained into SiO2 matrix	Not stated	Si nano sol added with UV absorber, coating of finished textile by sol gel process	A cross-linked grid with UV absorbers obtained with a layer of Nano porous SiO2

8.4.1.4.1   The Potential Area of Applications

There is no scheme for direct MedTech-associated commercial applications of UV-blocking textiles noted in any of the examined research papers. According to their added functionality the possible commercial applications demand combined sun protection, or sun shield or parasols production can be included; apparel and sportswear. Thus, it can serve well for treating patients having sensitive skin to safeguard them from sunburning.

8.4.1.4.2   Commercialized Products

The commercial applications noted in the scrutinized consumer records are briefed here. In case of the clothing and sports division, "NanoTsunami (2007) offers UV blocking bathing NanoTsunami." Additional commercial submissions were noticed in the auxiliary product ranges designed for the development of industry: nanogate and Tianjin Tianfang Investment Holding Co., proposing the production of textile materials capable of UV blocking using the coating systems designed for it. Luko International Technology on the other hand deals in direct trading of a fabric having equivalent properties and can be converted into shirts or pullovers. Nanogate (2007) has promoted an industrial coating agent for applying to textile fabric efficiently enough in causing UV blockage.

8.4.1.5   Clothing With Regulated Release of Active Drugs, Agents, or Fragrance

Nanoengineering serves as a tool to produce fibers empowered to release integrated species at a controlled rate by behaving as carriers for colognes, medicines, or any other active reagents. The preceding section has already summarized research projects involved in engineering antibacterial fabrics with the biocidal agents released in a metered manner. Thereby, in the present section only the projects having active species other than a biocide are accommodated. Persico et al. (2006) have designed nylon fibers by using a montmorillonite-nano clay to carry cosmetic jojoba oil elements, and they are expectedly fit for skin care products. Nanoclays and jojoba oil merger into the polyamide matrix originated by direct melt compounding. It is also

TABLE 8.6
Nanomaterials and techniques with controlled release of active agents for textiles

Nanoparticle	Textile medium	Production method	Amalgamation into the textile medium
Montmorillonite as embedded active agents with SiO2 matrix	Not demarcated	Active agents added to Si nano sol, finished textile coated through sol gel process	Cross-linked networking via nanoporous SiO2 coating
	PA	Melt-compounding	PA matrix with exfoliated nanoclay

possible to produce fibers capable of releasing various active reagents, viz., insect repelling fragrances, ethereal oils, or drugs etc., in precise amount by including them in a SiO2 nano sol coating in Table 8.6.

8.4.1.5.1 The Potential Area of Applications

Apparel, home furnishing materials, cosmetics, outdoor clothes, or medicinal appliances are few amongst the wide-span end use areas identified for the fibers having controlled release of oils, medicines, or fragrances. The plausible products cited in this regard are cosmetic pads with inbuilt skin care products, insect repellent textiles for clothing, therapeutical efficient medical textiles used mainly in wound dressings and drug-releasing, outdoor fabrics, or so-called fragrance emitting clothing as well as home textiles (Mankodi et al., 2017).

8.4.1.5.2 Commercialized Products

The cosmetic sector has emerged out with the predominant saleable products in this region. Woodrow Wilson International, Nano Gold Mask, and Aspen Aerogels (2007) offer facial masks with integrated cosmetics substances.

8.5 SUMMARY

The enormous monetary potential and exceptional characteristics of nanometal composite textiles and nanomaterials have fascinated all segments of society, starting from the common man, scientists, researchers, and industrialists to traders. According to the report given by the National Science Foundation, the nano-related articles and amenities will touch the magic figure of a trillion dollars market in the next 10 to 15 years. The collective trades of highly populated businesses like telecommunications and information technology have not even reached around this value to date. As per the forecast, a fast-growing market of nanotechnology in the forthcoming decade will expand further and cover a business span of several hundred billion Euros. Such rapidly growing universal yearly production requirements will invariably open the scope for none less than millions of new employment opportunities also.

The environment-conscious analysis also favors nanotechnology because it brings about almost identical or even better performance by utilizing only fewer resources. Thus, nanotechnology can save valuable raw materials and thereby supports environment preservation along with ensuring deliveries for a quality life.

REFERENCES

AgActive. (2007a). 100% cotton sheet sets, Available from www.agactive.co.uk/index.cfm/fuseaction/product.display/ProductID8/.htm.

AgActive. (2007b). Sports anklet sock, Available from www.agactive.co.uk/index.cfm/fuseaction/produ.

Ahmadi, S.J. (2004). Review synthetic routes, properties, and future applications of polymer-layered silicate nanocomposites. *J. Mater. Sci.*, 39, 1919–1925.

Amalvy, M.J. (2002). Polymer/Silica nanomaterial preparation, characterization, properties, and applications. *Mater. Chem.*, 12, 697.

Aspen Aerogels. (2007). Products. Available from www.aerogel.com/products/overview.html.

Bekaert, Innovative Textiles by Bekaert. 17.03.2004. [cited 9.05.2007], Available from www.bekaert.com/bft/Products/Innovative%20Textiles.htm.

Bozzi, A., Yuranova, T., Kiwi, J. (2005). Self-cleaning of wool-polyamide and polyester textiles by TiO_2-rutile modification under daylight irradiation at ambient temperature. *J. Photochem. Photobiol. a-Chem*, 172(1), 27–34.

Celzard, et al. (2002). Applications of the sol-gel process using well-tested recipes. *J. Chem. Educ.*, 79, 854–859.

Chattopadhyay, D.P., Patel, B.H. (2009). Improvement in physical and dyeing properties of natural fibres through pre-treatment with silver nanoparticles. *Indian J. Fibre Text. Res.*, 34, 368–373.

Chattopadhyay, D.P., Patel, B.H. (2014a). Functional properties of silver nano-sol treated wool and silk fabric. *Man-made Text. India*, 42(9), 340–344.

Chattopadhyay, D.P., Patel, B.H. (2014b). Nano metal particles: Synthesis, characterization, and application to textiles. *Manufacturing Nanostructures*, 184–215.

Chaudhari, S.B., Mandot, A.A., Patel, P.N., Patel, B.H. (2019). Studies on the thermal degradation behavior of nano-silica loaded cotton and polyester fabrics. *Man-Made Text. India*, 47(2), 55–58.

Daoud, W.A., Xin, J.H. (2004a). Low-temperature sol-gel processed photocatalytic titania coating. *J. Sol-Gel Sci. Technol.*, 29(1), 25–29.

Daoud, W.A., Xin, J.H. (2004b). Nucleation, and growth of anatase crystallites on cotton fabrics at low temperatures. *J. Am. Ceram. Soc.*, 87(5), 953–955.

Daoud, W.A., Xin, J.H., Zhang, Y.H. (2005). Surface functionalization of cellulose fibers with titanium dioxide nanoparticles and their combined bactericidal activities. *Surf. Sci.*, 599(1–3), 69–75.

Dubas, S.T., Kumlangdudsana, P., Potiyaraj, P. (2006). Layer-by-layer deposition of antimicrobial silver nanoparticles on textile fibers. *Colloids Surf. A Physicochem. Eng. Asp.*, 289(1–3), 105–109.

Eeon technology, EeonTexTM Conductive Textiles. [cited 22.08.2007], Available from www.eeonyx.com/prodsp.html.

Emergency Filtration Products Inc. (2007). Emergency filtration products. [cited 9.10. 2007], Available from http://www.Emergencyfiltration.com/Products/NanoMask.htm.

Francois, N.R.R., Jeanne, D.J., Freney, H. (2006). Evaluation of antimicrobial properties of a textile product with antimicrobial finish in a hospital environment. *J. Ind. Text.*, 36(1), 89.

Gao, Y., Cranston, R. (2008). Recent advances in antimicrobial treatments of textiles. *Text. Res. J.*, 78, 60.

Green Yarn Technology. (2007). Greenyarn technology: Weaving together a healthy tomorrow. [cited 9.10.2007], Available from www.Greenyarn.com/technology.htm.

Hegemann, D., Hossain, M.M., Balazs, D.J. (2007). Nanostructured plasma coatings to obtain multifunctional textile surfaces. *Prog. Org. Coat.*, 58(2–3), 237–240.

HeiQ Materials Ltd. (2007). St. Gallen, Microban, home products. [cited 10.10.2007], Available from https://www.microban.com/Americas/products/category.html?lang=en &CategoryID=1&SubcategoryID=200.

Home, I. (2002). Antimicrobials impart durable finishes. *Int. Dye*, 9–11.

Jeong, S.H., Yeo, S.Y., Yi, S.C. (2005). The effect of filler particle size on the antibacterial properties of compounded polymer/silver fibers. *J. Mater. Sci.*, 40(20), 5407–5411.

Lands End, ThermaCheck® Scarf [cited 22.08.2007], Available from www.landsend.com/cd/fp/prod/0,,1_2_1931_51997_151350_128897_5:view=-1,00. html?sid=0622107012275149920&CM_MERCH=SRCH.

Lee, H.J., Yeo, S.Y., Jeong, S.H. (2003). Antibacterial effect of nanosized silver colloidal solution on textile fabrics. *J. Mater. Sci.*, 38(10), 2199–2204.

Lubben, J. (2005). Funktionale fasern und textilien, tec21 [functional fibers and textiles.]: Fachzeitschrift fur Architektur, *Ingenieurwesen und Umwelt*, 41, 10–13.

Mahltig, B., Haufe, H., Bottcher, H. (2005). Functionalisation of textiles by inorganic sol-gel coatings. *J. Mater. Chem.*, 15(41), 4385–4398.

Mandot, A.A., Chaudhari, S.B., Patel, B.H. (2012). Nanocomposite: Manufacturing and applications in textiles. *Melliand Int.*, 18 (D 45169 F), 188–189.

Mankodi, H., Solanki, U., Patel, B. (2017). Characterization of colloidal solution for wound dressing using honey. *Int. J. Eng. Techniques*, 3(6), 482–487.

Murray, J. (2006). Introducing a novel nanosilver additive for antimicrobial textile functionality. In *Presentation at the Nano Europe Conference*. HeiQ Materials Ltd: St. Gallen.

Nanogate. [cited 8.10.2007], Functions, nanoparticles and commercial applications, Available from https://www.empa.ch/documents/56122/328606/NanoSafeTextiles_1. pdf/b2add656-265b-42df-9196-f2768d773748.

Nanoinfinity Nanotech. (2007). Healthy deodorant series products. [cited 9.10.2007], Available from www.nano-infinity.com.tw/product01.htm.

Nanopool. (2007). [cited 10.10.2007], Available from http://www.nanoingermany.com/smr/ content/company/company_id/88/exhibition_id/16/subexhibition/0/.

Nanotex, Fabric to the Next. [cited 22.08.2007], Available from www.nano-tex.com/index_ noflash.html.

NanoTsunami. (2007). Nanophase launches textile and non-woven nanoengineered products. [cited 9.10.2007], Available from https://www.voyle.net/Nano%20Textiles/2005%20 Textiles/Textiles-2005–0004.htm.

Nanover. (2007). NanoverWetWipes. [cited 9.10.2007], Available from www.nanogist.com/ English/products/tissue.htm.

Parkin, I., Palgrave, R. (2004). Self-cleaning clothes. *J. Mater. Chem.*, 15, 1689–1695.

Patel, B.H., Channiwala, M.Z., Chaudhari, S.B., Mandot, A.A. (2015a). Green synthesis of silver nano-sols by leaf extract of Ocimum sanctum and their efficacy against the human pathogenic bacterium. *J. Green Sci. Technol.*, 2(1), 1–6.

Patel, B.H., Channiwala, M.Z., Chaudhari, S.B., Mandot, A.A. (2016). Biosynthesis of copper nanoparticles, its characterization and efficacy against human pathogenic bacterium. *J. Environ. Chem. Eng.*, 4(2), 2163–2169.

Patel, B.H., Chaudhari, S.B., Mandot, A.A. (2017). Development and characterization of nano-silica cotton composite fabric. *Man-Made Text. India*, 45(5), 151–154.

Patel, B.H., Chaudhari, S.B., Mandot, A.A., Panchal, C.J. (2015b). Silica particles can improve the electrical conductivity of polyester and cotton. *Text. Asia*, 46, 39–41.

Patel, B.H., Patel, R.N. (2006). Plasma aided wet-chemical treatments, an update. *The Indian Text. J.*, 116, 31–34.

Patel, B.H., Tandel, M.G. (2005). Antimicrobial finishing for textiles: An overview. *Asian Dye*, 31.

Peltola, et al. (2001). Influence of sol and stage of spinnability on in vitro bioactivity and dissolution of sol-gel-derived SiO_2 fibers. *Biomaterials*, 22, 589–598.

Persico, P., Carfagna, C., Musto, P. (2006). Nanocomposite fibers for cosmetotextile applications. *Macromolecular Symposia*, 234, 147–155.

Qi, K.H., et al. (2006). Self-cleaning cotton. *J. Mater. Chem.*, 16(47), 4567–4574.

Russell, et al. (2002). Nanotechnologies and the shrinking world of textiles. *Text. Horiz.*, 10, 7–9.

Sensatex, Sensatex, Inc. Seamless Technology. [cited 22.08.2007], Available from www.sensatex.com.

Shaikh, T.N., Chaudhari, S., Patel, B., Patel, M. (2021). Gauging performance of biosynthesized silver nanoparticles loaded polypropylene nonwoven based textile electrodes for 3-lead health monitoring electrocardiogram on analogous system. *J. Ind. Text.*, 51(3), 4350S–4371S.

Shaikh, T.N., Chaudhari, S.B., Patel, B.H., Poonia, P. (2018). Biosynthesized nanoparticles based textile composite: Qualitative & quantitative impact analysis for end-use application. *Int. J. Eng. Sci. Res. Technol.*, 7, 524–531.

Song Sing Nanotechnology. (2007). Nano silver products. [cited 9.10.2007], Available from www.ssnano.net/ehtml/0418b.php.

Szymanowski, H., et al. (2005). Plasma enhanced CVD deposition of titanium oxide for biomedical applications. *Surf. Coat. Technol.*, 200(1–4), 1036–1040.

Vigneshwaran, N., et al. (2006). Functional finishing of cotton fabrics using zinc oxide-soluble starch nanocomposites. *Nanotechnology*, 17(20), 5087–5095.

Yadav, A., et al., (2006). Functional finishing in cotton fabrics using zinc oxide nanoparticles. *Bull. Mater. Sci.*, 29(6), 641–645.

Ye, W.J., et al. (2005). Novel core-shell particles with poly (n-butyl acrylate) cores and chitosan shells as an antibacterial coating for textiles. *Polymer*, 46(23), 10538–10543.

Yeo, S.Y., Lee, H.J., Jeong, S.H. (2003). Preparation of nanocomposite fibers for permanent antibacterial effect. *J. Mater. Sci.*, 38(10), 2143–2147.

Yuranova, T., et al. (2006). Performance, and characterization of Ag-cotton and Ag/TiO_2 loaded textiles during the abatement of E-coli. *J. Photochem. Photobiol. A-Chem*, 181(2–3), 363–369.

Zhang, J. (2008). Preparation and characterization of polymer/silica nanocomposites via double in Situ miniemulsion polymerization. *Chem. Rev.*, 108, 3893–3957.

Zou, H. (2008). Polymer/Silica nanocomposites: Preparation, characterization, properties, and applications. *Chem. Rev.*, 108, 3928–3947.

9 Superabsorbent Nanofibers Revolutionize in Feminine Hygiene Napkins and Incontinence Care

Arijit Das

9.1 INTRODUCTION

The present chapter deals with nanofibrous ultra-absorbent materials as an elementary component of feminine hygiene and incontinence care products. Nanotechnology has emerged as an interdisciplinary branch of science and engineering. The revolution-ized role of nanotechnology has been already established in various fields of applica-tions such as biomedical, textile, paints, agriculture, pollution control, bio-sensing, energy, etc. In recent years, the unique properties of hygienic textile nanomaterials have become one of the prime interests of researchers due to their superabsorption characteristics, antimicrobial function, and sustainability.

Cotton type fiber was used for its high absorbency, softness, and breathability prior to the application of the superabsorbent fibers. The usage of cotton is restricted for its poor mechanical strength, low durability, fibers' flammability, and ease of creasing (Yetisen et al., 2016). Disposable super absorption-based hygiene prod-ucts such as feminine pads, baby diapers, and adults' incontinence diapers are more effective than cloth diapers with respect to absorbency and safety aspects in regular usage. The rising female health consciousness and menstrual literacy rate through-out the world have spiked up feminine hygiene-related products sales within the last few years. In a survey, the global contribution of feminine hygiene products was around USD 37 billion in 2020 (www.fortunebusinessinsights.com/feminine-hygiene-products-market-103530, accessed Sep 25, 2022). The enhanced absorp-tion capacity of disposable hygiene products was achieved by the implementation of superabsorbent polymers (SAPs) (Bae et al., 2018; Counts et al., 2017). SAPs may be in the form of powder, granular and fibrous; the fibrous shape can retain water 100 times or even more of its own weight (Chinta et al., 2014). The enhanced functional properties such as higher surface-to-volume ratio, greater water retention capacity, smaller fiber diameter, and thin layers are coherently gained if the superabsorbent fibers are in nanoscale.

DOI: 10.1201/9781003331612-11

9.2 NANOTECHNOLOGY ON SUPERABSORBENT TEXTILE

9.2.1 NANOTECHNOLOGY

Nanotechnology is a branch of science and engineering that deals with substances within a range of 1 to 100 nm in length at least in one direction (1 billion nm = 1 m). The concept of nanotechnology was first proposed by Professor Richard Feynman in 1959 in a lecture at the California Institute of Technology titled 'There's Plenty of Room at the Bottom' (Feynman, 1960). In 1974, Japanese Professor Norio Taniguchi mentioned the term 'nanotechnology' at the International Conference on Manufacturing Engineering. He proposed a top-down strategy which is miniaturizing or breaking down bulk materials to yield nanosized substances, whereas the bottom-up approach is the building of nanomaterials from the atomic scale. The physical, chemical, and biological properties of nanomaterials drastically change from their bulk state due to a substantial increase in surface area-to-volume ratio as more atoms in the nanoparticles control the activity of the object. Nanomaterials may have different sizes such as nanoparticles, nanotubes, and nanosheets. Figure 9.1 shows the range of the fiber size used in the textile industries. Nanoparticles are mostly spherical or quasi-spherical in shape and considered as zero-dimensional. One-dimensional nanostructured materials are nanotubes, nanofibers, and nanowires. Nanofilms, nanolayers, and nanosheets have transverse dimensions of more than 100 nm, but the thickness is typically less than 5 nm. These are known as two-dimensional nanomaterials (Chimene et al., 2015). Three-dimensional nanomaterials have more than 100 nm in the x, y, and z dimensions. They include a bundle of nanotubes, nanowires, and nanocomposites.

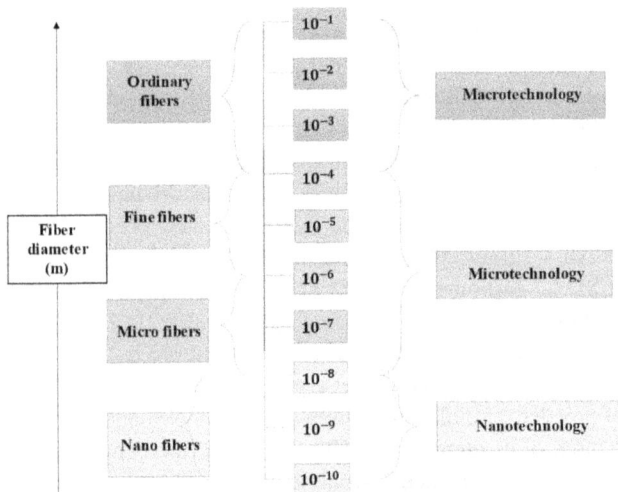

FIGURE 9.1   Size of macro to nanofibers and associated techniques

9.2.2 SUPERABSORBENT MECHANISM

By the definition of a superabsorbent, a polymer must be able to absorb at least 100 times of its initial volume in water (Sohn & Kim, 2003). SAPs are cross-linked polyelectrolytes that can be either natural or manufactured. The absorbent polymers may be non-ionic and ionic in nature. A few examples of non-ionic absorbent polymers are polyacrylamides, poly(ethylene oxide), poly(vinyl alcohol), and gelatin. All of them can be cross-linked to form absorbent materials, but none of them have enough absorption capacity to be regarded as the best substance for effective water absorption (Buchholz, 1997). When cross-linked, a number of cationic polymers can act as superabsorbents, namely poly(vinyl pyridine), poly(vinylbenzyltrimethylammonium salts), cationic starches, and hydrolyzed chitin (chitosan). Poly(acrylic acid) is one of the most widely used superabsorbent ionic polymers (Figure 9.2). Naturally occurring polysaccharides such as sodium carboxymethylcellulose (CMC) (from tree fiber), alginic acid (from brown seaweeds), carrageenans (from seaweeds), pectins (from plant extracts), and xanthan (from the microbial fermentation process) can be cross-linked for use as superabsorbents.

They have an insoluble polymer matrix that contains roughly 96% water and expand when they come into contact with water or aqueous solutions, eventually forming a rubbery hydrogel (Ucar & Kayaoglu, 2020; Gupta et al., 2011). Unlike ordinary water-absorbing materials, superabsorbents are capable of holding water under moderate pressure (Raju & Raju, 2001).

The association, dissociation, and binding of different ions to polymer chains allow them to expand or contract in aqueous solutions. When an equilibrium state is attained, SAPs may keep their original shape after swelling in water. The mechanical toughness, overall absorption, and swelling level of SAP are all directly impacted by the cross-linking level. High-density cross-linked polymer exhibits a stronger gel formation with reduced absorbent capacity, while low-density cross-linked SAP exhibits a soft and cohesive gel formation with high absorbent capacity (Ucar & Kayaoglu, 2020).

Acrylamide hydrogels have extensive commercial uses as absorbents in personal healthcare products. Figure 9.3 depicts a commercial cross-linked polyacrylic acid (PAA)-based SAP, where sodium hydroxide is used to partially neutralize the negative carboxylate groups. Hydration caused by the presence of hydrophilic chemical groups such as -OH, -COOH, -$CONH_2$, -CONH-, and -SO_3H, capillary regions, and variations in osmotic pressure inside and outside the gel are the key factors contributing to SAPs' tendency to expand (Elliott, 2004).

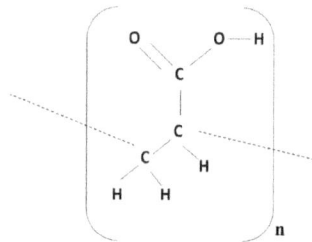

FIGURE 9.2   Structure of poly(acrylic acid)

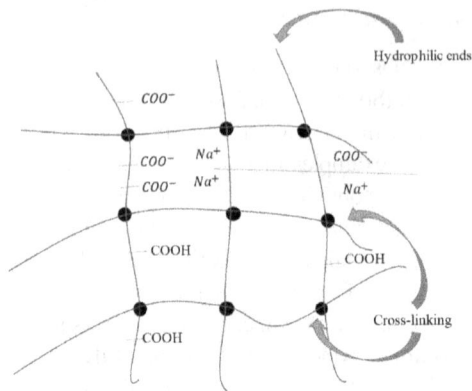

FIGURE 9.3   Cross-linking in a SAP network of polyacrylic acid during swelling

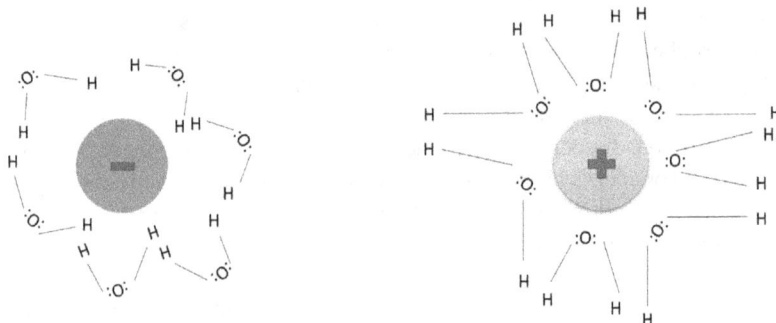

FIGURE 9.4   Pictorial presentation of hydration process

Hydration is the interaction of solute particles with dissolvable atoms, such as COO^- and Na^+ particles, which draw polar water atoms (Figure 9.4). Hydration of sodium ions decreases their attraction to the carboxylate ions and allows them to move freely throughout the network when a superabsorbent material comes into touch with water, which raises the osmotic pressure inside the gel (Elliott, 2004).

The gel formed by hydration is under light mechanical pressure. The pressure is 1–5 kPa in an adult diaper. The liquid is kept in a solid, rubbery condition by the swelling polymer gel, which also inhibits leakage. The presence of cross-links between polymer chains forming a three-dimensional network as well as both hydrophobic and electrostatic interactions are the forces that prevent hydrogel dissolution and aid in maintaining the integrity of superabsorbent material or controlling the degree of swelling when wet.

9.2.3   Layer Construction of Disposable Sanitary Pads and Diapers

The different layers of construction of disposable feminine hygiene pads and diapers are almost similar and mainly composed of four successive layers. Figure 9.5 shows

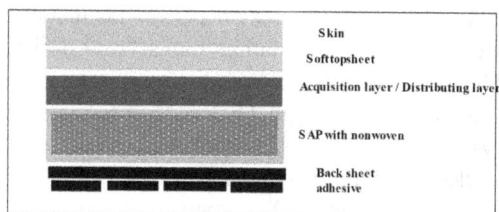

FIGURE 9.5 Layers of construction of disposable sanitary pads and diapers

the typical layers of hygiene pads and diapers. The perforated thin outer layer of polypropylene or polyethylene comes with skin contact which transfers the fluids into the inner layer by wicking action. The role of the superabsorbent layer is to hold the fluid. SAPs are used to compose this layer which is capable of holding fluids many times to its own weight. In between the top and core superabsorbent layer, an acquisition layer exists which mainly spreads the fluids evenly into the beneath layer. The back sheet layer is a water leakproof thin sheet made of polyethylene or polypropylene (Bae et al., 2018; Dey et al., 2016; Ajmeri & Ajmeri, 2010; Kosemund et al., 2009).

9.3 NANOFIBERS

The production of nanofibers was first reported by Formals in 1934 by using a cellulose acetate solution. But it took another 60–70 years to widen its scope in multidirectional applications in the textile industry. Owing to the unique characterizations like high aspect ratio (ratio of length to diameter >200), high surface area and porosity, as well as its range of dimensions covering nano and microscale, nanofibers are comprehensively applied in medical textiles (non-implantable and implantable), clothing, agriculture, etc. A variety of visco-elastic polymeric solutions, composites, metal, and metal oxide nanoparticles could be used as raw materials in nanofiber production. Moreover, the morphological and physico-mechanical properties can be tunable by controlling the operating parameters involved in production techniques to meet the desired specification (Bhardwaj & Kundu, 2010).

9.3.1 Nanofiber Synthesis

Nanofiber production can be achieved through various techniques such as electrospinning, wet spinning, dry spinning, drawing, phase inversion, etc. These are bottom-up approaches as the building of nanofibers from molecular interaction.

9.3.1.1 Electrospinning Process

Electrospinning (ES) is a simple, inexpensive, and popular method used to form nanofibers with fiber diameters between 10 nm and 10 μm (Cramariuc et al., 2013). ES was invented by Morton and Cooley in 1902. The main principle of the ES technique is that when a source of high electric voltage is applied to the tip of a suspended polymeric solution kept in a metallic needle, the droplets elongate and form very fine fibers from the tip. The fibers are collected on a grounded metallic collector. Various visco-elastic polymers and their combinations can achieve desired characteristics of nonwoven fibers. The electrospinning setup is easy to construct and found appropriate for producing continuous fiber length. Over the last few decades, several research and modifications were carried out on ES process.

The conventional electrospinning setup mainly comprises of four parts: a graduated syringe with a metallic needle (spinneret), a programable syringe pump, a high voltage power supply, and a grounded metal collector (Figure 9.6) (Rutledge & Fridrikh, 2007). Typically, 5 to 30 kV electric potential is applied to the spinneret which depends on the types of polymer solutions. The feed solution is filled inside the syringe which is then extruded at a constant flow rate through the spinneret by the control of syringe pump. If sufficient or no voltage is applied at the spinneret, the polymeric solution exits from the needle as a spherical droplet to minimize the surface tension (Williams et al., 2018). The nanofibers are collected on an earthed metal plate. Aluminium foil, aluminium foil covered with polyester netting, or metal mesh is usually used to deposit the fibers depending on the polymer's characteristics and fiber thickness. A rotating drum collector is more useful for continuous or scaling-up operations as it provides a larger area.

The high voltage causes protrusion of the feed solution through the syringe. More charges accumulate at the top of the protrusion, causing it to form a conical shape known as a Taylor cone. When the potential reaches a critical value, the repellent electrical force triumphs over the surface tension, and a jet of polymer solution is emitted from the tip of the Taylor cone. Once the jet is emitted, it elongates and gets thinner. Fiber jetting is induced due to the huge potential differences between charged solution in the spinneret and collector and a tensile force is developed in the jet (Nair et al., 2004). In between the distance of the Taylor cone and collector, the jet evaporates the solvent and reaches at the collector continuously as dry nonwoven

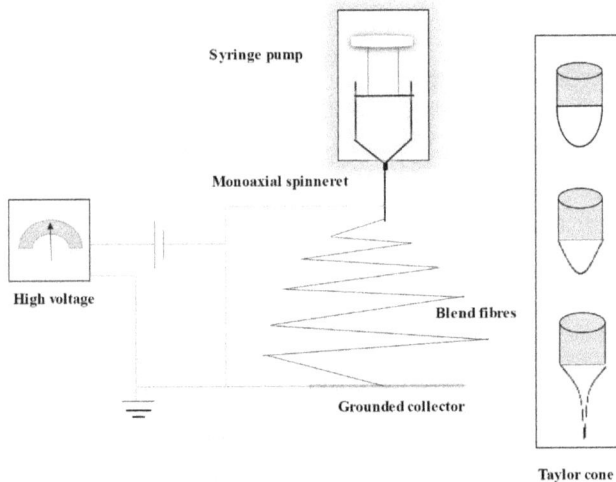

FIGURE 9.6　Schematic diagram of a conventional electrospinning process and shapes of Taylor cone

fibers. The distance of Taylor cone and the collector is maintained around 10–20 cm or even higher (Megelski et al., 2002). The fiber diameter generally decreases with increasing the distance between apex and the collector. The range of nanofiber diameter is quite broad; it is 60 to 5000 nm (Kramar & Gonzalez-Benito, 2002).

The employing of semi-conducting or insulating polymers could generate somewhat stable jets whereas utilizing highly conducting solutions result in very unstable streams that scatter in diverse directions when a high voltage is applied. The jet's instability is caused by repelling forces coming from the charge it contains. Another significant finding was that an unstable jet generates fibers with a wider variety of diameters (Hayati et al., 1987). It is worth mentioning that the electrospinning process is unaffected by the nature of the polarity of the potential; either positive or negative charge may be employed.

Electrospinning is a process that is frequently used to produce nanofibers, however there are few limitations to be solved. Conventional ES is a slow process. According to the Partheniadis et al. the nanofiber production rate is 0.01 to 0.1 g/h at standard laboratory conditions (2020). Also, volatile solvents cause health problems which narrow down the scope of scale-up operation. Needle clogging is another limitation of ES resulting in morphological changes in fibers. Various studies have been conducted to modify the traditional ES process in the last few years; some of the modified ES processes are briefly mentioned in Table 9.1.

TABLE 9.1
Types of electrospinning

Types	Working process	Remarks	Ref
Traditional ES	Polymer solution is dissolved in a volatile solvent. The solvent is placed in a programmable syringe pump. High voltage (5–30kV) is applied at the tip of the nozzle of the syringe pump. A charged jet of nanofibers ejects from the Taylor cone at the tip of the nozzle when electrostatic force exceeds the surface tension of the solution. Nanofibers are collected from a grounded collector by the rapid evaporation of the volatile solvent.	Morphology of the nanofibers is dependent on the concentration, viscosity, and flow rate of the polymeric solution, applied voltage, diameter of nozzle, distance between nozzle and collector, collector type etc.	(Li et al., 2007; Haider et al., 2018)
Multijet ES	Instead of single needle, this method employs multiple needles of multi-component polymers (not soluble in a single solvent) to get blend of nanofibrous mats. It may consist of 31–62 nozzles and metal collector of 50 cm wide.	Jet-jet repulsion of same charge causes loss of nanofibers deposition and inferior fiber quality. To overcome this drawback, metal collector is made opposite charged to that of spinneret and jets.	(Varesano et al., 2009, 2010)

TABLE 9.1 (Continued)
Types of electrospinning

Types	Working process	Remarks	Ref
Coaxial ES	Coaxial electrospinning is a variation on the traditional electrospinning procedure that involves setting up two or more solution feed systems to electrospin from coaxial capillaries simultaneously to form core-shell nanofibers. Due to the differences in surface charge of polymer solutions, shell layer forming polymer solution is lengthened and generate viscous stress which distributed to the core layer forming polymer solution is promptly stretched.	If the solvents of the polymer solutions are completely immiscible or miscible, there is no intervening interaction which causes perfect coaxial fiber formation. Core/shell solutes may precipitate out of solution at the nozzle tip when solvents are miscible, but their solutes are not soluble in the solvent of the opposite layer, leading to an unstable coaxial electrospinning process.	(Bayrak, 2022)
Melt ES	Unlike conventional ES, melt ES is performed by polymer at its molten state. Melt ES process employs a heat source like heating coil, lasers, etc. to keep the polymer in molten state. Nanofibers are obtained by cooling.	Melt ES does not require any solvent to dissolve polymer. Due to higher viscosity of the polymer, enhanced potential is required to initiate jets and wide fiber diameter is observed. Fiber diameter could be reduced by 50% if the voltage is doubled.	(Bayrak, 2022; Brown et al., 2016)
Centrifugal ES	It works on the principle of high centrifugal force instead of electric potential to form nanofibers. The polymeric solution jet ejected from the orifices in the spinneret and fiber is collected on fast evaporation of the solvent.	Fiber quality and morphology is controlled by rotational speed, nozzle design, collector type, etc. Nonconductive polymers can be electrospun.	(Bayrak, 2022)
Magnetic field-assisted ES	Magnetic field is induced at the collector zone of traditional electrospinning configuration. Two permanent magnets are placed 0.5–4 cm apart and 0.2 Tesla of magnetic field is maintained between the magnets.	Fiber uniformity is observed in MFAES. Fiber diameter is smaller. Polymer solution susceptible to magnetic field is used in MFAES.	(Bayrak, 2022; Liu et al., 2010)
Needleless ES	Needleless ES setup consists of metallic slow rotating fiber generator, solution container, high voltage power supply, and an earthed rotating drum collector. High voltage is applied at the bottom of the solution container (60kV) to attract the polymer jets into nanofibers. Nanofibers are collected on the surface of rotating drum collector. Electrospinning is often upward direction to prevent flaws in the nanofibrous mat by dripping solution onto it.	Increase the rate of production due to the formation of multiple jets. Improved fiber deposition compared to multiple needle ES.	(Niu et al., 2012)

9.3.1.2 Wet Spinning

When melt spinning is not an option for non-thermoplastic and temperature-sensitive polymers, solution spinning is often employed. Wet spinning employs a variety of polymers including natural polymers like alginate, chitosan, gelatin, collagen, etc. (Arafat et al., 2015). In the wet spinning process, continuous fibers are created by passing a polymer solution through a syringe into a coagulation or cross-linking solution bath (Figure 9.7). Depending on the properties of the polymer, the coagulation or cross-linking solution contains a solvent/non-solvent mixture or a poor solvent. The polymer solution coagulates to form fibers as a result of the mutual diffusion of the solvent and non-solvent. The concentration of polymer solution can vary from 1–25% (w/v) which depends on type of solvents, polymer chain length, and design of spinneret. The chains are normally free to entangle, detangle, and move in relation to one another once they have been dissolved in solution. The fibrous material is cleansed of its solvent while the fiber filament is passed through a bath during the wet spinning process. At temperatures between 140 and 180°C, the solvent that had become trapped in the coagulated filaments is first released, and the filaments are then stretched out to several times their original length. The diameter of the fiber can be adjusted by altering the flow rate of polymeric solution and needle size (Puppi & Chiellini, 2017).

Wet spinning setup mainly consists of a needle attached with syringe pump, a coagulation bath, and a rotating collector. The needle is kept immersed into the coagulating solvent to initiate fiber formation. The fiber spun using this technique in the highest quantity is viscose rayon. Other fibers in this group include polyvinyl chloride and calcium alginate. Wet spinning is used for most acrylic fibers like acrilan and courtelle. Superabsorbent fiber from cross-linked polyacrylate solution was spun by wet spinning process. The water absorbance capacity was reported up to 200 times of its own weight (Ucar & Kayaoglu, 2020).

9.3.1.3 Dry Spinning

In dry spinning process, the fiber formation is achieved by evaporating a high vapour-pressure polymeric solution in the spinline. The polymer solution is made using a volatile solvent, then the solution is allowed to eject through a spinneret into an evaporating chamber to blow out the volatile solvent by means of hot air or hot gases. The diluent

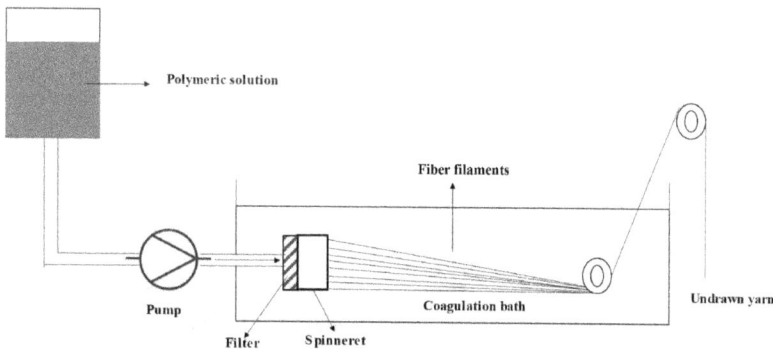

FIGURE 9.7 Schematic diagram of components of wet spinning

solution is fed at the fixed and controllable rate by a gear pump through jet nozzles (Figure 9.8). The formation of the filaments (fiber) occurs as soon as the solvent evaporates. The evaporated solvent is recycled after purifying it. This is a fast process compared to wet spinning. The heat and mass transfer and stress on the fiber control the rate of fiber formation. The fiber is drawn to improve its orientation prior to wind up on a drawing roller. When the stress imparted to the spinning filament is insufficient to drag the fiber to a smaller diameter, the spinning fiber reaches its terminal velocity (Imura et al., 2014). The cellulose acetate (CA), cellulose triacetate (CTA), and acrylic fibers are the most significant of the dry spun fibers. the choice of solvents must be made judiciously for non-toxicity, lower boiling point, thermal stability, and inertness.

9.3.1.4 Drawing

The drawing process is only applied to viscoelastic polymers capable of significant distortion while yet staying flexible enough to withstand the built-up tension during pulling. A conventional drawing process is simple and inexpensive; it consists of a micropipette, micropipette controller, and silicon oxide surface. The micropipette tip with a few micrometers diameter is soaked into a polymer solution droplet close to the contact surface. Then the micropipette is withdrawn from the solution at a speed of 100 μm/s by micropipette controller to form nanofibers (Almetwally et al., 2017). The pulled nanofibers are dumped on the silicon surface by touching it with the edge of the micropipette (Figure 9.9). The process is repeated several times for each droplet to form a fiber network.

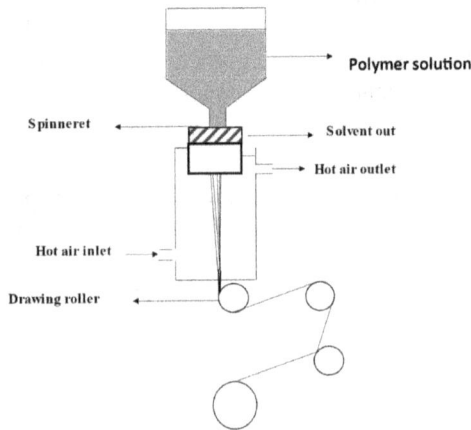

FIGURE 9.8   Schematic representation of dry spinning

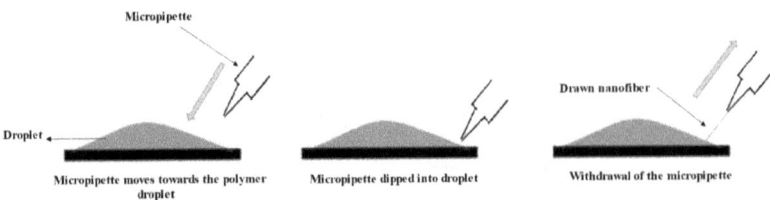

FIGURE 9.9   Schematic of drawing technique

During the withdrawl of the micropipette, the solvent evaporate and solid nanofiber are formed. The pulling of micropipette results formation of tensile stress in the fiber which a viscoelastic material only can survive. Drawing technique produces a single nanofiber at a time, so it prevents the process to be scaled up (Jayaraman et al., 2004).

9.3.1.5   Phase Separation

Phase separation technique can be employed for creating a 3-D nanoscale matrix. It was first developed by Zhang and Ma by thermally induced liquid-liquid phase separation. Phase separation of polymer solution creates polymer enrich and porous phases due to the dissolved polymers' sensitivity to temperature. Solvent removal causes the solidification of polymers. The process is completed in five stages: polymer dissolution, gelation, solvent extraction, freezing, and freeze-drying (Figure 9.10). The process requires minimal apparatus and is relatively simple. The phase separation can be induced either by changing the temperature or adding a non-solvent to the polymer solution. Polymer concentration, types of solvent, and freezing temperature determine the scaffold's morphology and porosity (Shah & Halacheva, 2016). Nanofiber 3-D matrix is obtained directly by this method but only appropriate for certain polymers (polylactide, polyglycolide, etc.) which are agreeable to phase separation (Sharma et al., 2015).

9.3.1.6   Template Synthesis

The template synthesis method uses nanoporous membranes as a template to create nanofibers of conductive polymers, metal, ceramic semiconductors, etc. The

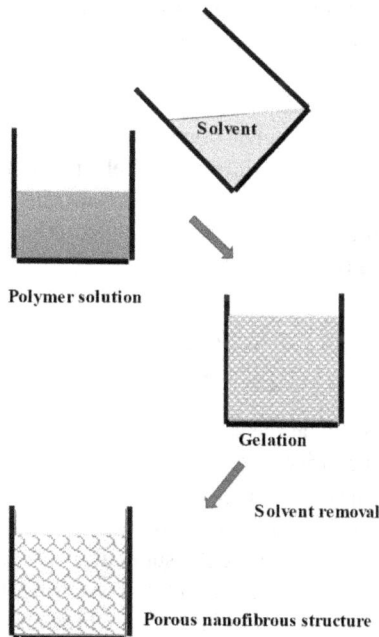

FIGURE 9.10   Schematic of phase separation technique

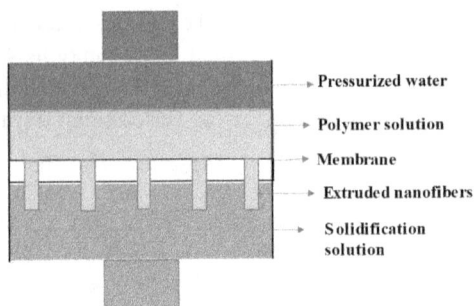

FIGURE 9.11 Schematic of template synthesis

membrane of metal oxide with a pore size range in the nanoscale is employed as a template or mold. These nanopores allow to form of nanofibers. Figure 9.11 shows the template synthesis process. The extrusion of the polymer through a nanoporous membrane is initiated by the pressure of water. During the extrusion, polymer solution comes into contact with a solidifying solution and provides a nanofiber. With this process fibers of desired diameter may be achieved by varying template pore size (Liu et al., 2020). The significant drawback of this method is that it lacks the production of continuous and lengthy fibers.

9.3.2 Parameters Affecting the Electrospinning Process

Since electrospinning is widely practiced for producing nanofibers, the dependency of nanofiber properties on its operating parameters has also been extensively studied. The morphology of the nanofibers produced in the electrospinning process depends on several process parameters. These parameters or process variables fall into two categories, namely, process and solution. Concentration, viscosity, molecular weight of the polymer, conductivity, dielectric constant, and volatility of the solution come in solution parameter, whereas, the intensity of electric potential, the gap distance between Taylor cone apex and collector, solution flow rate, the temperature of solution, and humidity are the process parameters. The effect of these parameters is tabulated in Table 9.2 briefly.

9.4 CHARACTERISTICS OF SUPERABSORBENT NANOFIBERS AND MODIFIED HYGIENE PRODUCTS

There are hundreds of studies on the superabsorbent nanofibers' characteristics produced by different spinning processes. The nanofibers so produced require examination of their morphology, absorption capacity, absorbency under load (AUL), residual test, etc. Different types of superabsorbent polymers and their fabrication processes have been modified in order to improve the super absorptivity.

The term 'free absorbency test' refers to freely swelling the sample with distilled water. There is no pressure to apply on the sample. Free absorbency test is simple to

TABLE 9.2
Electrospinning parameters and their effect on nanofibers

Parameters	Effects on fibers	Ref
Concentration and viscosity	Viscosity and concentration of solution are interrelated. In general, higher the polymer concentration, higher the viscosity and larger the fiber diameter. Fiber diameter follows the power law relationship with polymer concentration. At lower viscosity, formation of braided fiber is observed.	(Doshi & Reneker, 1995; Fong et al., 1999; Deitzel et al., 2001)
Electrical conductivity	Addition of salts into polymer solution increases the charge density on the jet surface. The jet radius and cube root of electrical conductivity are inversely proportional. Majority of the polymer solutions are conductive enough. An increase in conductivity increases the charge density in jet causing higher tensile forces on the jet and results in decrease of bead occurrence and finer fibers.	(Fong et al., 1999; Zong et al., 2002)
Solvent volatility	Solvent volatility is an extremely significant parameter. Studies on different solvents revealed that increase in solvent volatility resulted in smaller fiber diameters. Lower boiling point of solution is preferred as it allows fast solvent evaporation rate in fiber formation stage under ambient conditions. However, extremely volatile solvent often clogs the spinneret due to rapid evaporation of the solvent.	(Lee et al., 2002; Wannatong et al., 2004)
Molecular weight of polymer	High molecular weight polymer signifies intense polymer chain entanglement. The morphology and diameter of fiber can correlate with Berry number which is a product of intrinsic viscosity and concentration of polymer. Higher molecular weight of polymer forms a larger fiber diameter. Aqueous solution of PVA of various molecular weight (9000–186000 g/mol) was electrospun. Lower molecular weight and Berry number (<9) fibers exhibit a circular cross-section. At higher molecular weight and Berry number (>9) formed flat fibers with wider diameter.	(Koski et al., 2004)

TABLE 9.2   (Continued)
Electrospinning parameters and their effect on nanofibers

Parameters	Effects on fibers	Ref
Dielectric constant	Dielectric constant is a property of a substance to hold charge in an electric field. An increase in dielectric constant of a solvent fiber diameter is reported to decrease due to elongation by repulsive force. The choice of solvent with higher dielectric constant or its proportion leads to finer fiber formation.	(Almetwally et al., 2017)
Electric potential	An increase in voltage will speed up the polymer jet, which might lead to more solution being pulled from the needle's tip. According to Wu et al., the fiber diameters were observed to reduce to a minimum as the voltage increased, then the fiber diameters increased as the voltage increased further. Megelski et al. demonstrated that a reduction in PS fiber size from 20 to 10 μm when voltage increased from 5 to 12 kV.	(Lee et al., 2004; Wu et al., 2012; Megelski et al., 2002)
Gap between spinneret and collector	Evaporation time of solvent and distance to elongate of solution jet are dependent on spinning distance. Regardless of the concentration of the solution, higher spinning distance produces finer fiber; while a shorter gap results in wet fiber and a flat fiber structure. Less volatile solvent needs a more extended gap than a high vapor pressure solvent since longer evaporation time is required.	(Buchko et al., 1999)
Feed rate	Since higher amount of solution is extruded from the electrospun needle at increased feed rate keeping the viscosity constant, drying of fibers is troublesome during flight. As a consequence, fiber diameter increases and beaded morphology is larger. Lower feeding rate produces fewer and finer fiber diameter. Maintaining the feed rate of polyvinyl acetate solution less than 1mL/hr, fiber diameter of 24.83 nm was fabricated.	(Veerabhadraiah et al., 2017)
Relative humidity	Higher relative humidity of air inhibits the evaporation rate of solvent which yields coalescence of fibers on the collector plate. The solvent inside the core of the fiber subsequently evaporates and produces porous structure.	

conduct with high precision using centrifuge method, tea-bag method, Sieve method, etc. The AUL test is carried out under low pressure (0.3, 0.6, and 0.9 psi) using 0.9% saline solution unless specifying its swelling (Zohuriaan-Mehr & Kabiri, 2008). Another important characteristic of nanofiber is the residual test. The permissible limit of synthetic polymers (acrylic acid based) has been dropped to 300 ppm from 1000 ppm. Nanofiber synthesized by different methods showed remarkable water retention capacities. As for examples, superabsorbent fibers of aqueous polyacrylate solution showed absorbency of 200 and 60 g per gram in distilled and NaCl solution (Ucar & Kayaoglu, 2020); polyacrylic-based nanofibers by solvent spinning had maximum swelling capacity of 117 g/g (Liu et al., 2014); electrospinning nanofiber from natural polysaccharide swelling were 143.42g/g in aqueous solution and 39.75 g/g in standard saline solution (Islam et al., 2015).

In a study of swelling test of electrospun cellulose acetate nanofibers, 1963, 1800, and 2500% free absorbency were reported using distilled water, 0.9% saline water, and synthetic urine at 20 sec, respectively. In the same study, AUL value of CA nanofiber was measured around 962% under load $50g/cm^2$ and equilibrium absorbency around 2300% (Yadav et al., 2016). The cellulose-base nanofiber from wheat straw prepared by electrospinning technique showed mean diameter less than 100 nm. Xylan rich cellulose fibers were reported 132 g/g free absorbency and AUL as 83 g/g (Petroudy et al., 2021).

There are several studies on physico-mechanical properties of nanofibers. These studies can be broadly categorized as properties of nanofibers synthesized from synthetic (petrochemical based) and natural polymers. Salts of acrylic acid and acrylamide are extensively used as synthetic SAPs and cellulose based (polysaccharides and polypeptide) superabsorbent as natural source becomes popular nowadays for its non-toxic and environmental benign nature.

Zhou et al. reported the characteristics of electrospun cellulose acetate-trifluoroacetic acid solution (2011). The fiber diameter was found within a range of 100–300 nm with high surface-to-volume ratio of 2.02×10^7 m^2/m^3 and 87% porosity. The fibers showed less tensile stress (100 cN/mm^2) and large elongation ration of 40% before break.

Reshma et al. showed in a study that sodium carboxymethyl cellulose and starch blend membrane can be used as a core layer in sanitary napkins (2020). The optimal phase inversion membrane executed good mechanical characteristics. The tensile stress was observed as 25 ± 2 MPa with elongation $7 \pm 4\%$ at break point. The good flexibility of membrane also contained high absorbance capacity value of 25.5 ± 2.51 g/g.

Superabsorbent materials are used with other fluff pulps materials at the core layer of hygiene products. The desired functionality of SAPs may vary slightly in different hygiene products, mainly the swelling properties. The density of cross-linking in the superabsorbent polymers determines the swelling behavior. The fine-tuning in the polymer solutions is required to evaluate its properties for selective applications. For example, for adult diapers high absorption under load is desirable which could be obtained in dense cross-link polymers but absorption capacity decreases. Faster sorption rate requires larger specific surface area of SAPs that can be obtained by using porous small particles or by employing wrinkled particles (Jassal, 2011).

Sanitary pads receive menstrual discharge fluid that contains salts, biological cells, and water. The larger size of cells generally absorbs at the surfaces of SAPs due to lower diffusibility. Surface coating and neutralizing of superabsorbents may help to increase blood dispersibility. The addition of 3-dimethyl (methacryloyloxyethyl) ammonium propane sulphonate (DMAPS), trimethyl methacrylamidopropyl ammonium iodide (TMMAAI), etc. co-monomers increases the physiological fluid absorption which may be used in baby and adult diapers. Several metal nano particles possess antibacterial properties and are utilized as sterile hygiene products (Jassal, 2011). Constant research is still going on to improve the design and performance of the final absorbable sanitary products.

9.5 CONCLUSION

Superabsorbent polymers are extensively used in feminine hygiene and other incontinence care products in the form of nano or microfibers mainly. Cross-linked copolymers in nanofiber form can absorb and retain body fluids several times of their weight excellently through the formation of hydrogel under low to moderate pressure. The absorption rate, retention capacity, and deformability of the hydrogel is dependent on the degree of cross-linking. The superabsorbent nanofibers are mixed with other fibers and fluff in the hygiene products for higher holding capacity, and thinner and lighter products.

This chapter comprised the superabsorbency mechanism, different spinning techniques to fabricate nanofibers, the controlling parameters involved in spinning processes and properties of nanofibers. Almost all the properties of nanofibers synthesized by spinning methods are tunable. The chapter briefly discussed these critical parameters of electrospinning to tune the fiber morphology: applied potential, gaps between spinneret and grounded collector, viscosity, concentration of spinning solution, molecular weight of polymers, etc. Mechanical properties and fiber absorbency of nanofibers created from both synthetic and natural superabsorbent polymers were also cited.

REFERENCES

Ajmeri, J.R., Ajmeri, C.J. (2010). Nonwoven personal hygiene materials and products. In R.A. Chapman (Ed.), *Applications of Nonwovens in Technical Textiles* (pp. 85–102). Cambridge, UK: Woodhead Publishing.
Almetwally, A.A., El-Sakhawy, M., Elshakankery, M.H., Kasem, M.H. (2017). Technology of nano-fibers: Production techniques and properties-Critical review. *J. Text. Assoc.*, 78, 5–14.
Arafat, M.T., Tronci, G., Yin, J., Wood, D.J. Russell, S.J. (2015). Biomimetic wet-stable fibres via wet spinning and diacid-based crosslinking of collagen triple helices. *Polymer*, 77, 102–112.
Bae, J., Kwon, H., Kim, J. (2018). Safety evaluation of absorbent hygiene pads: A review on assessment framework and test methods. *Sustainability*, 10, 4146.
Bayrak, E. (2022). Nanofibers: Production, characterization, and tissue engineering applications. In P.V. Pham (Ed.), *21st Century Nanostructured Materials: Physics, Chemistry, Classification, and Emerging Applications in Industry, Biomedicine, and Agriculture.* London: IntechOpen.

Bhardwaj, N., Kundu, S.C. (2010). Electrospinning: A fascinating fiber fabrication technique. *Biotechnol. Adv.*, 28, 325–347.

Brown, T.D., Dalton, P.D., Hutmacher, D.W. (2016). Melt electrospinning today: An opportune time for an emerging polymer process. *Prog. Polym. Sci.*, 56, 116–166.

Buchholz, F.L. (1997). Absorbency and superabsorbency. In F.L. Buchholz, A.T. Graham (Eds.), *Modern Superabsorbent Polymer Technology* (p. 27). New York John, NY: Wiley & Sons.

Buchko, C.J., Chen, L.C., Shen, Y., Martin, D.C. (1999). Processing and microstructural characterization of porous biocompatible protein polymer thin films. *Polymer*, 40, 7397–7407.

Chimene, D., Alge, D.L., Gaharwar, A.K. (2015). Two dimensional nanomaterials for biomedical applications: Emerging trends and future prospects. *Adv. Mater.*, 27, 7261–7284.

Chinta, S.K., Mhetre, S.B., Daberao, A.M. (2014). Superabsorbent fibers and antimicrobial activity: A textile review. *Man-Made Text. India*, 42, 13–17.

Counts, J., Weisbrod, A., Yin, S. (2017). Common diaper ingredient questions: Modern disposable diaper materials are safe and extensively tested. *Clin. Pediatr (Phila)*, 56(5_suppl), 23S–27S.

Cramariuc, B., Cramariuc, R., Scarlet, R., Manea, L.R., Lupu, I.G., Cramariuc, O. (2013). Fiber diameter in electrospinning process. *J. Electrost.*, 71, 189–198.

Deitzel, J.M., Kleinmeyer, J., Harris, D.E.A., Tan, N.B. (2001). The effect of processing variables on the morphology of electrospun nanofibers and textiles. *Polymer*, 42, 261–272.

Dey, S., Kenneally, D., Odio, M., Hatzopoulos, I. (2016). Modern diaper performance: Construction, materials, and safety review. *Int. J. Dermatol.*, 55, 18–20.

Doshi, J., Reneker, D.H. (1995). Electrospinning process and applications of electrospun fibers. *J. Electrost.*, 35, 151–160.

Elliott, M. (2004). Superabsorbent Polymers, BASF Aktiengesellschaft.

Feminine hygiene products market. The feminine hygiene products market size, share & COVID-19 impact analysis, by product type (Menstrual care products and cleaning & deodorizing products), distribution channel (Hypermarkets/supermarkets, convenience stores, drug stores and others), and regional forecast, 2021–2028. Accessed 25 Sep. 2022 from www.fortunebusinessinsights.com/feminine-hygiene-products-market-103530.

Feynman, R.P. (1960). There's plenty of room at the bottom. *Eng. Sci. Mag.*, 23, 22–36.

Fong, H., Chun, I., Reneker, D.H. (1999). Beaded nanofibers formed during electrospinning. *Polymer*, 40, 4585–4592.

Gupta, B., Agarwal, R., Alam, M.S. (2011). Hydrogels for wound healing applications. In S. Rimmer (Ed.), *Biomedical Hydrogels: Biochemistry, Manufacture and Medical Application* (pp. 184–227). Cambridge, UK: Woodhead Publishing.

Haider, A., Haider, S., Kang, I.K. (2018). A comprehensive review summarizing the effect of electrospinning parameters and potential applications of nanofibers in biomedical and biotechnology. *Arab. J. Chem.*, 11, 1165–1188.

Hayati, I., Bailey, A.I., Tadros, T.F. (1987). Investigations into the mechanisms of electrohydrodynamic spraying of liquids: I. Effect of electric field and the environment on pendant drops and factors affecting the formation of stable jets and atomization. *J. Colloid Interface Sci.*, 117, 205–221.

Imura, Y., Hogan, R.M.C., Jaffe, M. (2014). Dry spinning of synthetic polymer fibers. In D. Zhang (Ed.), *Advances in Filament Yarn Spinning of Textiles and Polymers* (pp. 187–202). Cambridge, UK, NY: Woodhead Publishing.

Islam, M.S., Rahaman, M.S., Yeum, J.H. (2015). Electrospun novel super-absorbent based on polysaccharide-polyvinyl alcohol-montmorillonite clay nanocomposites. *Carbohydr. Polym*, 115, 69–77.

Jassal, M. (2011). The design of novel hygiene textile products. In B.J. McCarthy (Ed.), *Textiles for Hygiene and Infection Control* (pp. 3–13). Cambridge, UK, NY: Woodhead Publishing.

Jayaraman, K., Kotaki, M., Zhang, Y., Mo, X., Ramakrishna, S. (2004). Recent advances in polymer nanofibers. *J. Nanosci. Nanotechnol.*, 4, 52–65.

Kosemund, K., Schlatter, H., Ochsenhirt, J.L., Krause, E.L., Marsman, D.S., Erasala, G.N. (2009). Safety evaluation of superabsorbent baby diapers. *Regul. Toxicol. Pharmacol.*, 53, 81–89.

Koski, A., Yim, K., Shivkumar S.J.M.L. (2004). Effect of molecular weight on fibrous PVA produced by electrospinning. *Mater. Lett.*, 58, 493–497.

Kramar, A., Gonzalez-Benito, F.J. (2002). Cellulose-based nanofibers processing techniques and methods based on bottom-up approach—A Review. *Polymers*, 14, 286.

Lee, J.S., Choi, K.H., Ghim, H.D., Kim, S.S., Chun, D.H., Kim, H.Y., Lyoo, W.S. (2004). Role of molecular weight of atactic poly (vinyl alcohol)(PVA) in the structure and properties of PVA nanofabric prepared by electrospinning. *J. Appl. Polym. Sci.*, 93, 1638–1646.

Lee, K.H., Kim, H.Y., La, Y.M., Lee, D.R., Sung, N.H. (2002). Influence of a mixing solvent with tetrahydrofuran and N, N-dimethylformamide on electrospun poly (vinyl chloride) nonwoven mats. *J. Polym. Sci. B: Polym. Phys.*, 40, 2259–2268.

Li, W.J., Shanti, R.M., Tuan, R.S. (2007). Electrospinning technology for nanofibrous scaffolds. In C. Kumar (Ed.), *Tissue Engineering, Nanotechnologies for the Life Sciences Series*. New York, NY: Wiley VCH.

Liu, H., Zhang, Y., Yao, J. (2014). Preparation and properties of an eco-friendly superabsorbent based on flax yarn waste for sanitary napkin applications. *Fibers Polym.*, 15, 145–152.

Liu, S., Shan, H., Xia, S., Yan, J., Yu, J., Ding, B. (2020). Polymer template synthesis of flexible SiO2 nanofibers to upgrade composite electrolytes. *ACS Appl. Mater Interfaces*, 12, 31439–31447.

Liu, Y., Zhang, X., Xia, Y, Yang, H. (2010). Magnetic field assisted electrospinning of aligned straight and wavy polymeric nanofibers. *Adv. Mater.*, 22, 2454–2457.

Megelski, S., Stephens, J.S., Chase, D.B., Rabolt, J.F. (2002). Micro-and nanostructured surface morphology on electrospun polymer fibers. *Macromolecules*, 35, 8456–8466.

Nair, L.S., Bhattacharyya, S., Laurencin, C.T. (2004). Development of novel tissue engineering scaffolds via electrospinning. *Expert. Opin. Biol. Ther.*, 4, 659–668.

Niu, H., Wang, X., Lin, T. (2012). Upward needleless electrospinning of nanofibers. *J. Eng. Fibers Fabr.*, 7, 17–22.

Partheniadis, I., Nikolakakis, I., Laidmae, I., Heinamaki, J. (2020). A mini-review: Needleless electrospinning of nanofibers for pharmaceutical and biomedical applications. *Processes*, 8, 673.

Petroudy, S.R.D., Kahagh, S.A., Vatankhah, E. (2021). Environmentally friendly superabsorbent fibers based on electrospun cellulose nanofibers extracted from wheat straw. *Carbohydr. Polym.*, 251, 117087.

Puppi, D., Chiellini, F. (2017). Wet spinning of biomedical polymers: From single fibre production to additive manufacturing of three dimensional scaffolds. *Polym. Int.*, 66, 1690–1696.

Raju, K.M., Raju, M.P. (2001). Synthesis and swelling properties of superabsorbent copolymers. *Adv. Polym. Technol.*, 20, 146–154.

Reshma, G., Reshmi, C.R., Nair, S.V., Menon, D. (2020). Superabsorbent sodium carboxymethyl cellulose membranes based on a new cross-linker combination for female sanitary napkin applications. *Carbohydr. Polym.*, 248, 116763.

Rutledge, G.C., Fridrikh, S.V. (2007). Formation of fibers by electrospinning. *Adv. Drug Deliv. Rev.*, 59, 1384–1391.

Shah, T., Halacheva, S. (2016). Drug-releasing textiles. In L.V. Langenhove (Ed.), *Advances in Smart Medical Textiles* (pp. 119–154). Cambridge, UK, NY: Woodhead Publishing.

Sharma, J., Lizu, M., Stewart, M., Zygula, K., Lu, Y., Chauhan, R., Wei, S. (2015). Multifunctional nanofibers towards active biomedical therapeutics. *Polymers*, 7, 186–219.

Sohn, O., Kim, D. (2003). Theoretical and experimental investigation of the swelling behavior of sodium polyacrylate superabsorbent particles. *J. Appl. Polym. Sci.*, 87, 252–257.

Ucar, N., Kayaoglu, B. K. (2020). Superabsorbent fibers. In J. Hu, B. Kumar, J. Hu (Eds.), *Handbook of Fibrous Materials* (pp. 315–334). New York, NY: Wiley.

Varesano, A., Carletto, R.A., Mazzuchetti, G. (2009). Experimental investigations on the multi-jet electrospinning process. *J. Mater. Process. Technol.*, 209, 5178–5185.

Varesano, A., Rombaldoni, F., Mazzuchetti, G., Tonin, C., Comotto, R. (2010). Multi-jet nozzle electrospinning on textile substrates: Observations on process and nanofibre mat deposition. *Polym. Int.*, 59, 1606–1615.

Veerabhadraiah, A., Ramakrishna, S., Angadi, G., Venkatram, M., Ananthapadmanabha, V.K., NarayanaRao, N.M.H., Munishamaiah, K. (2017). Development of polyvinyl acetate thin films by electrospinning for sensor applications. *Appl. Nanosci.*, 7(7), 355–363.

Wannatong, L., Sirivat, A., Supaphol, P. (2004). Effects of solvents on electrospun polymeric fibers: Preliminary study on polystyrene. *Polym. Int.*, 53, 1851–1859.

Williams, G.R., Raimi-Abraham, B.T., Luo, C.J. (2018). *Nanofibres in Drug Delivery.* London, UK, NY: UCL Press.

Wu, C.M., Chiou, H.G., Lin, S.L., Lin, J.M. (2012). Effects of electrostatic polarity and the types of electrical charging on electrospinning behavior. *J. Appl. Polym. Sci.*, 126, E89–E97.

Yadav, S., Illa, M.P., Rastogi, T., Sharma, C.S. (2016). High absorbency cellulose acetate electrospun nanofibers for feminine hygiene application. *Appl. Mater. Today*, 4, 62–70.

Yetisen, A.K., Hang, Q., Manbachi, A., Butt, H., Dokmeci, M.R., Hinestroza, J.P., Skorobogatiy, M., Khademhosseini, A., Yun, S.H. (2016). Nanotechnology in textiles. *ACS Nano.*, 10, 3042–3068.

Zhou, W., He, J., Cui, S., Gao, W. (2011). Studies of electrospun cellulose acetate nanofibrous membranes. *Open Mater. Sci. J.*, 5, 51–55.

Zohuriaan-Mehr, M.J., Kabiri, K. (2008). Superabsorbent polymer materials: A review. *Iran. Polym. J.*, 17, 451–447.

Zong, X., Kim, K., Fang, D., Ran, S., Hsiao, B.S., Chu, B. (2002). Structure and process relationship of electrospun bioabsorbable nanofiber membranes. *Polymer*, 43, 4403–4412.

Part 3

Applications of Biotextiles for Medical Implants

10 Drug-Releasing Property Using Nanotechnology in Biotextiles

Rashmi Bhushan, Ruchi Pandey, Sachindra Kumar, Khushboo Choudhary, and Nitesh Kumar

10.1 INTRODUCTION

A drug-releasing system is created by integrating polymer science, pharmaceutical science, biochemistry, molecular biology, and other emerging analytics. For effective achievement, new resources, technological advancements, and measures are needed. Biotextile and textile technologies offer new methodologies, approaches, and advantages over pharmaceutical materials and technology (Dash & Cudworth, 1998).

Biotextiles have emerged as new technology and gained popularity in the latest years, with advancements in bioengineering, polymer science, pharmaceutics as well as textile technologies. It has been defined as structured textile fibres, particularly designed to perform under biological surroundings, and its efficiency will be expressed in terms of biostability as well as biocompatibility which can be measured through its interaction potential with cellular as well as biological fluids (Fialho & da Silva Cunha, 2005). Different drug delivery systems (DDS) which are composed of discrete medicated fibres, braided, woven, or composite fabrics, or mono or multifilament yarns are all categorized as biotextiles. These biotextile compounds have been modified in different forms to closely resemble the extracellular matrix, interconnective tissues, and perhaps even organs to ensure an efficient DDS either through topical or systemic routes. Over the last 50 years, routes of administration for biotextiles have evolved from systemic to nano-capsulation, implantable devices, and many more from the most common wounds, burns, and dermatosis (Rabin et al., 2008). These biotextile-based DDS promote controlling deliverance, active site or microorganism, sustain local and even raise smart release by local stimuli. They can be administered transdermally or topically, or be implantable. Recently, newly designed electrospun fibres made through the electrospinning technique (which produces up to 100 nanometers diameter fibres) have been developed which entrap the effectively proven therapeutic active compound against microbial infection and restrict microbial colonization and also promote wound healing. The primary, considerable requirement of DDS is to maintain the level of therapeutically active drug for a prolonged duration while still enabling "dosing-on-demand", regarded as an efficient tool (Schlesinger et al., 2016). To achieve desired results in various

DOI: 10.1201/9781003331612-13

biomedical contexts, advanced manufacturing procedures are being developed to build fibrous scaffolds with suitably textured fibre meshes. Indeed, various strategies for incorporating biomolecules into thermoplastic solutions have been optimized, either through direct (like co-axial spinning) or indirect (such as co-spinning) encapsulation (Colaris et al., 2017).

For instance: Polacco et al. designed a fibre loaded with multiple drugs by combining different technologies, i.e. wet spinning as well as nanotechnology. The designed biotextiles were carrying hollow microfibres that were loaded with the nanoparticles containing drug. In order to facilitate the simultaneous release of various types of drugs, the implantable DDS used hollow fibres and nanoparticles synthesized from biodegradable type polymers. After the medications' function was accomplished, biotextiles were removed without surgery (De Witt et al., 2004).

The ease of production, high surface area for drug release, and variety of possible structures are major advantages of drug-loaded fibres. Drug-loaded polymer nanofibres produced by electrospinning have diameters ranging from some nanometers to more than a metre (more commonly 50–500 nm) and have distinctive characteristics such as an extremely high surface area per unit mass (for instance, nanofibres with a diameter of 100 nm have a specific surface of 1000 m^2/g), together with remarkable highly porous, excellent structural mechanical characteristics, high axial strength combined with extreme flexibility, and low basis weight (Nunes-Pereira et al., 2015).

10.2 PRODUCTION OF NANO-BIOTEXTILES: FIBRE TECHNOLOGIES

Currently, a variety of fabrication techniques has been evolved and implemented to turn polymers into fibres. The resulting fibres can be used to make mono- or multifilament yarns that can be divided into various short-staple fibres and bonded with native fibres like cotton or wool, or they can be used by themselves to make scaffolds. The resulting fibres can be used to make mono- or multifilament yarns that can be divided into various short-staple fibres and bonded with native fibres like cotton or wool, or they can be used by themselves to make scaffolds (Shastri, 2003). A few of the technologies to achieve so are mentioned in the following.

10.2.1 Fibre Extrusion Spinning

A specialized form of extrusion known as spinning employs a spinneret to create mono or multiple filaments in a continuous manner. It is considered to be a multidisciplinary method because it brings together concepts from the fields of engineering and materials science. The spinning technique for the production of fibres initially involves the formation of the spinnable and processable form of polymer. Thermoplastic polymers could be transformed into fluid as well as a melted spun form while in a suitable solvent system, other polymers can dissolve or be altered chemically to form soluble or thermoplastic derivatives, and then they can be spun at the nanoscale using wet-spinning, dry-spinning, or electrospinning techniques (Zur et al., 2011; Kumar & Pillai, 2018; Martínez-Rus et al., 2012).

10.2.1.1 Electrospinning

It is defined as a method by which fibrous structures are produced in the range of nanometers (40–2000 nm) by exposing a fluid jet to a strong electric field (Claes & Ignatius, 2002). The traditional method of spinning fibres relies on the idea that a viscous polymer can be extruded under pressure into fibres with diameters ranging from 10 to 500 μm (Tian et al., 2016). The emergence of a viable technique of electrospinning used for the production of nanofibres was previously tracked since when Formhals filed his first patent for a method and apparatus for creating artificial filaments with electric charges in 1934 (Kleiner et al., 2014). A variety of fibres, polymers, and particles can be laced together using this cutting-edge electrospinning technique to create ultra-thin layers. The polymer solution can be added with the insoluble small particles which were encapsulated in the form of dry nano fibres while bacterial agents and soluble drugs can also be added, electrospun, and transformed into new nonwoven mats (Jacob et al., 2018).

The electrospinning technique has received a lot of attention in the field of biomedicine due to the inherent characteristics of the resulting nanofibres such as its high porosity, large surface areas along with continuous three-dimensional web structure (Herrlich et al., 2012; Verma, 2002; Kutz, 2009). In an effort to aid in the regeneration and repair of numerous human tissues and organs, such as the skin, bone, blood vessels, kidneys, and liver, nanofibrous scaffolds have demonstrated great potential as well as effectiveness (Gulati et al., 2016). Schematic drawing of the electrospinning setup is presented in Figure 10.1.

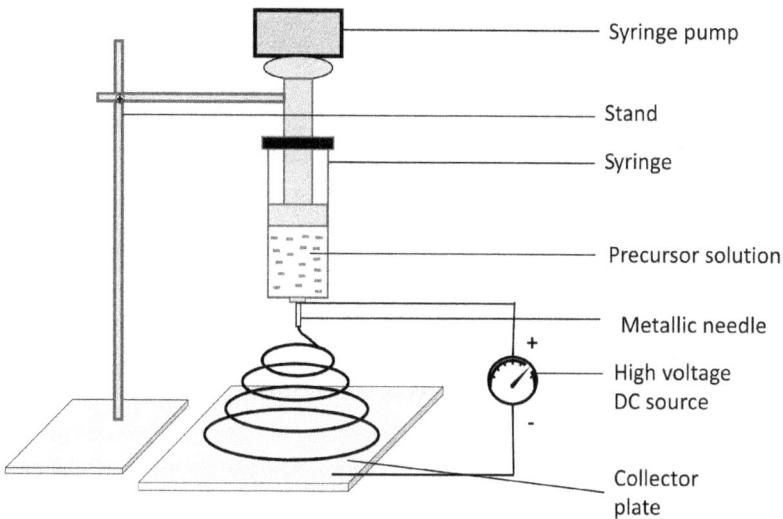

FIGURE 10.1 Electrospinning

10.2.1.2 Wet Spinning

The wet-spinning technique involves the formation of continuous fibres by passing a solution of polymer via syringe through a syringe pump into a coagulation or cross-linking solution which contains a non-solvent and/or a poor solvent (based on the characteristics of polymer). This method allowed the generation of fibrous scaffolds with a variety of morphologies and relatively large pore sizes (250–500 m) with optimum fibre thicknesses (30–600 μm). The development of fibres from a variety of polymers, including natural polymers like chitosan, alginate, silk, collagen, and gelatin along with synthetic polymers like polycaprolactone (PCL) and PEG, could be accomplished using the wet-spinning technique (Pillai & Panchagnula, 2001). Principle and components of wet spinning are shown in Figure 10.2.

Therefore, with the aid of this method, fibres of comparatively large diameters (in the nano- to micrometer ranges) can be created. Also, the generation of architectures with an open-interconnected pore structure along with high porosity could be achieved which are better for cell adhesion, proliferation, and penetration (Fu & Kao, 2010).

10.2.1.3 Dry Spinning

In this method, the polymer is being dissolved in a suitable solvent media and this solution is then forced via a spinneret, which was further passed across a heating column from where solvents get evaporated and leave dry fibres behind (requires highly volatile oil). This method is appropriate for fibres that need specific surface characteristics and for polymers that are susceptible to thermal degradation however

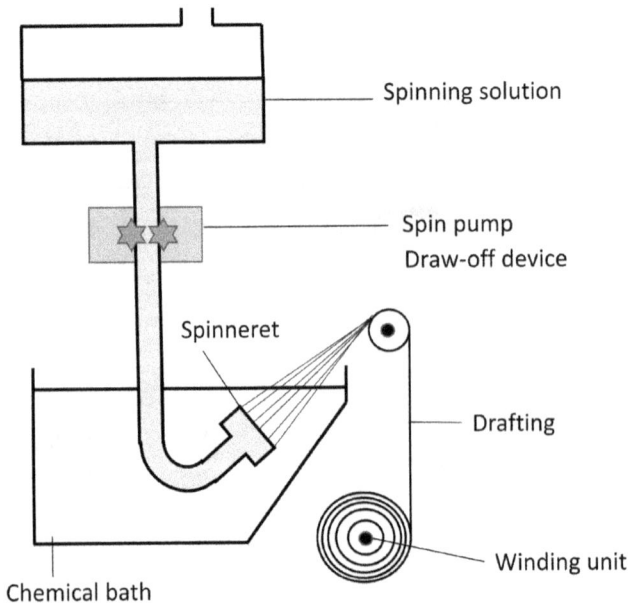

FIGURE 10.2 Principle of wet spinning

cannot form viscous melts. Traditional dry-spinning methods have been used to process a number of polymer fibres, including some variants of acrylics and modacrylics, acetate and triacetate, spandex fibres and aramid fibres (Siepmann & Siepmann, 2008; Lin et al., 1985). For instance, gelatin-loaded nanoparticles (GNPs) carrying bovine serum albumin (BSA) in poly(ε-caprolactone) (PCL) fibres were designed utilizing this dry-spinning technique. Numerous biomedical applications, including surgical sutures, controlled release systems, and bioactive scaffolds for tissue engineering, could be found for such a system (Ulery et al., 2011). A dry-spinning device is shown in Figure 10.3.

10.2.1.4   3D Printing

Within the biomedical and pharmaceutical industries, three-dimensional (3D) printing is a rapidly increasing and expanding technology (Verma et al., 2002). In this technique, materials such as metal, plastic, powders, ceramics, liquids, or living cells are fused or deposited in layers to create a three-dimensional item (Yang et al., 2006; Jerzewski & Chien, 1992; Rao et al., 2001). This methodology is implied by which micro- and nanoparticles can be easily prepared and also customized with desired properties as these particles are further combined with specific functional antibodies

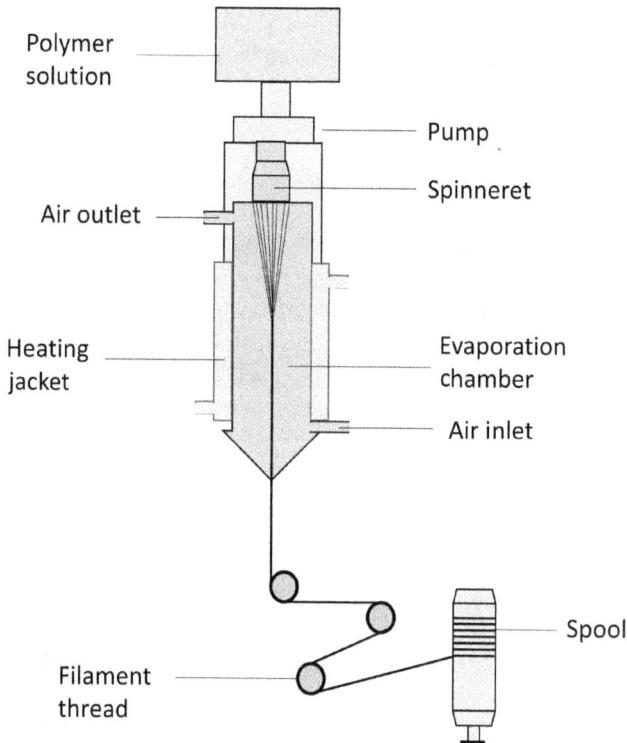

FIGURE 10.3   Dry spinning of cellulose acetate fibres

in a continuously mixed process as per the requirements (Verma et al., 2002). 3D printing enables the synthesis of oral dosage forms with distinct dimensions as well as geometries. The initial component for the process of 3D screen printing was generated for the model of paracetamol (acetaminophen) to ensure controlled release. Therefore, this 3D printing technique ensures the production as well as utilization of different nano-biotextiles in a variety of biomedicals devices such as implants, nanofibres, controlled delivery systems, thermoresponsive hydrogels, nanocapsules, and many others (Santus & Baker, 1995; Verma & Garg, 2004).

10.3 DRUG RELEASING PROPERTIES OF IMPLANTS

Active implants and passive implants are the two primary categories that can be used to describe the broad categories of implantable medication delivery systems. The first category contains the two most common kinds of implants, which are biodegradable and non-biodegradable, respectively. On the other side, active systems rely on energy-dependent processes to govern drug release. This is because active systems are more dynamic. These methods provide the driving power necessary to operate the system. The second category contains a variety of different types of drives, including electromechanical and osmotic pressure gradients (Eckenhoff et al., 1981).

The release profile can be controlled by modifying a variety of parameters, such as the kind of drug and its concentration, the type of polymer, the implant design, and its surface qualities. There are two primary categories that can be applied to passive implants: non-biodegradable and biodegradable system (Thombre et al., 2004).

10.3.1 Non-biodegradable Implantable Systems

Polymers such as silicones, poly(urethanes), and poly(acrylates), or copolymers such as poly (ethylene vinyl acetate) are typically used in the preparation of non-biodegradable implants (Kaushal & Garg, 2003). This category of an implant may take the form of a monolithic or reservoir-type device, shown in Figure 10.4. Implants of the monolithic kind are fabricated using a polymer matrix that has the medication disseminated uniformly throughout it (Li & Jasti, 2006). On the other hand, reservoir-type implants have a densely packed drug core that is surrounded by a membrane that is both permeable and non-biodegradable. The rate of medication release can be controlled by altering factors such as the thickness of the membrane and the drug's permeability through the membrane (Verma & Mishra, 1999).

For the delivery of contraceptives, non-biodegradable implanted drug delivery methods have seen extensive application (Migliaresi & Motta, 2014). Over the course of their existence, these devices maintain their structural integrity and robustness. Accordingly, the most significant disadvantage of non-biodegradable implants is that they have to be removed when the drug load they contain has been used up. Even if the components utilized to make these devices have a high level of biocompatibility over the long term, there is still a possibility that they could result in infections, tissue damage, or cosmetic deformity (Zhu & Yu, 2013). As a consequence of this, once all of the medicine has been released, it is customarily removed so that any negative consequences can be avoided.

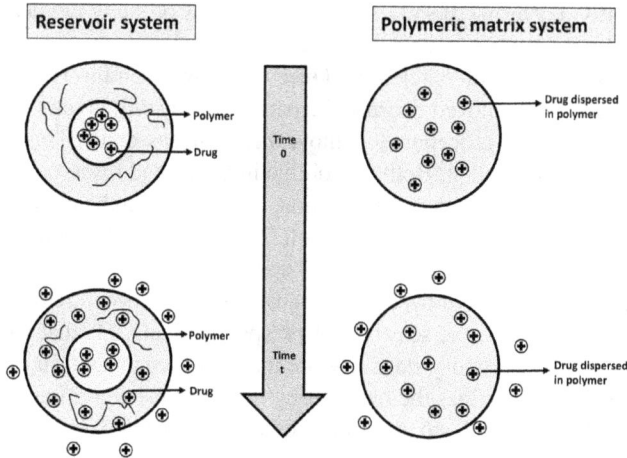

FIGURE 10.4 Reservoir and matrix system showing diffusion of drug across the polymer

Although there are numerous kinds of non-degradable implants that are accessible for purchase, the membrane-enclosed reservoir and matrix-controlled varieties are the ones that are utilized the vast majority of the time (Zhu & Yu, 2013). The primary mechanism of solute transfer for these implants that do not degrade is called passive diffusion.

Reservoir-type devices separate a diffusional barrier polymer membrane from a drug compartment (Gajjar & King, 2014). These processes have the advantage of upholding a constant release rate, which is most likely determined by the thickness and permeability of the rate-controlling polymeric membrane (zero-order release) and is not influenced by concentration gradient (Mirabedini et al., 2016). In matrix-type systems, the drug is uniformly dissolved or dispersed, and half-order drug release corresponds to matrix desorption (Nayak et al., 2010). The drug release in the latter systems is primarily facilitated by Fickian dispersal, which is influenced by the incline of concentration, the distance of diffusion, and the degree of swelling (Nayak & Padhye, 2017). In order to maintain the drug release, these methods offer a gradual diffusion of the medication through the polymeric substance. However, the release from matrix-type systems is exactly proportional to the amount of drug encapsulated within the matrix because the release kinetics of these systems depends on the percentage by volume of the agent present in the matrix (Teixeira et al., 2020).

10.3.2 MATRIX DEGRADATION (BIODEGRADABLE IMPLANTS)

In order to address the limitations posed by non-biodegradable implants, matrix-degradable alternatives have been created. These devices are fabricated utilizing polymers or block copolymers that have the capability of being shattered into smaller fragments, which can then be expelled or absorbed by the body (You et al., 2018). Polymers such as poly (lactic acid) (PLA) poly(caprolactone) (PCL), or poly (lactic-co-glycolic acid) (PLGA) are used in the production process the majority of the time

(Narayan, 2019). There has been a significant amount of study conducted on these materials, and it is simple to adjust their breakdown dynamics in order to change the rate at which the medication is released. Once they have been inserted in the patient, they do not need to be removed because the patient's body will break them down over time. This means that the procedure to remove them is not essential. This is the primary benefit of this kind of implant. Both monolithic implants and reservoir-type implants, which were described in the preceding section, can be used in the manufacturing process to create these devices (Puppi & Chiellini, 2017). The development of this particular kind of gadget is more difficult than the development of non-biodegradable ones, which is one of the device's drawbacks. Because the material will remain in the body after it has been removed, the selection of prospective materials that can be utilized is narrowed, and the regulatory standards are made more stringent. In conclusion, the primary factor that determines the rate of drug release is the deterioration of the polymeric matrix. On the other hand, this varies quite a little from patient to patient. After being implanted in the desired region of the body, the polymer will break down over time, causing the medicine to be released at a rate that has been previously specified. The rate of drug release from a reservoir system can be controlled in one of three ways: by the rate at which the polymer wall degrades; by the rate at which the drug dissolves into the polymer wall; or by a combination of these two factors. Diffusion, swelling, or erosion can be used to control the amount of medicine that is released from a drug-polymer mixture. The drug's capacity to dissolve and pass through the polymer as well as its permeability, the amount of drug loaded onto the system, and the rate at which the polymer degrades in vivo are the factors that will determine how much drug is released from the system (Gupta, 2013).

The degradation of the polymer and the subsequent release of the drug can take place as a result of one or more of the following processes: hydrolysis, which is the process by which bonds in the polymer backbone, such as ester bonds, are broken down; enzyme degradation, which is the process by which hydrolytically vulnerable bonds, such as amide bonds, demonstrate degradation in the presence of a catalyst; and photodegradation, which is the process by which light is absorbed by the polymer and converted into energy. Oxidation and physical deterioration involve the breaking of bonds, either due to chemical reactions, such as oxidation, or physical pressures such as swelling or mechanochemical reactions (Gajjar & King, 2014). The amount of time it takes for polymers to degrade might vary greatly depending on characteristics such as the mass of the polymer and its surface qualities. The release of any medicine that is contained within a formulation will be impacted as a direct result of this. In addition, the rate of disintegration will be determined by elements in the living organism, such as the pH and the temperature (Azimi et al., 2016).

10.3.3 OSMOTIC PUMPING

The most promising strategy-based systems for regulated medication delivery are osmotic devices. Osmosis refers to the process in which water diffuses over a membrane that allows certain molecules to pass through but not others. This movement is driven by a differential in the osmotic pressure on each side of the membrane, arising from variations in solute concentration. This enables the passage of water while obstructing the majority of solute molecules or ions. The development of an optimal regulated medicine delivery system makes use of osmosis as a delivery mechanism. The osmotic pressure that is generated by the osmogene is employed as the driving mechanism for these systems so that the medicine can be released in a regulated manner (Schubert et al., 2014).

These systems are versatile enough to be utilized for either the oral or the implantation mode of delivery. When compared to alternative regulated medication delivery methods, the usage of an osmotic pump has various benefits. These advantages include the ease with which they can be formulated and operated, increased patient compliance with decreased dosing frequency and increased consistency, and a prolonged therapeutic effect with uniform blood concentration (Science & society, 2013).

In most cases, osmotic drug-delivery systems that are designed to be taken orally consist of a compacted tablet core that is covered with a semipermeable membrane coating. This coating has one or more delivery ports that allow for a solution or suspension of the drug to be permitted to be gradually discharged over the course of time. An osmotic agent and a water-swellable polymer are both components of the medication formulation that make up the core of the device. The osmotic pressure that is produced by the components of the core, as well as the permeability of the membrane coating, both have a role in determining the pace at which the core absorbs water. The core engrosses water, which causes it to expand in volume. This causes the drug solution or suspension inside the tablet to be forced out of the tablet through one or more delivery ports (Figure 10.5) (Lipson, 2013).

Osmotic drug delivery systems are distinguished from other techniques used in controlled-release compositions by the fact that the rate at which they release the drug is not affected by the pH or hydrodynamics of the medium through which it is

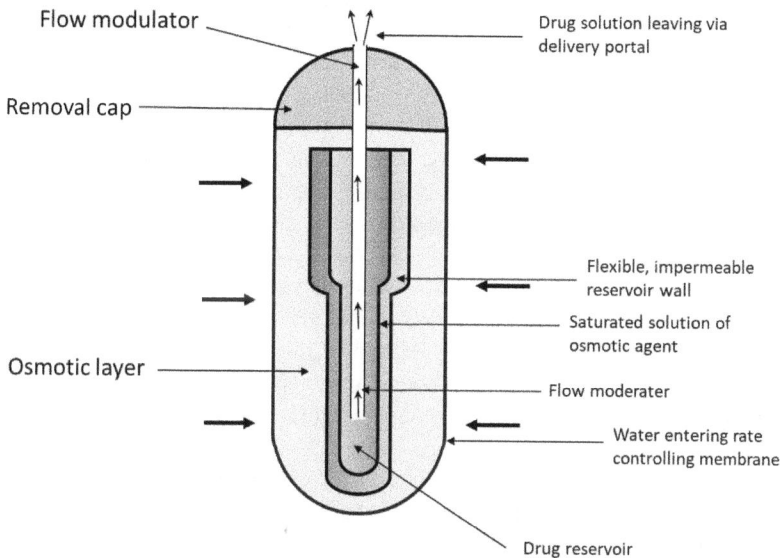

FIGURE 10.5 Illustration of design elements of osmotic pump devices

dissolved in the body (Jain et al., 2021). This is the defining characteristic of osmotic drug delivery systems. The end result is a dependable dosage form for which the rate of medication released *in vitro* is equivalent to the rate *in vivo*, resulting in an outstanding correlation between in vitro and in vivo testing results. One other important benefit of the existing osmotic systems is that they can be utilized with a variety of different medications having varying degrees of aqueous solubility (Ventola, 2014).

10.4   ROLE OF BIOTEXTILES AS NANOFORMULATION

With appropriate biocompatibility along with biodegradability, nanoparticles as well as nanofibres both are useful for applications in drug transport, medicines, and tissue engineering (Boland et al., 2006). Numerous polymers have been electrospun effectively and employed in biomedical applications as nonwoven mats. Biodegradable polycaprolactone (PCL) was employed in electrospinning by Yoshimoto et al., who also determined its potential in reference to bone tissue engineering (Ma et al., 2003). They discovered that the PCL scaffolds offer a setting that promotes the production of mineralized tissue and may be applied to the repair of bone deformities. Other nanofibres, which are electrospun type silk fibroin, have been shown to promote the spreading of type I collagen and better cell adhesion as its 3D structure, high surface area-to-volume ratio, and wide range of pore size distribution-like features support its better adhesion with cells (Hadjiargyrou & Jonathan, 2008). The degummed type silk fibroin which is a nonwoven nanofibre is used in wound dressing and was also found to be advantageous for cell adhesion, growth as well as proliferation and thus found beneficial for wound dressing as well as tissue engineering (Ignatious et al., 2010). Another reported study is by Xie and Hsieh in which they synthesized fibres being loaded with enzyme through the electrospinning approach where a solution carrying PEO/PVA as well as enzyme was used and discovered that the enzyme had improved its reactivity up to six folds (Son et al., 2014).

Many researchers have also studied drug-loaded nanofibre stents due to their membranous nature and ability to build a coating on the surface of traditional stents. In addition to being sprayed directly onto conventional stents, electrospray nanoparticles can also be administered orally, topically, and intravenously (Sridhar et al., 2015). Recent research has resulted in the development of sirolimus-encapsulated PDLLA nanoparticles, which were then deposited onto stents to ensure a sustained biomolecule release (Zhao et al., 2018). They were generated utilizing the traditional emulsion solvent evaporation approach. Studies using fashioned stents in cell culture showed that these could slow the growth of smooth muscle cells while elevating the endothelial cells. This revealed the potential of these modified stents in lowering the incidence of both, i.e. acute thrombosis and in-stent restenosis (Li et al., 2012). A study by Li et al. has submitted a report in which they have synthesized oxygen-releasing fabricated core-shell microparticles through electrospraying which were used along with cardiosphere (being derived from cells) as well as poly(hydroxyethyl methacrylate/oligo-hydroxybutyrate) made thermosensitive hydrogels used for cardiac regeneration (Jayasinghe, 2011).

The establishment of cell electrospinning (i.e., electrospinning/electrospraying of living cells into a biopolymer matrix) is an exciting method that could potentially increase the biomedical value of electrospun nanofibres (Jayasinghe, 2013). Recently, in a study, human blood was electrosprayed to test the viability of electrospinning or electrospraying for biomedical uses (Mongkoldhumrongkul et al., 2009). Along with these applications, drug release in a controlled manner would also be a positive aspect of electrospinning. For example, Norouzi et al. electrospun PLGA and gelatin nanofibres to achieve the desired bioactivity with hemostasis of the fibrous scaffolds in a regulated protein release manner (Norouzi et al., 2015a). An epidermal growth factor (EGF) loaded PLGA nanofibre has also been electrospun producing appropriate bioactive as well as biocompatible scaffolds with controlled EGF release (Norouzi et al., 2015b).

The human nervous system is an intricate network of neurons that lacks its own regenerative property. Therefore, it's a need for the restoration of neurons' functionality using biological or synthetic tools. To ensure the successful generation of a nano-fibrous porous scaffold using poly(L-lactic acid) PLLA for supporting nerve stem cell differentiation and neurite outgrowth, illustrating their ability as cell carriers in nerve tissue engineering (Yang et al., 2004). Also, by using straightforward plasma treatment, Prabhakaran et al. modified the surface of constructed PCL nanofibres. Several studies have shown that nanofibrous scaffolds made of PCL and gelatin have been reported to aid neurite outgrowth and improve neuronal differentiation as well as proliferation. One more time, the alignment of the nanofibres was followed by nerve cell elongation, demonstrating the appropriateness of this biocomposite for nerve regeneration (Ghasemi-Mobarakeh et al., 2008).

REFERENCES

Azimi, B., et al. (2016). Application of the dry-spinning method to produce poly (ε-caprolactone) fibers containing bovine serum albumin laden gelatin nanoparticles. *Journal of Applied Polymer Science*, 133, 48.

Boland, E.D., Pawlowski, K.J., Bowlin, Barnes, C.P., Simpson, D.G., Bowlin, G.L., et al. (2006). Electro spinning of bioresorable polymers for tissue engineering scaffolds. *Polym Nanofibers*, 188–204.

Claes, L., Ignatius, A. (2002). Development of new, biodegradable implants. *Chirurg*, 73, 990–996.

Colaris, M.J.L., de Boer, M., van der Hulst, R.R., Cohen Tervaert, J.W. (2017). Two hundreds cases of ASIA syndrome following silicone implants: A comparative study of 30 years and a review of current literature. *Immunol. Res.*, 65, 120–128.

Dash, A., Cudworth G. (1998). Therapeutic applications of implantable drug delivery systems. *J. Pharmacol. Toxicol. Methods*, 40, 1–12.

De Witt, D., Finley, M., Lawin, L., Dewitt, D.M., Finley, M.J.L., Laurie, R. (2004). A blends comprising ethylene-vinyl acetate copolymer and poly (alkyl (meth) acrylates or poly (aromatic (meth) acrylates); implantable medical device; permit stents releasing the bioactive agent over time in vivo; provide clear coats, durability, biocompatibility, and release kinetic. *Drug Delivey Device*. Application No. 11/099,997. U.S. Patent.

Eckenhoff, B., Theeuwes, F., Urquhart, J. (1981). Osmotically actuated dosage forms for rate-controlled drug delivery. *Pharmaceutical Technology*, 5(1), 35–44.

Fialho, S.L., da Silva Cunha, A. (2005). Manufacturing techniques of biodegradable implants intended for intraocular application. *Drug Deliv.*, 12, 109–116.

Fu, Y., Kao, W.J. (2010). Drug release kinetics and transport mechanisms of non-degradable and degradable polymeric delivery systems. *Expert Opin. Drug Deliv.*, 7, 429–444.

Gajjar, C.R., King, M.W. (2014). Biotextiles: Fiber to fabric for medical applications. In *Resorbable Fiber-Forming Polymers for Biotextile Applications* (pp. 11–22). Basel, Switzerland: Springer.

Ghasemi-Mobarakeh, L., Prabhakaran, M.P., Morshed, M., Nasr-Esfahani, M.-H., Ramakrishna, S. (2008). Electrospun poly (ε-caprolactone)/gelatinnanofibrous scaffolds for nerve tissue engineering. *Biomaterials*, 29, 4532–4539.

Gulati, K., Kogawa, M., Prideaux, M., Findlay, D.M., Atkins, G.J., Losic, D. (2016). Drug-releasing nano-engineered titanium implants: Therapeutic efficacy in 3D cell culture model, controlled release and stability. *Mater. Sci. Eng. C*, 69, 831–840.

Gupta, B.S. (2013). Manufacture, types and properties of biotextiles for medical applications. In M.W. King, B.S. Gupta, R. Guidoin, (Eds.). *Biotextiles As Medical Implants* (pp. 3–47). Cambridge, UK: Woodhead Publishing.

Hadjiargyrou, M., Jonathan B.C. (2008). Enhanced composite electrospunnanofiber scaffolds for use in drug delivery. *Expert Opinion on Drug Delivery*, 5(10), 1093–1106.

Herrlich, S., Spieth, S., Messner, S., Zengerle, R. (2012). Osmotic micropumps for drug delivery. *Adv. Drug Deliv. Rev.*, 64, 1617–1627.

Ignatious, F., et al. (2010). Electrospunnanofibers in oral drug delivery. *Pharmaceutical Research*, 27(4), 576–588.

Jacob, J., Haponiuk, J.T., Thomas, S., Gopi, S. (2018). Biopolymer based nanomaterials in drug delivery systems: A review. *Mater. Today Chem.*, 9, 43–55.

Jain, K., et al. (2021). 3D printing in development of nanomedicines. *Nanomaterials*, 11(2), 420.

Jayasinghe, S.N. (2011). Bio-electrosprays: From bio-analytics to a generic tool for the health sciences. *Analyst*, 136(5), 878–890.

Jayasinghe, S.N. (2013). Cell electrospinning: A novel tool for functionalising fibres, scaffolds and membranes with living cells and other advanced materials for regenerative biology and medicine. *Analyst*, 138(8), 2215–2223.

Jerzewski, R., Chien, Y. (1992). Treatise on controlled drug delivery: Fundamentals, optimization, application: Marcel Dekker. *Osmotic drug delivery*, 225–253.

Kaushal, A.M., Garg, S. (2003). An update on osmotic drug delivery patents. *Pharmaceutical Technology*, 38–44.

Kleiner, L.W., Wright, J.C., Wang, Y. (2014). Evolution of implantable and insertable drug delivery systems. *J. Control. Release*, 181, 1–10.

Kumar, A., Pillai, J. (2018). Implantable drug delivery systems. In A.M. Grumzescu (Ed.), *Nanostructures for the Engineering of Cells, Tissues and Organs* (pp. 473–511). Amsterdam, Netherlands: Elsevier.

Kutz, M. (2009). *Biomedical Engineering and Design Handbook*. New York, NY: McGraw-Hill.

Li, X., Jasti, B.R. (2006). Osmotic controlled drug delivery systems. In X. Li, B.R. Jasti (Eds.), *Design of Controlled Release of Drug Delivery Systems* (pp. 203–229). New York, NY: McGraw Hill.

Li, Z., Guo, X., Guan, J. (2012). An oxygen release system to augment cardiac progenitor cell survival and differentiation under hypoxic condition. *Biomaterials*, 33(25), 5914–5923.

Lin, S.B., Hwang, K.S., Tsay, S.Y., Cooper, S.L. (1985). Segmental orientation studies of polyether polyurethane block copolymers with different hard segment lengths and distributions. *Colloid Polym. Sci.*, 263, 128–140.

Lipson, H. (2013). New world of 3-D printing offers "completely new ways of thinking:" Q & A with author, engineer, and 3-D printing expert Hod Lipson. *IEEE Pulse*, 4(6), 12–14.

Ma, H., Zeng, J., Realff, M.L., et al. (2003). Processing, structure, and properties of fibers from polyester/carbon nanofiber composites. *Composites Sci. Technol.*, 63, 1617.

Martínez-Rus, F., Ferreiroa, A., Özcan, M., Bartolomé, J.F., Pradíes, G. (2012). Fracture resistance of crowns cemented on titanium and zirconia implant abutments: A comparison of monolithic versus manually veneered all-ceramic systems. *Int. J. Oral Maxillofac. Implants*, 27, 1448–1455.

Migliaresi, C., Motta, A. (2014). *Scaffolds for Tissue Engineering: Biological Design, Materials, and Fabrication*. Singapore: Jenny Stanford Publishing.

Mirabedini, A., Foroughi, J., Wallace, G.G. (2016). Developments in conducting polymer fibres: From established spinning methods toward advanced applications. *RSC Adv.*, 6, 44687–44716.

Mongkoldhumrongkul, N., Best, S., Aarons, E., Jayasinghe, S.N. (2009). Bio-electrospraying whole human blood: Analyzing cellular viability at a molecular level. *J. Tissue Eng. Regener. Med.*, 3, 562–566.

Narayan, R. (2019). *Encyclopedia of Biomedical Engineering* (pp. 330–344). Oxford, UK: Elsevier.

Nayak, R., Padhye, R. (2017). Nano fibres by electro spinning: Properties and applications. *J. Text. Eng. Fash. Technol*, 2(5), 486–497.

Nayak, R., Padhye, R., Lyndon, A. (2010). Recent advancements in electro spinning process. *Melliand International*, 9(3), 17–18.

Norouzi, M., Shabani, I., Ahvaz, H.H., Soleimani, M. (2015a). PLGA/gelatin hybrid nanofibrous scaffolds encapsulating EGF for skin regeneration. *J. Biomed. Mater. Res. A*, 103, 2225–2235.

Norouzi, M., Shabani, I., Atyabi, F., Soleimani, M. (2015b). EGF-loaded nanofibrous scaffold for skin tissue engineering applications. *Fiber Polym.*, 16, 782–787.

Nunes-Pereira, J., Ribeiro, S., Ribeiro, C., Gombek, C.J., Gama, F.M., Gomes, A.C., Patterson D.A., Lanceros-Méndez, S. (2015). Poly(vinylidene fluoride) and copolymers as porous membranes for tissue engineering applications. *Polym. Test*, 44, 234–241.

Pillai, O., Panchagnula, R. (2001). Polymers in drug delivery. *Curr. Opin. Chem. Biol.*, 5, 447–451.

Puppi, D., Chiellini, F. (2017). Wet-spinning of biomedical polymers: From single-fibre production to additive manufacturing of three-dimensional scaffolds. *Polym. Int.*, 66, 1690–1696.

Rabin, C., Liang, Y., Ehrlichman, R.S., Budhian, A., Metzger, K.L., Majewski-Tiedeken, C., Winey, K.I., Siegel, S.J. (2008). In vitro and in vivo demonstration of risperidone implants in mice. *Schizophr. Res.*, 98, 66–78.

Rao, B.S., Kumar, N.R., Madhuri, K., Narayan, P.S., Murthy, K.V.R. (2001). Osmotic drug delivery systems. *The Eastern Pharmacist*, 521, 21–28.

Santus, G., Baker, R.W. (1995). Osmotic drug delivery: A review of the patent literature. *Journal of Controlled Release*, 35(1), 1–21.

Schlesinger, E., Johengen, D., Luecke, E., Rothrock, G., McGowan, I., Van der Straten, A., Desai, T., Tunable, A. (2016). Biodegradable, thin-film polymer device as a long-acting implant delivering tenofovir alafenamide fumarate for HIV pre-exposure prophylaxis. *Pharm. Res.*, 33, 1649–1656.

Schubert, C., van Langeveld, M.C., Donoso, L.A. (2014). Innovations in 3D printing: A 3D overview from optics to organs. *Br J Ophthalmol.*, 98(2), 159–161.

Science and Society. (2013). Experts warn against bans on 3Dprinting. *Science*, 342(6157), 439.

Shastri, V.P. (2003). Non-degradable biocompatible polymers in medicine: Past, present and future. *Curr. Pharm. Biotechnol.*, 4, 331–337.

Siepmann, J., Siepmann, F. (2008). Mathematical modeling of drug delivery. *Int. J. Pharm*, 364, 328–343.

Son, Y.J., Kim, W.J., Yoo, H.S. (2014). Therapeutic applications of electrospun nanofibers for drug delivery systems. *Archives of Pharmacal Research*, 37(1) 69–78.

Sridhar, R., et al. (2015). Electrosprayed nanoparticles and electrospun nanofibers based on natural materials: Applications in tissue regeneration, drug delivery and pharmaceuticals. *Chemical Society Reviews*, 44(3), 790–814.

Teixeira, M.A., Amorim, M.T.P., Felgueiras, H.P. (2020). Poly (vinyl alcohol)-based nanofibrous electrospun scaffolds for tissue engineering applications. *Polymers*, 12, 7.

Thombre, A.G., Appel, L.E., Chidlaw, M.B., et al. (2004). Osmotic drug delivery using swellable-core technology. *Journal of Controlled Release*, 94(1), 75–89.

Tian, W., Mahmoudi, M., Lhermusier, T., Kiramijyan, S., Chen, F., Torguson, R., Suddath, W.O., Satler, L.F., Pichard, A.D., Waksman, R. (2016). The influence of advancing age on implantation of drug-eluting stents. *Catheter. Cardiovasc. Interv.*, 88, 516–521.

Ulery, B.D., Nair, L.S., Laurencin, C.T. (2011). Biomedical applications of biodegradable polymers. *J. Polym. Sci. Part B Polym. Phys.*, 49, 832–864.

Ventola, C.L. (2014). Medical applications for 3D printing: Current and projected uses. *Pharmacy and Therapeutics*, 39(10), 704.

Verma, R.K. (2002). Formulation aspects in the development of osmotically controlled oral drug delivery systems. *J. Control. Release*, 79, 7–27.

Verma, R.K., Garg, S. (2004). Development and evaluation of osmotically controlled oral drug delivery system of glipizide. *European Journal of Pharmaceutics and Biopharmaceutics*, 57(3), 513–532.

Verma, R.K., Krishna, D.M., Garg, S. (2002). Formulation aspects in the development of osmotically controlled oral drug delivery systems. *Journal of Controlled Release*, 79(1–3), 7–27.

Verma, R.K., Mishra, B. (1999). Studies on formulation and evaluation of oral osmotic pumps of nimesulide. *Pharmazie*, 54(1), 74–75.

Yang, F., Murugan, R., Ramakrishna, S., Wang, X., Ma, Y.-X., Wang, S. (2004). Fabrication of nano-structured porous PLLA scaffold intended for nerve tissue engineering. *Biomaterials*, 25, 1891–1900.

Yang, X.G., Zhang, G.H., Li, W., Peng, B., Liu, Z.D., Pan, W.S. (2006). Design and evaluation of jingzhiguanxin monolithic osmotic pump tablet. *Chem Pharm Bull (Tokyo)*, 54(4), 465–469.

You, M.-H., Wang, X.-X., Yan, X., Zhang, J., Song, W.-Z., Yu, M., Fan, Z.-Y., Ramakrishna, S., Long, Y.-Z. (2018). A self-powered flexible hybrid piezoelectric—Pyroelectricnanogenerator based on non-woven nanofiber membranes. *J. Mater. Chem. A*, 6, 3500–3509.

Zhao, J., Mo, Z., Guo, F., Shi, D., Han, Q.Q., Liu, Q. (2018). Drug loaded nanoparticle coating on totally bioresorbable PLLA stents to prevent in-stent restenosis. *J. Biomed. Mater. Res. B.*, 106, 88–95.

Zhu, L.-M., Yu, D.G. (2013). Drug delivery systems using biotextiles. *Biotextiles as Medical Implants*, 213–231.

Zur, G., Linder-Ganz, E., Elsner, J.J., Shani, J., Brenner, O., Agar, G., Hershman, E.B., Arnoczky, S.P., Guilak, F., Shterling, A. (2011). Chondroprotective effects of a polycarbonate-urethane meniscal implant: Histopathological results in a sheep model. *Knee Surg. Sports Traumatol. Arthrosc.*, 19, 255–263.

11 A Critique

Advancement and Applications of Surgical Sutures in Medical Implants

Shovan Ghosh, Vivek Dave,
Prashansa Sharma, and Pranay Wal

11.1 INTRODUCTION

Sutures, which look like threads and provide tissue strength, blood vessel compression, natural healing, and other benefits, are one of the most commonly implanted devices in humans. They can be used in muscle, organs, vessels, skin, and bone for the purpose of skin wound closure; different surgeries like vascular, ocular, and neuro; plastic surgery; surgery of the musculoskeletal system; intestinal anastomoses; etc. The ideal suture should be able to maintain a suitable level of strength during the healing process as well as extend to accommodate wounds that have dropped and shrunk back to their former size as a result of retraction of the wound. After the injury has completely recovered, the foreign body might be absorbed and destroyed by the body on its own, leaving no trace. Sutures are commonly treated for non-carcinogenicity, reduced inflammation, and minimal irritation through processes such as dye application, sterilization, and other appropriate treatments. Ideal sutures can tie a secure, solid knot, which is easy to create, inexpensive, and capable of mass production (Gierek et al., 2018; Pacer et al., 2020).

Sutures are specialized threads that are used in the medical field to control bleeding during surgical procedures. They are capable of holding the tissues that surround the wound together or constricting the blood vessels in order to achieve hemostasis. This wound repair device utilized in connective tissue (skin, bone, tendon, cartilage, and muscle) must be highly elastic and flexible (Lekic & Dodds, 2022). Ideal sutures produce a very minimal toxic or allergic response and provide a wound-healing environment. As a result, a surgical suture is considered optimal for use in medical practice if it has qualities such as ease of handling, minimal tissue reaction, ease of sterilization, lack of support for bacterial growth, sufficient tensile strength, non-carcinogenicity, and so on (Balaji, 2013; Pillai & Sharma, 2010).

11.1.1 HISTORY

The term "suture" is derived from the Latin sutura, "a sewn seam." Techniques for suturing have been used for more than 4,000 years. They have been utilized for wound healing and closure since the beginning of time. Ancient Egypt and India were the birthplaces of sutures, where natural fiber materials like cotton, silk, and grass were combined with animal tissue and hair. Suture use in surgery was initially documented in prehistoric Egypt around 3000 BC, but the first example of suturing ever found was in a mummy that dated back to roughly 1100 BC. Sushruta, an Indian philosopher and healer, wrote a detailed description of the materials used in the process of suturing on different wounds in 500 BC. Suture processes were described by Hippocrates, the Greek father of medicine, and later Roman Aulus Cornelius Celsus. Galen, a 2nd-century Roman physician, introduced suturing through catgut around 175 CE. Until the 20th century, silk, cotton, and catgut were commonly used as suturing materials, but after the 1930s, acceptance of synthetic materials increased, and materials like polypropylene, polyethylene terephthalate, and nylon are commonly used (Pillai & Sharma, 2010; Muffly et al., 2011; Balaji, 2013). Non-resorbable sutures were first proposed in the 1940s, and polyglycolic acid was first introduced as a resorbable suture in the 1960s.

For improving infection resistance in sutures, Lord Joseph Lister promoted sterilizing all suture threads. He initially began sterilizing products in the 1860s with "carbolic catgut," and two decades later, he sterilized them with chromic acid. Lord Moynihan discovered "chromic" catgut to be perfect due to its non-irritating qualities, twice the tensile strength of catgut, and its ability to be sterilized. Finally, sterilization through iodine treatment became the standard method in 1902 under Claudius.

11.2 PROPERTIES OF SUTURES

The performance of any suture is determined by the properties of the suture material, though single suture materials are insufficient to meet those requirements. Suture material performance is determined by its mechanical, physical, handling, biological, and biodegradation properties. These materials must be sterile, nonallergenic, noncarcinogenic, nonferromagnetic, and have viscoelasticity, among other essential properties, and their function is dependent on those properties, such as the bacteria-transport ability of sutures, which is based on capillarity, and handling properties such as pliability, which is based on modulus of elasticity. The four essential properties of sutures are described in Table 11.1.

11.2.1 MECHANICAL AND PHYSICAL PROPERTIES

This is the most essential quality required for suture function which includes following.

11.2.1.1 Tensile Strength

The most commonly used calculation to find out the physical and mechanical properties of sutures, as described by the US Pharmacopeia, is the weight required to break a suture divided by the suture's cross-sectional area. Tensile strength plays an essential role in wound healing rate and in fulfilling other clinical needs and specific purposes. Both wet and dry sutures can be used for measuring tensile strength, but the tensile strength of wet sutures is prominent because of their implantation into

TABLE 11.1
Properties of surgical sutures

Mechanical and physical properties	• Tensile strength
	• Elasticity
	• Knot strength and security
	• Elasticity
	• Plasticity
	• Capillarity
	• Swelling
	• Stiffness
	• Stress relaxation and creep
Biocompatibility	• Carcinogenicity
	• Calculi formation
	• Inflammatory reaction propensity
	• Allergy
Biodegradation	• Biocompatibility of degradation products
	• Tensile breaking strength and mass loss profile
Handling	• Knot security
	• Knot slippage
	• Pliability
	• Tissue drag

tissue and inner organs filled with extracellular fluid. Effective tensile strength is another parameter that changes with suture materials and knot and is used for the evaluation of the tensile strength of looped and knotted sutures (Khiste et al., 2013; Dart & Dart, 2011).

11.2.1.2   Knot Strength and Security

This is one of the most reliable components of any suture. Knot security describes secure holding and safety. Knot strength and coefficient of friction are directly proportional to each other; they can be measured by counting the force required to break or slip a knot. The friction between the knots determines how they are tied. A suture with a high coefficient of friction provides good knot security, but its abrasiveness causes unwanted resistance when pulling with tissue.

Knot efficiency depends on intrinsic and extrinsic factors in sutures: extrinsic factors like knot type, number of throws in knots, size of suture, applied tension, etc.; and intrinsic factors like coefficient of friction, chemical composition, physical configuration, and surface treatment of sutures.

11.2.1.3   Plasticity and Elasticity

Those are closely interrelated. Because of elasticity, sutures come back to their original length after the reduction of edema and maintained proper holding. This desirable property allows for proper stretching and tissue apposition so that sutures can hold swollen tissue without damaging its structure or preventing proper healing. Plasticity is the property due to which suture material cannot be stretched back to its original length when edema subsides.

11.2.1.4 Coefficient of Friction

Friction is the resistance created by sutures. The coefficient of friction has to be measured in a suture to know the amount of trauma it creates when it passes through a tissue. Smooth sutures pass through the skin more easily and cause less trauma than rough ones; they are especially important for delicate tissue.

11.2.2 HANDLING CHARACTERISTIC

These properties are interconnected with mechanical properties and are related to surgeons' feelings and experiences while suturing. Sutures are characterized by their pliability, ease of knotting, tissue drag, surface friction, knot security, viscoelasticity, and package memory. There is a direct or indirect connection between the mechanical, physical, and surface aspects.

11.2.2.1 Bending Stiffness

This property is related to the handling characteristic of sutures, which comes from the modulus of elasticity, which was further acquired from the tensile test as well. Stiffness depends on knots and modules of elasticity. Research shows that non-coated sutures have less stiffness than coated ones, and braided sutures are more fixable than monofilament. Suture mobility may be reduced as a result of coating due to an increase in binding force. Binding stiffness also depends proportionally on the size of the suture and the chemical structure that expresses the increase in magnitude.

11.2.2.2 Suture Compliance

This mechanical property is based on the elongation of sutures under tensile force. It is very useful in cases of surgery where tubular anastomosis is present, like a vascular graft, and it also creates a compliance mismatch at the anastomotic site.

11.2.2.3 Packaging Memory

The gentleness of sutures depends upon this handling property, which can easily be calculated by taking note of the amount of time required to get a kink out of sutures dangling in the air. Suture knotting is dependent on packaging memory; a high packaging memory makes handling properties and knotting difficult. Sutures with a high packaging memory tend to return as kinks in the knot, so use them sparingly. Braided sutures have lower packaging memory than monofilament sutures in general (exceptions: Biosyn, Monocryl, Gore-Tex).

11.2.2.4 Knot Security and Tie-Down

This is related to the mechanical and surface properties of sutures; this property talks about the slipping tendency of the suture knot. Sutures with a rough surface show lower knot tie-down (uncoated braided) than sutures with a smooth surface, like coated braided or monofilament sutures.

This handling property is affected by another physical property, the coefficient of friction, which has a relationship that is linear with regard to knot security. Sutures with a high coefficient of friction display better knot security because they produce additional frictional force but hamper the knot tie-down process.

11.2.3 BIOLOGICAL CHARACTERISTIC

Sutures immediately cause an inflammatory reaction since they are foreign substances in the body. The suture's composition, design, and size, as well as its stiffness and tension in place, all affect the severity and length of this reaction. The anatomical setting in which it is located within the human body also has a crucial influence on determining the pH and enzymatic activity (King et al., 2013).

The term "biocompatibility of suture materials" refers to the relationship between the qualities of sutures, which are foreign to the body, and the surrounding tissues. The concept of biocompatibility works in both directions. In absorbable sutures, the degree to which sutures cause a response in the tissue is primarily determined by breakdown products and chemical composition. Synthetic sutures elicit a less intense tissue reaction than natural sutures (silk, catgut) due to their enzymatic activity. Different degrees of tissue reactivity have been attributed not only to chemical considerations but also to the suture materials' physical characteristics, such as their shape, quantity, and stiffness. A knot formed by cutting a strong suture, for instance, would have protruding ends that were equally stiff. Monofilament sutures, rather than braided multifilament sutures, manifest stiff ends that might cause mechanical irritation to the surrounding tissues. A modest drop in diameter leads to a substantial reduction in buried suture volume; hence, a smaller suture that supports wounds and doesn't cut tissue is desired. The basic characteristics for determining biocompatibility of suture materials are cellular response and enzyme histochemistry. The concepts of enzymatic histo-chemistry state the involvement of enzymatic activity with exogenous material, which can be determined by cryostat sectioning and microscopic photometry. This process is more consistent, quantitative, and reproducible than the cellular technique, making it useful for biodegradation studies of absorbable sutures, though it requires more resources, time, and experience to perform. The tissue reaction to sutures differs depending on the type of suture and the stage of healing: polymorphonuclear leucocyte infiltration was involved in the first stage, then an acute response was developed by lymphocytes and monocytes for the next three to four days, fibroblasts and macrophages from four to seven days, and fibrous connective tissue formed with chronic inflammation between seven and 10 days.

11.2.4 DEGRADATION CHARACTERISTIC

Absorbable sutures should have biodegradation and absorption properties. The presence of those features in absorbable sutures reduces the production of chronic inflammation as occurs in non-absorbable sutures, and the rate of absorption also alters the degree of scar formation. Biocompatibility, strength, and mass loss are the most crucial aspects of absorbable sutures with regards to absorption and biodegradation. Mass loss of absorbable sutures is a slower process than strength reduction, so after the complete loss of suture strength, some amount of suture mass is still present in the tissue. We didn't see a parallel profile between mass loss and strength loss in ideal sutures, which we expected. This profile varies due to different intrinsic and extrinsic factors like stress, pH, temperature, type of tissue, microorganisms, electrolytes, etc., along with chemical factors (Dennis et al., 2016).

Absorbable sutures undergo natural degradation over a certain time, making their biodegradation profile significant. Conversely, non-absorbable sutures require removal post-recovery, often accompanied by noticeable inflammatory reactions. The rate of absorption of absorbable sutures has been discovered to be proportional to the degree of scar development (Dennis et al., 2016). Furthermore, the absorption process varies among different types of absorbable sutures. An ideal absorbable suture should exhibit a similarity between the profile of mass and strength loss. However, the majority of marketed sutures are not able to fulfill these criteria, many demonstrate a quicker strength loss than mass loss.

11.3 CLASSIFICATION OF SUTURES

11.3.1 Suture Classification According to Degradation

According to the way of degradation or the way of strength loss inside the body, sutures are divided into two categories: absorbable and non-absorbable are shown in Figure 11.1.

11.3.1.1 Absorbable Sutures

After implantation, these sutures break down and decompose, either as a result of enzyme breakdown and subsequent hydrolysis or simple hydrolysis on its own. During the crucial wound healing time or in areas where removal is challenging, absorbable sutures are typically utilized for temporary deep tissue repair (Pillai &

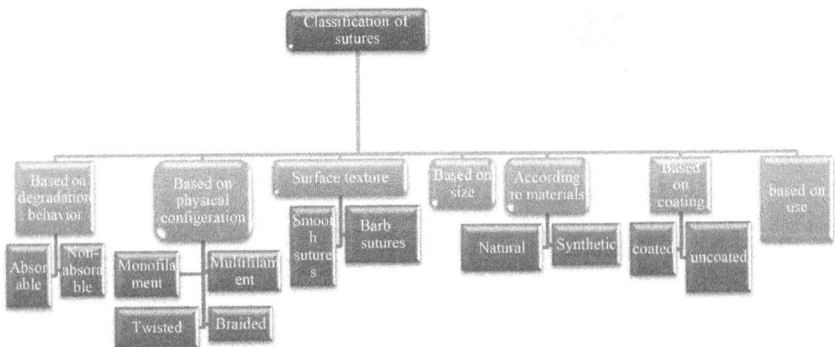

FIGURE 11.1   Classification of sutures

Sharma, 2010). If they are used topically, they might result in more inflammation and scarring. If absorbable sutures are to be applied superficially, a rapid-absorbing suture is advised. However, it is important to keep in mind that more recent absorbable sutures could last for a long time.

They further classify as natural and synthetic absorbable sutures. Sutures made of natural materials degrade primarily through enzymatic action, whereas those made of synthetic materials are absorbed through hydrolysis. When water permeates the suture strands, the polymer structure of the filament is broken down, a process known as hydrolysis. Treatments and chemical structuring, which extend absorption time, have helped to maintain the equilibrium between quick absorption and the extension of tensile strength.

Normal absorbable suture wound closure results in a progressive, linear decline in tensile strength throughout the first few weeks. A leukocyte cellular response is mounted at this time to clear away physical suture material and cell debris. This phase overlaps with the second stage, during which the majority of the suture mass is removed. Infection and protein deprivation can have an impact on either of these stages, causing tensile strength to deteriorate too quickly and clinically evident wound dehiscence. Compared to the enzymatic breakdown process, hydrolysis causes a lower level of tissue response. Benefits of the absorbable suture are speedy re-epithelization, maximal tensile strength during the early phases of healing, low scar development with rapid absorbable sutures, and reduced risk of infection with mono-filament synthetic absorbable sutures. They are also beneficial for short-term utilization and in anatomical positions where removal of sutures is difficult. The absorbable suture materials are as follows:

11.3.1.1.1 Surgical Gut

These are pure connective tissue-based, natural absorbable multifilament sutures that are made from either the serosal layer of bovine intestines or the submucosa of sheep intestines. Sutures are made by twisting together strands of collagen that have been mostly purified. Surgical gut was formerly a standard in surgery but has since lost favor since its tensile strength and knot security are inferior to more modern synthetic suture materials. Due to the possibility of contracting bovine spongiform encephalitis, it is no longer used in Europe. Surgical gut is available in a wide range of styles, including plain, chromic, and quick absorption. Despite the fact that collagen is a major component, surgical gut causes some inflammation. This inflammatory response is presumably brought on by a variety of muscle fibers and mucoproteins present in the surgical gut. By combining enzymatic breakdown and phagocytosis, it disintegrates quickly (Scott Taylor & Shalaby, 2013).

11.3.1.1.2 Polyglycolic Acid

This is the first created absorbable synthetic, also known as Dexon and Dexon II, and is composed of a glycolic (hydroacetic) homopolymer (Scott Taylor & Shalaby, 2013). In its initial stage, it is stronger than suture gut but has less tensile strength than other synthetic sutures. At seven days, it still has 89% of its tensile strength, but in 14 and 21 days, it retains just 63% and 17%, respectively, and 90–120 days later, it has lost all of it (Dart & Dart, 2011).

11.3.1.1.3   Vicrylpolyglactin 910 (Coated Vicoatedvicryl Vicryl Rapide, and Coated Vicryl Plus)

This synthetic absorbable suture material is called polyglactin 910, and it is a copolymer made up of 10% L-lactide and 90% glycolide. The first synthetic absorbable suture to be created was called Dexon, and the second was polyglycolic acid (Munton et al., 1974).

Coated Vicryl is braided sutures coated with calcium stearate, and ethylene oxide sterilizes Vicryl. Both transparent and colored varieties are available. Many of Vicryl's traits resemble those of Dexon. Although it is just slightly stronger than Dexon, the initial tensile strength of this material is greater than that of surgical gut (Dart & Dart, 2011). Clinically, this difference is not substantial. At two weeks, Vicyl still contained 50–65% tensile strength, but it was completely gone in three weeks (Dart & Dart, 2011). It only slightly increases the inflammatory response, taking 60 to 90 days for hydrolysis to reach full absorption. Because of its outstanding handling qualities and strength-to-size ratio, it is applicable to a wide variety of tissues, including infected wounds, among others (Gómez-Alonso et al., 2007).

The antibacterial triclosan is coated on Coated Vicryl Plus, the purpose of which is to prevent germs from colonizing the braided suture and to minimize the discomfort caused by subclinical infection (Dart & Dart, 2011). Because of its antimicrobial characteristics, which lessen the effects of pain on infants, it is frequently utilized in pediatric surgery.

Vicryl Rapide is an absorbable synthetic multifilament suture that is produced from partly hydrolyzed polyglactin 910. This gamma-sterilized synthetic material shows a higher rate of absorption. About 66% of the original tensile strength of coated Vicryl is possessed by this material. It has a substantially higher rate of tensile strength loss than Vicryl does, and it is used in the oral cavity since it flakes away after seven to 10 days. By seven to 14 days, the body's other tissues begin to lose their strength, and after 21 days, absorption is complete (Dart & Dart, 2011).

11.3.1.1.4   Caprosyn

To create caprosyn, a synthetic polyester called Polyglytone 6211 is utilized. This quickly absorbable suture material is composed of trimethylene carbonate, lactide, glycolide, and caprolactone. At five days after implantation, a minimum of 50–60% caprosyn knot strength was retained, and a minimum of 20–30% knot strength was seen at 10 days (Dart & Dart, 2011). After 56 days, it had completely absorbed and lost all of its tensile strength. Caprosyn has significantly improved tissue handling qualities. Absorption of chromic gut and caprosyn are similar, but caprosyn has more infection resistance, and it is mainly used in urology, gynecology, and plastic surgery (Joseph et al., 2017).

11.3.1.1.5   Polydioxanone (PDS II)

Sutures made of polydioxanone (PDS) or poly-p-dioxanone are "monofilaments" that are progressively absorbable and made of polyester (poly-p-dioxanone). This monofilament has less tissue drag than multifilament materials and is stronger than monofilament nylon and polypropylene. It retains its strength well, losing only 20% after two weeks and 60% after eight. It can be challenging to control at times because of its memory and propensity to coil, or "pig-tail." After the end of a continuous suture line, seven throws are suggested because knot security can be relatively low. It takes about 200 days for hydrolysis to complete the absorption process.

11.3.1.1.6   *Polyglyclide-Trimethylene Carbosnate (Maxon)*

Absorbable and synthetic, Maxon is a copolymer of glycolide and trimethylene carbonate. It's easier to work with than polydioxanone and polyglactin 910, but harder to work with than polypropylene. Reportedly, Maxon offers more reliable knot security than PDS II. Although its initial tensile strength after implantation is higher than that of most other absorbable sutures, its tensile strength drops by 81% after 14 days, 59% after 28 days, and 30% after 42 days, making it equivalent to PDS II. Maxon has a tensile strength retention time of 42–92 days, but PDS II only has 64–80 days. Like the other synthetic absorbable sutures, it is broken down by hydrolysis, and like PDS II, it loses its tensile strength before its bulk is appreciably diminished. Absorption is complete after six months (Dart & Dart, 2011).

11.3.1.2   Non-absorbable Suture Materials

Non-absorbable suture materials are those whose deterioration is minimal upon implantation. When extra support is needed, these sutures are typically employed. Though those sutures provide long-term support, they have to be removed after healing, which can be problematic, and they also increase the chance of tissue scarring (Li et al., 2021). Natural fibers are more reactive; they can produce a more inflammatory response than synthetic fabrics, so they are typically not preferred. There are many synthetic materials used as sutures; a few of those are also included in this chapter.

11.3.1.2.1   *Silk*

It is a natural, non-absorbable braided suture made of protein filaments and created by silkworm larvae. These are colored for better visibility and braided for convenience of handling, but they can produce an inflammatory reaction and capillary action as well. The coating of silk sutures was done by submerging them in silicone, wax, or oil (Hochberg et al., 2009). Silk that has been coated has less capillarity but less secure knots. Silk has exceptional handling qualities, and other suture materials are measured against it in comparison. Silk has higher initial tensile strength as compared to gut, but the risk of infection is very high (Swanson & Tromovitch, 1982); however, most synthetic sutures are stronger. At one year, it retains 50% of its tensile strength, and by two years, it may have completely absorbed the material (Dart & Dart, 2011; Wu et al., 2016).

To enhance knot security and lessen tissue drag, it can be soaked in sterile saline prior to use, although doing so may somewhat diminish its tensile strength. As silk might exacerbate infection by trapping bacteria in its braiding, it is not advised to use it on hollow viscera or infected wounds. Because of its calculogenic potential, it cannot be used in urinary tract surgery and gallbladder surgery, like with other multifilament materials. Its braided design makes it susceptible to infection and tissue ingrowth by allowing blood and serum to build up between its threads. It has also been shown to accelerate the development of Staphylococcal spp. infection by up to 1000 times, in addition to causing an inflammatory response (Wu et al., 2016; Rodeheaver et al., 1983; Huang et al., 2018).

11.3.1.2.2 Nylon

Hexamethylenediamine and adipic acid are used to create the chemically inert polyamide thermoplastic known as nylon, a synthetic, nonabsorbable monofilament. Both types of sutures, monofilament and multifilament, are available in this category. Monofilament (Ethilon, Monosof) is much more prevalent and less prone to infection. Immediately upon implantation, the tensile strength of monofilament is maintained at 72%, and then the deterioration stabilizes. Progressive hydrolysis over time will cause it to lose 30–50% of its tensile strength by the end of the second year. Nylon sutures cause less inflammation than polyglycolic acid sutures because of their gradual hydrolysis and chemical inertness. After being implanted in tissue, a sufficient elasticity level is maintained, which is crucial to take into account if tissue edema and inflammation occur. Nylon is the most commonly used skin suture material because of its benefits. Nylon's biggest shortcomings are its poor handling capabilities and inadequate knot security. Alcohol shock improved the handling characteristics of monofilament (Mohammadi et al., 2020; Mahesh et al., 2019; Asher et al., 2019).

11.3.1.2.3 Polyester

This multifilament suture is made up of condensation-polymerized material that is non-absorbable. It is available in two categories: coated (with polybutilate) and uncoated, which have a high coefficient of friction. The coated version was created to solve this issue, although it has been shown that the covering cracks after implantation and can trigger inflammatory responses. Polyester sutures were developed in order to minimize tissue reaction while maintaining positive handling characteristics. Polyester sutures are not as inert as other synthetic materials, despite having less tissue reactivity than other multifilament sutures. In general, they exhibit weak knot security, specially coated types. Only metal sutures are stronger than polyester braided when it comes to tensile strength, making them stronger than silk or gut. Over time, they suffer minimal tensile strength loss. They are more expensive than the majority of sutures, so they are less frequently used. Utilizing braided polyesters in a contaminated or infected environment is not advised because bacteria have the potential to become trapped inside the fibers and become separated from phagocytic cells, which can lead to sinus drainage tracts (Dart & Dart, 2011).

11.3.1.2.4 Polypropylene

A common type of synthetic monofilament suture made of polymerized polypropylene is called polypropylene. It is frequently used in cardiovascular surgery on people since it is non-thrombogenic. It is offered as an implantable mesh material. If the sutures are properly tightened, polypropylene's high plasticity—the ability to change shape under tension—significantly aids in the material's good knot security. Due to its memory and propensity to break if handled aggressively, this material might be challenging to handle for some surgeons. After implantation, there is no discernible tensile strength reduction. After application on day 28 in the feline oral cavity, polypropylene was still intact, and a visual examination revealed that it had the least amount of tissue reactivity of any suture material examined (Veleirinho et al., 2014; France & Fancey, 2021).

11.3.1.2.5   Stainless steel

This natural alloy is the strongest suture that is available in monofilament or braided multifilament form. And it is biologically inert and easily sterilizable through autoclaving. It causes little tissue reaction aside from mechanical discomfort at the ends. Though this material shows good knot security, knot making is tricky. If this type of suture is allowed to become loose, it can migrate and break if bent repeatedly. If overtightened, then it can cause tissue damage through cutting or ripping. This material is mostly used as staples and clips rather than sutures because of its challenging handling features, but it has a wide range of applications in clips and staples. Steel suture is still routinely employed in the treatment of sternotomy wounds in dogs because of its better stability-providing capabilities than PDS II.

11.3.2   CLASSIFICATION BASED ON PHYSICAL CONFIGURATION

According to the physical arrangement of the thread's sutures, they can be divided into the following categories:

11.3.2.1   Monofilament Sutures

Monofilament spinning and polymer extrusion are used to create monofilament sutures, which are single threads. When compared to multifilament sutures, they provide a smooth surface that reduces surface friction, which minimizes tissue reactivity, limits tissue stress during suturing, and significantly decreases the probability of bacterial development due to their tiny contact area. It is relatively simple to tie a knot during surgery because of the single filament. Monofilament sutures can have certain disadvantages: they can only be knotted with a low knotting force; otherwise, they are easily broken due to their low knot security, and because of their lower fixability, handling this type of suture is also difficult. Monofilament sutures also have a memory that keeps the shape of the package because of the thickness of their filament, which adds to the knotting issues (Deng et al., 2021). Additionally, the resistance encountered when going through the tissue is lower, causing less harm to the tissue; that's why they are appropriate for treating infected wounds (Deng et al., 2021). Polyethylene terephthalate (PET or polyester), polyglycolic acid (PGA), and polylactic acid (PLA), as well as polypropylene, stainless steel, and polydioxanone, are being used to make monofilament sutures.

11.3.2.2   Multifilament Sutures

Multiple filaments are braided or twisted together to form multifilament sutures as like Figure 11.1. Nonwoven sutures have less tissue reaction and scarring than braided sutures, but they are more flexible and have superior tensile strength (Joseph et al., 2017). Twisted multifilament catgut (reconstituted collagen), cotton, and stainless steel are available, while polyesters, polyamides, and silks are frequently utilized to make braided sutures. Multifilament sutures, as opposed to monofilament sutures, are simpler to handle and offer greater knot security. Suturing by this method causes tissue pull, stress, and injury to the surrounding tissue because of their rough and uneven surface, which can be minimized by the application of coatings that reduce surface friction (Deng et al., 2021). Monofilament sutures are less likely to cause harm to the tissue around them as a result of this (Reinbold et al., 2017).

Additionally, microcapillaries arise as a result of structural micro-voids in multifilament sutures, aiding in the wicking of fluid into these void spaces. Multifilament sutures may become contaminated with infectious germs due to the buildup of fluid around wounds. Multifilament sutures also cause several inflammatory tissue reactions and infections. To reduce those problems, pseudo-monofilament sutures are developed by coating multifilament sutures with a thin polymer, and they will also minimize the chance of bacterial growth by preventing the capillary action and fluid imbibition (Chellamani et al., 2013; Zhukovskii et al., 2015; King et al., 2013).

When active pharmaceutical ingredients are wrapped in the structural gap between multifilament, a wider band is visible, which provides insight into the drug delivery role of sutures. In braided multifilament sutures, coating became necessary, so in that case, surface coating with therapeutic ingredients therefore offered a wider chance of loading full doses of therapeutic ingredients like antioxidants, antibacterials, anti-inflammatory agents, etc.

11.3.2.3 Barb Suture

This type of surgical suture contains barbs on the surface, which allow for easy tissue penetration and wound closure without the need for knotting. These sutures are known as barb sutures. Barb sutures are less knotted than conventional monofilament and multifilament sutures. They come in absorbable and non-absorbable varieties and have barbs that can penetrate tissue to repair it. Without the requirement for knotted sutures, unidirectional barb sutures have a much higher tensile strength while also having less tissue reaction. Barb sutures are therefore used as a substitute for regular sutures, mainly in soft tissue (Dennis et al., 2016; Umranikar et al., 2017).

Clinical application of barb sutures is very common because this type of suture effectively restricts the chance of microorganism growth and prevents

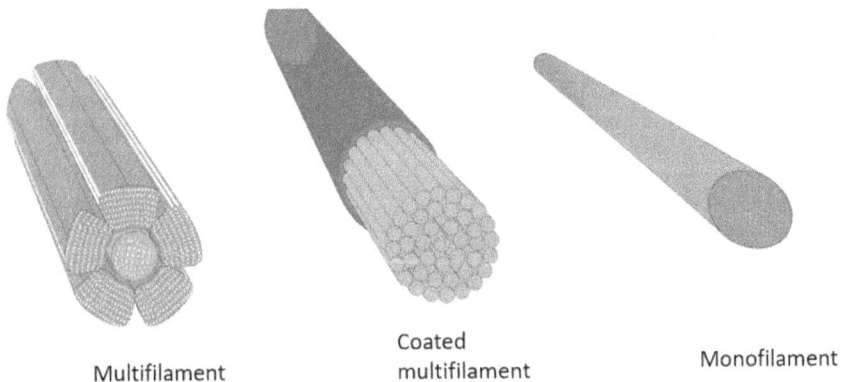

Multifilament   Coated multifilament   Monofilament

FIGURE 11.2   Suture filament

inflammation, knot-related problems, and other wound issues like wound healing promotion by antibacterial activity (Zaruby et al., 2011). However, because of the barb design, which can mistakenly pierce the surgical gloves, those sutures can indirectly spread infection, which is one of the main disadvantages of barb sutures.

11.3.3 CLASSIFICATION OF SUTURES BASED ON SIZE

According to the thread's diameter, sutures are divided into various sizes. Currently, the USP (United States Pharmacopeia) and EP (European Pharmacopeia) standards are used to characterize size. The USP is most commonly used when the size is denoted by two Arabic numbers, one between 1 and 9, and another zero, as in 3–0. The suture material becomes finer as the first number increases, and 1 through 9 are used to indicate sizes greater than 0 (1/0), though these vary depending on the suture material type. The EP standard uses a code between 0.1 and 10. By multiplying the code number by 10, it is simple to determine the equivalent minimum diameter (mm). Unlike USP, EP Standard does not distinguish between natural and synthetic absorbable sutures (Byrne & Aly, 2019). Table 11.2 displays the size-based classification of sutures.

11.3.4 CLASSIFICATION OF SUTURES BASED ON COATING

According to their coating, they are classified as coated sutures and non-coated sutures. PGA sutures, polydioxanone, polyglactin 910, braided and twisted sutures,

TABLE 11.2
Size-based classification

USP size code	Metric gauge	Diameter	EP size code	Diameter (mm)
9–0	0.3	0.030–0.039	0.1	0.01–0.019
8–0	0.4	0.040–0.049	0.2	0.02–0.029
7–0	0.5	0.050–0.069	0.3	0.03–0.039
6–0	0.7	0.070–0.099	0.4	0.04–0.049
5–0	1	0.100–0.149	0.5	0.05–0.069
4–0	1.5	0.150–0.199	0.7	0.07–0.99
3–0	2	0.200–0.249	1	0.10–0.14
2–0	3	0.300–0.349	1.5	0.15–0.19
0	3.5	0.350–0.399	2	0.20–0.24
1	4	0.400–0.499	2.5	0.25–0.29
2	5	0.500–0.599	3	0.30–0.39
3	6	0.600–0.699	4	0.40–0.49
4	6	0.600–0.699	5	0.50–0.59
5	7	0.700–0.799	6	0.60–0.69
6	8	0.800–0.899	7	0.70–0.79
7	9	0.900–.0999	10	1.00–1.09

and chromic catgut are examples of coated sutures, and polypropylene, nylon, PVDF, and stainless steel are available as uncoated sutures in the market.

Some suture types come with particular surface coatings to improve qualities including knotting, simple tissue passage, and reduced tissue response. Typically, braided sutures rather than monofilament sutures are coated. Compared to mono-filaments, braided sutures are simpler to coat with substances like calcium stearate, silicon, wax, PTFE, and chromium salt. Compared to traditional coating materials such as chromium salts, beeswax, paraffin, gelatin, etc., polymeric coating materials are recognized to be more biocompatible. New functional coatings have been added to monofilament and multifilament sutures, such as antibacterial or antimicrobial coatings and stem cell coatings, to enhance their ability to heal. To decrease the risk of infection at the surgical site and promote wound healing, any suture may receive an antimicrobial surface coating such as chlorhexidine, triclosan, or silver ions in addition to the standard coating materials (Abhari et al., 2017).

11.3.5 Classification Based on Use

In accordance with their use or application, sutures are further divided into numerous sorts. Sutures can be divided into general sutures, cardiovascular sutures, valve sutures, orthopedic sutures, dental sutures, gynecological, veterinary, cosmetic surgery, ophthalmology, and other sutures. Depending on the needs, a range of suture materials may be employed for a certain application. However, for a specific application, the suture diameters, lengths, needle profiles, etc., will be somewhat altered.

11.3.6 Classification Based on Origin

On the basis of origin, sutures can classify as natural sutures and synthetic sutures. Natural sutures further classify as plant based natural sutures like cotton, silk, and animal origin based natural sutures like catgut. Natural sutures are more unpredictable in their biodegradation aspect, and they produce inflammatory reaction as well. Synthetic sutures, such as polydioxanone (PDO), are known for their high mechanical strength and polytrimethylene carbonate (PTMC) is another biodegradable polymer that is occasionally used in medical applications, and these typically induce fewer inflammatory reactions. That is why their acceptance rates are higher.

11.4 SELECTION OF APPROPRIATE SUTURE MATERIAL

If the suture material is not strong enough, it may cause the wound to break down. Suture material with high memory, on the other hand, may cause knots to unravel unless the surgeon is aware of this property and adds additional throws to the knot to compensate. Suture material with insufficient strength may cause wound deterioration. Suture material with an excessively large diameter weakens the knot, increasing knot insecurity and the amount of foreign material at the surgical site. It is best to choose sutures with a small diameter—the smallest diameter suture material that can hold the healing tissue securely.

The surgeon selects the suture material by thinking about a variety of things, like the age of the patient, health status and disease condition, site of injury, thickness, inflammatory reaction, healing speed and flexibility, and depth of tissue. At the time of selection, they also take care of the sterility, pliability, and acceptance of the tissue (Celeste, 2016).

Natural sutures sometimes produce an inflammatory reaction, and their absorption at the application site can vary, but in synthetic materials, the rate of absorption is more predictable. Due to the larger friction coefficient of multifilament suture material, it often has greater strength than monofilament and provides superior knot security. On the other hand, multifilament material, especially if dry, can generate drag that can harm sensitive tissue and cause iatrogenic injury due to suture pullout by the surgeon. Additionally, multifilament suture material contains fissures that might act as breeding grounds for germs and has a larger surface area for bacterial penetration. Coating multifilament and braided sutures alleviate these issues.

Fast-absorbing sutures known as the "rapid range" and the "Plus" range of sutures, which are resistant to bacterial penetration, are two examples of modified generic sutures. Triclosan, an inhibitor of bacterial fatty acid production, has been shown to have great antibacterial effectiveness, and it has been applied to the "Plus" family of sutures (Polyglactin 910, Polydioxanone, and Poliglecaprone).

11.5 PREPARATION OF SURGICAL SUTURES

Sutures are generally prepared by using electrospinning, melt extrusion, and coating techniques. These sutures are applied on the wound side, so their effectiveness to reduce wound site infection, the healing process, and pain is important. The application of electrospinning is wide in terms of nanofiber preparation because of its ability to incorporate drug molecules like antibiotics and anticancer agents and its sustained release ability, which has a specific treatment advantage (Stojanov et al., 2020; Sa'adon et al., 2021; Sivan et al., 2022; Wang et al., 2020; Yu & Lv, 2022).

A high-pressure generator, spinneret, collector, and syringe pump (one or more) are organized together in an electrospinning device that produces multiple interactions between the working fluid and electrostatic energy. Polymeric solution is taken in a syringe and placed in a high voltage power field where the solution starts spinning from the tip of syringe and develops "Taylor cone" to overcome the surface tension of the polymeric solution (Xu et al., 2022). At this point, the voltage will be constantly raised. The solution may be sprayed in the form of a trickle when the electric field is strong enough, and while it is being sprayed, the solvents in the solution continue to evaporate and the solution continues to solidify. Finally, a fibrous web that resembles a nonwoven fabric is dropped onto the collector (Xu et al., 2022; Aidana et al., 2022; Shepa et al., 2021). Though this process concept is octogenarian, it is used in several scientific fields with minor modifications and is known as single-fluid electrospinning, double-fluid electrospinning, and multi-fluid electrospinning (Weldon et al., 2012).

Emulsion electrospinning, suspension electrospinning, and blend electrospinning are all examples of single-fluid electrospinning. The oldest technique of creating nanofibers among them is blend electrospinning; in this technique, sutures hold polymers dissolved in a suitable solvent to create a spinning fluid. Sometimes bioactive ingredients are added to provide them with particular functionalities, which are optional. Different nanoparticles and drug materials can be incorporated, and controlled drug release sutures can be prepared by using this technique (Song et al., 2021, 2022; Liu et al., 2022; Ning et al., 2021; Rasekh et al., 2021; Kesici Güler et al., 2019).

11.5.1 Double-Fluid Electrospinning

In this process, a double fluid system is used for the formation of a double layer in contrast to the single-fluid electrospinning technology (Yu & Lv, 2022). The inner layer and outer layer are separated by a certain amount to allow for easy passage of the polymer solution. Nanofibers with a core-sheath structure are then produced. Coaxial electrospinning is one of the various electrospinning processes that is often used to create nanofibers with core-sheath structures. With the help of this preparation technique, the performance of the medical suture nanofibers may be altered by moving the bioactive ingredient around inside them. For example, if bioactive substance is added to the sheath solution, then the duration of action is reduced due to the direct contact and quick release of medicaments at the application site. And, as shown in coaxial spinning, adding bioactive materials to the core solution results in prolonged and controlled release (Xu et al., 2021; Zhao et al., 2021; Rathore & Schiffman, 2021; Lv et al., 2021).

11.5.2 Multi-Fluid Electrospinning

Multi-fluid electrospinning is clearly superior to the dual-fluid electrospinning technique. Both the number of fluids and the spinneret structure are altered in this case. This spinning technique allows for the incorporation of polymers and bioactive compounds with a wide range of characteristics. As a result, nanofibers with improved functionality and structural complexity are developed. In the area of medical sutures, it is possible to obtain the sustained release of medications, antibacterial activity, scar removal, and biodegradation at the application site.

11.5.3 In Situ Electrospinning

In situ electrospinning is one of the various electrospinning technologies that have emerged in order to employ medicinal materials that are practical and can be modified to fit wounds. Electrospinning is used to make wound dressings, but it is only employed in vitro. A new study deposited nanofibers directly on real tissues to achieve wound hemostasis. Zhang et al. embedded the long needle into the laparoscopic tube using long-needle electrospinning and minimally invasive surgery. Laparoscopy might create electrospun nanofibers and place them on live organs. It shows that rapid hemostasis reduces surgical inflammation and speeds recovery.

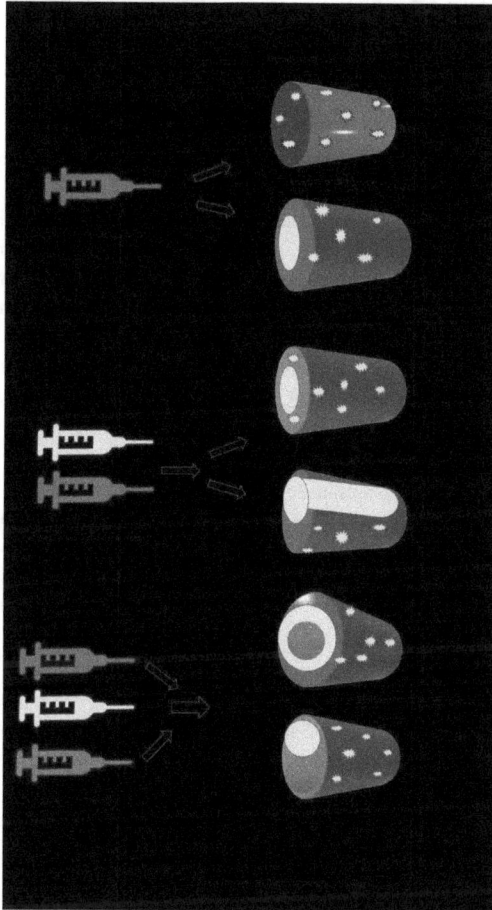

FIGURE 11.3 Electrospinning process

11.6 SUTURE SELECTION FOR SPECIFIC TISSUES

TABLE 11.3
Suture selection by organ

Organ	Preferable suture
Blood vessel and nerve	For its low thrombogenicity, polypropylene sutures come highly recommended. There have also been applications of nylon and coated polyester. The lowest tissue reactivity is achieved using nylon and polypropylene.
Muscle	It is possible to employ synthetic absorbable or nonabsorbable sutures. For usage in heart muscle, nylon and polypropylene are advised due to their higher mechanical qualities. Ex. polyglycolic acid, glycomer 631, polyglactin.

TABLE 11.3   (Continued)
Suture selection by organ

Organ	Preferable suture
Tendon	Slowly absorbable or strongly non-absorbable are preferable. Common suggestions are nylon and stainless steel.
Skin	Nonabsorbable sutures made from a single strand are preferred. When suture removal is likely to be challenging, longer-retained monofilament absorbable sutures like polydioxanone or polyglycolide-trimethyl carbonate would be a better option (Dart & Dart, 2011).
Fascia	Sutures that are synthetic and absorbable are advised, but in case of long-term need nonabsorbable can be utilized; However if contaminated, they run the danger of suture sinus development (Dart & Dart, 2011). Facial suture should be arranged in such a way that they can be quickly removed if necessary.
Subcutis	Sutures made of synthetic absorbable materials. Polyglycolic acid and polyglactin 910 are typically utilized when tissue approximation is desired for a short period of time. Polyglycolide-trimethylene carbonate or polydioxanone may be employed where extended retention time is required for slower healing tissues (Dart & Dart, 2011).
Parenchymal organ	Absorbable monofilament like poliglecaprone, glycomer 631 are commonly used.
Infected or contaminated wounds	Absorbable sutures are preferrable (Polyglactin, Poliglecaprone). Avoid using catgut, which absorbs quickly, or braided nonabsorbable sutures, which can fistulate.
Subcutaneous	Absorbable sutures like polyglytone, polyglactin are preferable.

11.7   IMPROVEMENT OF SUTURE PERFORMANCE BY DYES AND COATINGS

Because this foreign body is directly placed at the site of injury, its surface is extremely important. Coating was invented in the late 1960s to improve handling properties (primarily knot making and tissue drag reduction) as well as identification and tissue drag reduction. Suture coating's primary goal is to promote biological healing, reduce surgical site infection, and make handling easier.

Coating material can be divided into two categories, as nonabsorbable coating materials like silicone, paraffin wax, Teflon, etc. are traditionally used. The majority of newly used coating materials are absorbable and thus more biocompatible with the body. Absorbable suture material can be categorized into water-soluble and insoluble types. Insoluble materials generally having similar chemical characteristics like sutures that break down in the body through hydrolysis, like polyhydroxybutyrate and polyglactin 370, are generally used. After the incision has been closed, the uncoated suture quickly dissolves due to the water-soluble covering (poloxamer 188).

Sutures can be coated in a variety of ways; in the case of dip coating, sutures are immersed in a concentrated solution of various factors; the concentration of the solution determines the type of coating. Drip coating is done by dripping a polymeric solution onto the sutures. Another method is spraying, where coating materials are sprayed over sutures. Different types of growth factors are used as coating materials for improving the tissue healing property in suturing areas, like vascular endothelial growth factor, recombinant human growth and differentiation factor-5, bone morphogenetic protein-12, basic fibroblast growth factor, arginine-glycine-aspartic acid, etc. Except for all those, a coating of an antimicrobial agent is used to minimize the chance of infection by preventing microbial growth. Antimicrobial sutures can be made by coating an antimicrobial agent over sutures, by graft polymerization followed by immobilization of an antimicrobial agent, or by incorporation and blending of an antimicrobial agent (like iodine, silver, or polyglycolic acid).

The Food and Drug Administration (FDA) approves many different dyes for use in sutures, including the violet-colored logwood extract, the brownish-green ferric ammonium citrate, and the blue chromium-cobalt-aluminum oxide.

11.8 APPLICATION OF SUTURES

Sutures are one of the most commonly used surgical materials, and they are used to close wounds and hold tissues together until they have healed enough to withstand the stresses of daily life without tearing. They can be used as wound closers in tendon repair, bone surgery, cervical correction, internal organ invasive surgery, strabismus surgery, cosmetic and reconstructive surgery, and drug delivery as well (Li et al., 2021; Yuan et al., 2022).

11.8.1 Drug Delivery

Delivery of drug (mainly anti-bacterial and anti-inflammatory agent) in surgical site is always a concern which can be resolved by incorporating or coating active therapeutic molecules in sutures. Those biologically active sutures can develop as a drug delivery device. The development of self-healing sutures by incorporating therapeutic ingredients inside the sutures, which release medications to speed up the healing process without sacrificing suture quality, has exploded recently to provide direct medication where the medication process is challenging (Kulshreshta & Mahapatro, 2008; Dumitriu et al., 2001; Champeau et al., 2017). In this regard, active pharmaceutical ingredient (API)-infused sutures, also referred to as medication-eluting sutures, have been produced (Dennis et al., 2016). Sutures are used for medication delivery because their controlled release mechanisms are capable to produce effective drug concentration in surgical site without producing excessive systemic drug concentration. Since sutures are used in practically all surgical operations, using them to deliver medications eliminates the need to implant a foreign object in the wound bed, which could delay healing or lead to infection.

Controlled release and site-specific drug delivery can be developed by using prominent surface and bulk property of sutures polymers, recent researches used for therapeutic molecules, antibiotics, protein, stem cell delivery in suturing site. Using sutures for releasing different natural extracts is also getting good response recently, like propolis extract (caffeic acid phenethyl ester) and grape seed extract.

11.8.2 ORAL AND PERIODONTAL SURGERY

In periodontal surgery, a dentist uses sutures to correct gum disease, reduce a gap between two teeth or sometimes to stop bleeding. Selection of periodontal sutures depends upon the anatomical injury, and simple interrupted technique is followed for suturing. Suturing and removal process in oral surgery leads towards infection, so antibacterial coating can be a good option. Silk, polytetrafluoroethylene, polyglactine 910, polyglycolic acid, polypropylene, nylon, and catgut are generally selected as periodontal and oral sutures (Meghil et al., 2015).

11.8.3 COSMETIC AND CUTANEOUS SURGERY

In cosmetic and cutaneous surgery, the purpose of sutures is to both seal a wound and encourage healthy wound healing, all while producing desirable cosmetic outcomes. Many different kinds of suture materials have been created for this purpose. Different types of suture material (polypropylene, nylon, surgical silk, polyglactic acid, polydioxanone) are available, and they are selected on the basis of wound location, infection risk, cost, etc.

11.8.4 SUTURES FOR TENDON REPAIR

Tendon sutures are one of the major sutures used in musculoskeletal injury where repair is dependent upon the link between suture and tendon, bone interface, and cuff muscle. Selection of particular suture material for tendon surgery is also important, surgeon preferred material having high mechanical strength with better absorption rate. Stainless-steel suture contains high mechanical strength but its preference is low because of its absorption and handling characteristic like knot making, though strength of this suture can be utilized by minimizing the handling difficulties through a knotless anchoring device known as Teno Fix (Seo et al., 2016; Zhang et al., 2020).

11.8.5 OPHTHALMIC APPLICATION

Approximately 12 million sutures are used every year in ophthalmic surgeries (Kashiwabuchi et al., 2017). For the ophthalmic sutures preparation, highly biocompatible materials which are uniform and delicate and have much less inflammation producing capacity are selected. On behalf of those criteria, anti-inflammatory or antibacterial molecule incorporated sutures with sufficient mechanical strength should be a good option. In Table 11.4 we included some ophthalmic sutures which are available in market (Parikh et al., 2021).

TABLE 11.4
Few ophthalmic sutures

Sutures type	Commercial name	Material	Application area
Absorbable sutures	CARESORB	Polyglactin 910	Conjunctiva, eye muscle, sclera
Non-absorbable sutures	PROTIBOND	Polyester	Retinal surgery, eye muscle, plomb fixation
	CARELON	Nylon	Iris, sclera, eyeball
	TRUSTILENE	Polypropylene	Eyeball fixing, sclera, cornea, iris
	CARESILK	Silk	Eyeball fixing, corneal operation

11.9 CONCLUSION

Although surgical sutures have been used for 3000 years, their use in injury management is indispensable. There are various types of materials, and they are chosen based on their properties and capabilities. Coating sutures became important for smooth handling and to reduce the coefficient of friction and the delivery of drug materials as well. The electrospinning process was also modified by researchers, which has a high impact on incorporating bioactive materials in sutures. This process can also create sutures that can deliver local and systemic drug delivery with controlled drug release.

REFERENCES

Abhari, R.E., Martins, J.A., Morris, H.L., Mouthuy, P.A., Carr, A. (2017). Synthetic sutures: Clinical evaluation and future developments. *J. Biomater. Appl.*, 32(3), 410–421.

Aidana, Y., Wang, Y., Li, J., Chang, S., Wang, K., Yu, D.-G. (2022). Fast dissolution electrospun medicated nanofibers for effective delivery of poorly water-soluble drug. *Curr. Drug Deliv.*, 19, 422–435.

Asher, R., Chacartchi, T., Tandlich, M., Shapira, L., Polak, D. (2019). Microbial accumulation on different suture materials following oral surgery: A randomized controlled study. *Clin. Oral Investig.*, 23, 559–565.

Balaji, S.M. (2013). *Textbook of Oral and Maxillofacial Surgery*. Chennai: Elsevier.

Byrne, M., Aly, A. (2019). The surgical suture. *Aesthetic Surgery Journal*, 39, S67–S72.

Celeste, C. (2016). Selection of suture materials, suture patterns, and drains for wound closure. *Equine Wound Management*, 173–199.

Champeau, M., Thomassin, J.M., Tassaing, T., Jerome, C. (2017). Current manufacturing processes of drug-eluting sutures. *Expert Opinion Drug Delivery*, 14(11), 1293–1303.

Chellamani, K.P., Veerasubramanian, D., Balaji, R.V. (2013). Surgical sutures: An overview. *Journal of Academia and Industrial Research*, 1(12), 778–782.

Dart, A.J., Dart, C.M. (2011). Suture material: Conventional and stimuli responsive. *Comprehensive Biomaterials*, 573–587.

Deng, X., Qasim, M., Ali, A. (2021). Engineering and polymeric composition of drug-eluting suture: A review. *J. Biomed. Mater. Res.*, 109, 2065–2081.

Dennis, C., Sethu, S., Nayak, S., Mohan, L., Morsi, Y.Y., Manivasagam, G. (2016). Suture materials—Current and emerging trends. *J. Biomed. Mater. Res.*, 104(6), 1544–1559.

Dumitriu, S. (2001). *Polymeric Biomaterials* (Revised and expanded, 2nd ed.). New York: CRC Press.

France, L.A., Fancey, K.S. (2021). Visco elastically active sutures—A stitch in time? *Mater. Sci. Eng.*, 121, 111695.

Gierek, M., Kuśnierz, K., Lampe, P., Ochała, G., Kurek, J., Hekner, B., Merkel, K., Majewski, J. (2018). Absorbable sutures in general surgery—Review, available materials, and optimum choices. *Pol. J. Surg.*, 90, 34–37.

Gómez-Alonso, A., García-Criado, F.J., Parreño-Manchado, F.C., García-Sánchez, J.E., García-Sánchez, E., Parreño-Manchado, A., Zambrano-Cuadrado, Y. (2007). Study of the efficacy of coated VICRYL Plus® antibacterial suture (coated polyglactin 910 suture with triclosan) in two animal models of general surgery. *Journal of Infection*, 54(1), 82–88.

Hochberg, J., Meyer, K.M., Marion, M.D. (2009). Suture choice and other methods of skin closure. *Surg. Clin. N. Am.*, 89, 627–641.

Huang, W., Ling, S., Li, C., Omenetto, F.G., Kaplan, D.L. (2018). Silkworm silk-based materials and devices generated using bionanotechnology. *Chem. Soc. Rev.*, 47, 6486–6504.

Joseph, B., George, A., Gopi, S., Kalarikkal, N., Thomas, S. (2017). Polymer sutures for simultaneous wound healing and drug delivery—A review. *Int. J. Pharm.*, 524, 454–466.

Kashiwabuchi, F., Parikh, K.S., Omiadze, R., Zhang, S., Luo, L., Patel, H.V., Xu, Q., Ensign, L.M., Mao, H.-Q., Hanes, J., et al. (2017). Development of absorbable, antibiotic-eluting sutures for ophthalmic surgery. *Transl. Vis. Sci. Technol.*, 6, 1.

Kesici Güler, H., Cengiz Çallıoğlu, F., Sesli Çetin, E. (2019). Antibacterial PVP/cinnamon essential oil nanofibers by emulsion electrospinning. *J. Text. Inst.*, 110, 302–310.

Khiste, S.V., Ranganath, V., Nichani, A.S. (2013). Evaluation of tensile strength of surgical synthetic absorbable suture materials: An in vitro study. *J. Periodontal Implant Sci.*, 43(3), 130–135.

King, M.W., Gupta, B.S., Guidoin, R. (2013). *Biotextiles as Medical Implants*. Cambridge, NY: Woodhead Publishing.

Kulshreshta, A.S., Mahapatro, A. (2008). Polymers for biomedical applications. *American Chemical Society*, 1, 1–7.

Lekic, N., Dodds, S.D. (2022). Suture materials, needles, and methods of skin closure: What every hand surgeon should know. *J. Hand Surg.*, 47, 160–171.

Li, J., Guan, S., Su, J., Liang, J., Cui, L., Zhang, K. (2021). The development of hyaluronic acids used for skin tissue regeneration. *Curr. Drug Deliv.*, 18, 836–846.

Liu, Y., Chen, X., Liu, Y., Gao, Y., Liu, P. (2022). Electrospun coaxial fibers to optimize the release of poorly water-soluble drug. *Polymers*, 14, 469.

Lv, H., Guo, S., Zhang, G., He, W., Wu, Y., Yu, D.-G. (2021). Electrospun structural hybrids of acyclovir-polyacrylonitrile at acyclovir for modifying drug release. *Polymers*, 13, 4286.

Mahesh, L., Kumar, V.R., Jain, A., Shukla, S., Aragoneses, J.M., Martínez González, J.M., Fernández-Domínguez, M., Calvo- Guirado, J.L. (2019). Bacterial adherence around sutures of different material at grafted site: A microbiological analysis. *Materials*, 12, 2848.

Meghil, M.M., Rueggeberg, F., El-Awady, A., Miles, B., Tay, F., Pashley, D., Cutler, C.W. (2015). Novel coating of surgical suture confers antimicrobial activity against porphyromonas gingivalis and enterococcus faecalis. *J. Periodontol.*, 86, 788–794.

Mohammadi, H., Alihosseini, F., Hosseini, S.A. (2020). Improving physical and biological properties of nylon monofilament as suture by chitosan/hyaluronic acid. *Int. J. Biol. Macromol.*, 164, 3394–3402.

Muffly, T.M., Tizzano, A.P., Walters, M.D. (2011). The history and evolution of sutures in pelvic surgery. *Journal of the Royal Society of Medicine*, 104(3), 107–112.

Munton, C.G., Phillips, C.I., Martin, B., Bartholomew, R.S., Capperauld, I. (1974). Vicryl (Polyglactin 910): a new synthetic absorbable suture in ophthalmic surgery. A preliminary study. *Br J Ophthalmol*, 58(11), 941–947.

Ning, T., Zhou, Y., Xu, H., Guo, S., Wang, K., Yu, D.-G. (2021). Orodispersible membranes from a modified coaxial electrospinning for fast dissolution of diclofenac sodium. *Membranes*, 11, 802.

Pacer, E., Griffin, D.W., Anderson, A.B., Tintle, S.M., Potter, B.K. (2020). Suture and needle characteristics in orthopaedic surgery. *JBJS Rev.*, 8, e19.00133.

Parikh, K.S., Omiadze, R., Josyula, A., Shi, R., Anders, N.M., He, P., Yazdi, Y., McDonnell, P.J., Ensign, L.M., Hanes, J. (2021). Ultra-thin, high strength, antibiotic-eluting sutures for prevention of ophthalmic infection. *Bioeng. Transl. Med.*, 6, e10204.

Pillai, C.K.S., Sharma, C.P. (2010). Review paper: Resorbable polymeric surgical sutures: Chemistry, production, properties, biodegradability, and performance. *Journal of Biomaterials Applications*, 25(4), 291–366.

Rasekh, A., Raisi, A. (2021). Electrospun nanofibrous polyether-block-amide membrane containing silica nanoparticles for water desalination by vacuum membrane distillation. *Sep. Purif. Technol.*, 275, 119149.

Rathore, P., Schiffman, J.D. (2021). Beyond the single-nozzle: Coaxial electrospinning enables innovative nanofiber chemistries, geometries, and applications. *ACS Appl. Mater. Interfaces*, 13, 48–66.

Reinbold, J., Uhde, A.-K., Müller, I., Weindl, T., Geis-Gerstorfer, J., Schlensak, C., Wendel, H.-P., Krajewski, S. (2017). Preventing surgical site infections using a natural, biodegradable, antibacterial coating on surgical sutures. *Molecules*, 22, 1570.

Rodeheaver, G.T., Thacker, J.G., Owen, J., Strauss, M., Masterson, T., Edlich, R.F. (1983). Knotting and handling characteristics of coated synthetic absorbable sutures. *J. Surg. Res.*, 35, 525–530.

Sa'adon, S., Ansari, M.N.M., Razak, S.I.A., Anand, J.S., Nayan, N.H.M., Ismail, A.E., Khan, M.U.A., Haider, A. (2021). Preparation and physicochemical characterization of a diclofenac sodium-dual layer polyvinyl alcohol patch. *Polymers*, 13, 2459.

Scott Taylor, M., Shalaby, S.W. (2013). Sutures. *Biomaterials Science*, 1010–1024.

Seo, Y.-K., Kim, J.-H., Eo, S.-R. (2016). Co-effect of silk and amniotic membrane for tendon repair. *J. Biomater. Sci. Polym. Ed.* 27, 1232–1247.

Shepa, I., Mudra, E., Dusza, J. (2021). Electrospinning through the prism of time. *Mater. Today Chem.*, 21, 100543.

Sivan, M., Madheswaran, D., Valtera, J., Kostakova, E.K., Lukas, D. (2022). Alternating current electrospinning: The impacts of various high-voltage signal shapes and frequencies on the spinnability and productivity of polycaprolactone nano fibers. *Mater. Des.*, 213, 110308.

Song, X., Jiang, Y., Zhang, W., Elfawal, G., Wang, K., Jiang, D., Hong, H., Wu, J., He, C., Mo, X., et al. (2022). Transcutaneous tumor vaccination combined with anti-programmed death-1 monoclonal antibody treatment produces a synergistic antitumor effect. *Acta Biomater*, 140, 247–260.

Song, Y., Huang, H., He, D., Yang, M., Wang, H., Zhang, H., Li, J., Li, Y., Wang, C. (2021). Gallic acid/2-hydroxypropyl-_-cyclodextrin inclusion complexes electrospun nanofibrous webs: Fast dissolution, improved aqueous solubility and antioxidant property of gallic acid. *Chem. Res. Chin. Univ.*, 37, 450–455.

Stojanov, S., Berlec, A. (2020). Electrospun nanofibers as carriers of microorganisms, stem cells, proteins, and nucleic acids in therapeutic and other applications. *Front. Bioeng. Biotechnol.*, 8, 130.

Swanson, N.A., Tromovitch, T.A. (1982). Suture materials, 1980s: Properties, uses, and abuses. *Int. J. Dermatol.*, 21, 373–378.

Umranikar, S.A., Ubee, S.S., Selvan, M., Cooke, P. (2017). Barbed suture tissue closure device in urological surgery—A comprehensive review. *J. Clin. Urol.*, 10, 476–484.

Veleirinho, B., Coelho, D.S., Dias, P.F., Maraschin, M., Pinto, R., Cargnin-Ferreira, E., Peixoto, A., Souza, J.A., Ribeiro-do-Valle, R.M., Lopes-da-Silva, J.A. (2014). Foreign body reaction associated with PET and PET/Chitosan electro spun nanofibrous abdominal meshes. *PLoS One*, 9, e95293.

Wang, M., Yu, D.G., Li, X., Williams, G.R. (2020). The development and bio-applications of multifluid electrospinning. *Mater. Highlight*, 1, 1–13.

Weldon, C.B., Tsui, J.H., Shankarappa, S.A., Nguyen, V.T., Ma, M. (2012). Electro spun drug eluting sutures for local anaesthesia. *Journal of Control Reliability*, 161(3), 903–909.

Wu, D.-Q., Cui, H.-C., Zhu, J., Qin, X.-H., Xie, T. (2016). Novel amino acid based nanogel conjugated suture for antibacterial application. *J. Mater. Chem.* B, 4, 2606–2613.

Xu, H., Xu, X., Li, S., Song, W.-L., Yu, D.-G., Annie Bligh, S.W. (2021). The effect of drug heterogeneous distributions within core-sheath nanostructures on its sustained release profiles. *Biomolecules*, 11, 1330.

Xu, H., Zhang, F., Wang, M., Lv, H., Yu, D.G., Liu, X., Shen, H. (2022). Electrospun hierarchical structural films for effective wound healing. *Biomater. Adv.*, 212795.

Yu, D.-G., Lv, H. (2022). Preface-striding into nano drug delivery. *Curr. Drug Deliv.*, 19, 1–3.

Yuan, Z., Sheng, D., Jiang, L., Shafiq, M., Khan, A.U.R., Hashim, R., Chen, Y., Li, B., Xie, X., Chen, J., et al. (2022). Vascular endothelial growth factor-capturing aligned electrospun polycaprolactone/gelatin nanofibers promote patellar ligament regeneration. *Acta Biomater.*, 140, 233–246.

Zaruby, J., Gingras, K., Taylor, J., Maul, D. (2011). An in vivo comparison of barbed suture devices and conventional monofilament sutures for cosmetic skin closure: Biomechanical wound strength and histology. *Aesthet Surg J.*, 31(2), 232–240.

Zhang, Q., Mao, J., Li, C., Han, H., Lin, J., Wang, F., Wang, L. (2020). Bamboo-inspired lightweight tape suture with hollow and porous structure for tendon repair. *Mater. Des.*, 193, 108843.

Zhao, K., Lu, Z.-H., Zhao, P., Kang, S.-X., Yang, Y.-Y., Yu, D.-G. (2021). Modified tri—axial electrospun functional core—shell nanofibrous membranes for natural photodegradation of antibiotics. *Chem. Eng. J.*, 425, 131455.

Zhukovskii, V., Moskalyuk, O., Tsobkallo, E. (2015). Study of strength and relaxation properties of polyester surgical suture threads. *Fibre Chemistry*, 47(3), 202–206.

12 Nano-Biotechnology in Vascular Graft Implant and Heart Valve for Biotextile

Amisha Singh, Prashansa Sharma, and Vivek Dave

12.1 INTRODUCTION

Biotextiles or medical textiles, are fibrous textiles made from natural or synthetic materials that are commonly used to prevent, diagnose, and treat injury or disease. As a result of their versatility, biotextiles may be used in a variety of medical settings, including non-implantable materials (bandages, wound dressing), implantable medical devices for ex vivo cell administration, and tissue culture and in vitro experimentation. They are used inside (in contact with the circulating blood or wounds) as well as outside the body. Biotextiles have been classified on the basis of the type of constituent polymer (natural, synthetic biodegradable, and synthetic), manufacturing technique, and their application in the biomedical field, for example, in healthcare products such as sanitary napkins; surgical gowns; gloves; non-implantable materials such as gauze, plasters, and bandages; and implantable materials such as sutures, vascular grafts, stents, artificial joints, etc. So, the manufacturing technique and processing depend upon the desired property of the product.

The discipline of medical textiles involves the application of the principles and techniques of textile science and biomedical engineering to the enhancement of medicines and medicinal devices so as to improve and enhance the health condition, lifestyle, and quality of life of individual humans. The advancement in technology and upgrade in manufacturing methods have created an interdisciplinary approach involving tissue engineering, biotechnology, genetic science, medical science, physics, and chemistry to create new biotextiles with altered and requisite properties. One such discipline is nanotechnology. With the help of emerging techniques in nanotechnology, it is now possible to develop natural and synthetic biotextiles with tailored physical and biochemical properties. Nowadays, nanotechnology is readily used in engineering the desired attributes of biotextiles, such as high surface area, fabric softness, durability, porosity, flexibility, biodegradability, antimicrobial resistance, biocompatibility, anti-calcification property, etc.

The concept of nanotechnology was first developed by Nobel Laureate scientist Richard Feynman in his 1959 work "There's Plenty of Room at the Bottom." He

DOI: 10.1201/9781003331612-15

is known as the "Father of Nanotechnology." Nanotechnology is the science of all matter that exists in the "nano-dimension." Here, the word "nanoparticle" includes all the materials of size 1–100 nanometers (1 nanometer = 10^{-9} meters). Presently, this is the need of the hour to manufacture nano-sized fibers that provide greater surface area and are thin and porous, which are considered to be highly desirable for engineering vascular graft implants, bone grafts, heart valve sewing rings, endovascular stent grafts, tissue-engineered heart valves, etc. The most economic and accessible technique for manufacturing such nanofibers is electrospinning. In 1933, Darrel H. Reneker (Doshi & Reneker, 1995) produced fibers from an electrostatically charged mixture and termed the whole procedure "electrospinning." That is how the word "electrospinning" was first introduced to the world of science. The first medical application of electrospun fiber mesh was the fabrication of a wound dressing (Tucker et al., 2012).

Currently, cardiovascular diseases (CVDs) constitute the leading cause of mortality on a global scale. As per the fact sheet of the World Health Organization, roughly 17.9 million people died in 2019 due to CVDs, which represents 32% of the deaths all over the world. Of those deaths, 85% were caused by heart attacks and strokes. In the same year, the total count of premature deaths due to noncommunicable diseases reached 17 million; all of them were below the age of 70, out of which 38% were due to CVDs. By cardiovascular diseases, one means all the disorders of the heart and blood vessels, namely peripheral arterial disease, coronary heart disease, pulmonary embolism, deep vein thrombosis, and myocardial infarction (MI), all of which may result in ischemia, tissue occlusion, and tissue death. Among them, myocardial infarction and heart failure are the principal causes that result in death. In cardiovascular medicine, surgical approaches and transplantation are often the best treatments for patients with chronic diseases. As it has already been stated in the preceding paragraphs, nanotechnology may provide a more effective cure (i.e., vascular grafts, stents, heart valve prostheses, nerve guidance conduits) to cardiovascular diseases, severed nerves, etc., so as to enhance the efficacy of the treatment and to minimize the chances of vascular graft infection and thrombosis. In this review study, several major applications of biotextile in vascular graft implants will be discussed; furthermore, the techniques used to develop vascular graft implants and heart valves using nanotechnology will also be discussed in detail.

12.2 BIOTEXTILE

Biotextile refers to all products and structures that are made up of fibers (yarn, RN, or fabric). Medical application of those textile-made products is increasing gradually in medication delivery system and tissue engineering. The hygiene and healthcare sectors are the crucial and developing segment of the textile industry. Because of their adaptability to their environment (when used inside the body), biotextiles have emerged as an essential solution for implantable medical devices. Manufacturing technologies and new fibers with modified properties have emerged in the medical sectors as polymer science, nanotechnology, and related fields have advanced. The most promising approach for developing new medical textiles is to change the chemical and physical properties of the fiber structures, develop stimuli-responsive materials, and finish the textile material with multifunctional finishing.

12.2.1 CLASSIFICATION OF BIOTEXTILE

12.2.1.1 Non-implantable Materials

This refers to the class of materials that are applied externally to the body and do not necessarily lie close to the skin. Examples: gauzes, compression, plasters, wadding, lint, etc. in Figure 12.1.

12.2.1.2 Implantable Materials

This refers to the class of materials that are used to repair and treat any injury, such as sutures (which are used to close the wound) or vascular grafts, artificial ligaments, etc. (used in transplantation procedures). Examples: wound closure, orthopedic implants, soft tissue implants, cardiovascular implants, etc. (Figure 12.1). For a textile material to be implantable in a living body, it must be biocompatible and biostable. The following factors will influence the body's reaction to the implanted textile material:

    a. The most important physical property of a vascular graft or fabricated scaffold is its porosity. The porosity of the textile material determines the speed of tissue ingrowth and tissue regeneration, subsequently supporting or damaging the implanted material.

    b. As compared to large fibers with non-uniform cross-sections, small circular fibrous structures are a better encapsulating agent for human tissue. This means the fiber size should be small.

    c. The textile material must not contain any harmful substances, such as surface adulterants, lubricating agents, and sizing agents, so as to avoid any possibility of immunogenicity.

    d. The excellence of the artificial implant is based upon the biodegradability of the textile material used in its fabrication.

12.2.1.3 Extracorporeal Devices

This refers to the class of materials that are arranged extracorporeally (based on or occurring outside the living body) and applied to aid dysfunctional organs like a diseased kidney, heart, lung, etc. They function as mechanical devices that mimic natural organs, such as a dialyzer, an artificial liver, an artificial inhalator, and ECMO (Extracorporeal Membrane Oxygenation) in Figure 12.1. The textile materials used in these devices greatly affect their performance.

12.2.1.4 Healthcare and Hygiene Products

This refers to the class of materials that are used for health and hygiene purposes. For example, sanitary napkins, diapers, adult diapers, wipes, PPE kits, etc. in Figure 12.1. Though they may be used for many different things, their application in the medical field was enormous due to their natural capabilities. They are particularly useful in the medical field, where they are used to create surgical gowns, hair masks,

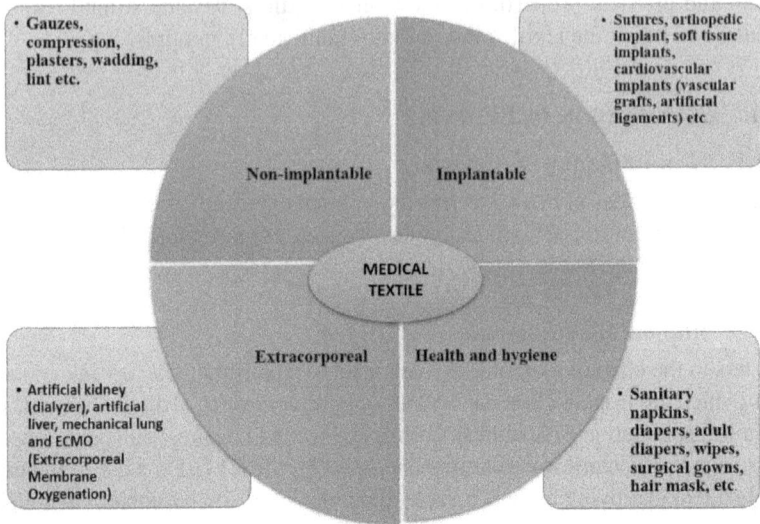

FIGURE 12.1 Medical textile classification

hygiene, and safety equipment for patients and hospital staff. Moreover, during the COVID-19 pandemic, PPE kits, masks, and gloves became a part of every individual's daily life (Shah et al., 2019).

12.2.2 NANOTECHNOLOGY IN BIOTEXTILES

In the manufacturing of a biomedical device with textile material, the most crucial task is to create a suitable fiber with the desired traits. Since the spinning technique affects the inherent properties (texture, cross-sectional shape, size, and surface-to-volume ratio, etc.) of the fibers and yarns, the choice of the spinning technique is of utmost importance. There are numerous methods to create textile fiber. To name a few, electrospinning, gel spinning, co-electrospinning, centrifugal electrospinning, hydrogel fiber spinning, 3D bioprinting, etc. (Calvin et al., 2020). Precisely, due to advancements in spinning technology, surface finishing, surface coating, and fiber assembly methods, the construction of new biotextile materials is much easier, more economical, and more efficient. Advancement in nanotechnology has paved the path to a new era of medicinal devices: now one can incorporate nanoparticles into fiber-forming polymers (natural or synthetic) before spinning into yarn; electrospinning facilitates the preparation of nanofibers from fiber-forming polymers; and nanofinishing treatments allow nanoparticles to be impregnated into fabrics (Morris & Murray, 2020). Various applications of nanotechnology in biotextile are shown in Figure 12.2. The following are the methods of production for biotextiles:

12.2.2.1 Melt Extrusion/Melt Spinning

In this method of spinning, the first step is to heat the polymer at a temperature exceeding the melting point of the same polymer; after that, the polymer is shaped using a spinneret. The structural design of the spinneret, which includes its shape and the

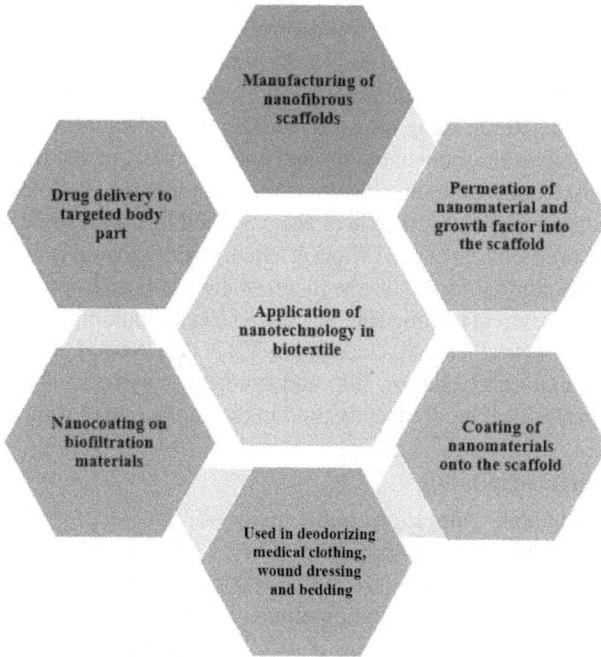

FIGURE 12.2 Application of nanotechnology in biotextile

dimensions of the holes, determines the physical and chemical characteristics of the fiber so formed, for instance, size, filament number (monofilament or multifilament), and structural orientation. Cross-sectional shape influences many physicochemical features of the fiber, namely the surface-to-volume ratio, twist, yield strength, shrinkage, and bending rigidity. The fabrication process through melt spinning is very fast, and it can work without solvent addition; however, melt spinning's application is limited to only thermoplastic materials. Another limitation of this process is the decomposition of materials at temperatures below their melting point (Miranda et al., 2020).

12.2.2.2 Wet or Gel Spinning

Wet spinning led the way to the convenient spinning of thermoplastic materials since they experience decomposition at elevated temperatures when processed through melt extrusion (as in the case of cellulose, chitosan, and alginate) (Gupta, 2013). Rayon was the first material to get spun through wet spinning (Miranda et al., 2020). This approach to spinning enables the formation of fibers in nano- as well as micrometer-scale dimensions, consequently resulting in highly porous and interconnected fibers, which are beneficial for cell embedding and cell proliferation (Miranda et al., 2020).

12.2.2.3 Electrospinning

Electrospinning is the most convenient and economic technique for producing fine fibers of varying sizes (from nanometers to micrometers). The process employs two major components: the spinneret and the collector plate (Wang & Zhao, 2019). Under a high potential difference between the spinneret and collector plate, the ejected polymer solution converts into nanofibers. The electrospinning process is capable to prepare continuous 3D structures with high porosity and surface area (Felgueiras & Amorim, 2017; Teixeira et al., 2020). Early research revealed that, when it comes to supporting the regeneration of various human tissues and organs, including the heart and liver as well as organs like bone, skin, and blood vessels, nanofibrous scaffolds offer a lot of promise and adaptability and researchers also reported that with biodegradable polymer they aid the proliferation of cell (Wang & Zhao, 2019; Agarwal et al., 2008; Qian et al., 2018). Electrospinning facilitates the incorporation of bioactive agents into vascular grafts through different techniques like coaxial electrospinning, blending, covalent and non-covalent binding, etc. (Rychter et al., 2017). Various organic and inorganic, natural (gelatin, chitosan, collagen, silk) and synthetic polymer (polyurethane, polylactide, polycaprolactone) are frequently used in electrospinning (Yang et al., 2018).

13.2.2.4   Coelectrospinning

One of the most notable innovations in the history of the electrospinning technique was the introduction of coaxial spinnerets. The coaxial spinneret is different from others because it has a core-shell nozzle that is connected to a double-compartment syringe and two separate pumps and pipelines. So, the coaxial spinneret can electrospin two different polymer solutions at different speeds, making nanofibers with a core and a shell. This method lets fibers made from polymers that aren't usually used in the electrospinning process of vascular grafts be made (Andrzej et al., 2017).

13.2.2.5   Centrifugal Electrospinning

This technique of spinning overcomes various drawbacks to the electrospinning technique, such as improved scalability and yield of production by using aligned fiber (Mehta et al., 2019). Employing a centrifugal electrospinning system, highly aligned fiber can be formed from different polymers (polyvinylidene fluoride, polyethylene, chitosan) (Wagner et al., 2020).

12.2.2.6   3D Printing

In recent decades, printing methods have been considered a quick and economical way of manufacturing. In the 1980s, 3D printing technology was initially developed as an additive manufacturing technique. After that, it influenced the medical field along with some other areas (Bishop et al., 2017). Applications for 3D printing complicated biomedical devices range from the regeneration of intricate organs with sophisticated 3D microarchitecture (such as the liver and lymphoid organs) to stem cell differentiation scaffolds (Chia & Wu, 2015). Another prospective application of this technique is in regenerative medicine using seeded stem cells and tissue replacement (Chia & Wu, 2015; Miranda et al., 2020).

12.2.2.7   Nanofibres

All the fibers with diameters less than 100 nanometers are classified as nanofibers. In comparison to bulk monofilaments, these fibers have higher flexibility, a high ratio of surface area to volume, structural similarity with extracellular matrix (ECM), and the provision for surface modification, which makes them a good fit in a variety of contexts, for example, the filtration of impurities (submicron particles) in industrial separation processes, wound dressing, tissue-engineered scaffolds, and blood vessel implants (Jyothirmai & Panda, 2021). Nanofibers are generally generated by the electrospinning technique (He et al., 2022). Nanofibers can be acquired from a variety of polymers, both natural and manmade, according to the needs of the experimenter (Matsuzaki et al., 2019). In an earlier study, the researcher transformed bundles of thousands of nanofibers into woven nanotextiles with the aid of an innovative robotic system, this is the exclusive method for producing seamless nanotextiles made of tubular nanofibers. Further investigation into the physical and biological characteristics of the woven nanotextile used in this work showed a striking and significant difference between the woven nanotextile and their nanofibrous counterparts. When placed within an artery, the nanotextile conduits might serve as an effective emboli, as they were found to be strong, suturable, kink-proof, and non-thrombogenic, according to in vivo tests carried out by the researchers (Joseph et al., 2018).

12.3 VASCULAR GRAFT IMPLANTS

12.3.1 VASCULAR GRAFT

Vascular bypass or vascular grafts (Figure 12.3) are utilized to replace any portion of a damaged artery that has developed an aneurysm or atherosclerosis. It

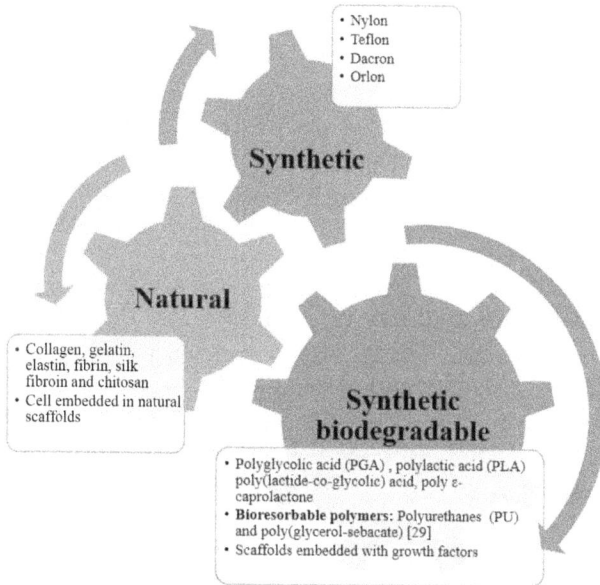

FIGURE 12.3   Vascular graft biotextile

can be either arteries, veins, capillaries, or tissue. In the early 1950s, Professor William Edward Shinn was the one to make the first arterial graft (a knitted artery) (King et al., 2013). The first commercial tube, a braided nylon tube, was introduced in 1956. It was further investigated that nylon was hydrostatically unstable, which made it ineligible for long-term implantation (King et al., 2013). Commonly, autograft—a graft of tissue from the same individual's vein—is the most suitable graft material for a bypass (Shah et al., 2019). The saphenous vein is the most prominent vascular graft due to its convenient detachment and patency of at least 10 years (Toong et al., 2020). However, for many patients, use of an autograft is not a feasible choice since they lack a proper blood vessel because of a size mismatch, pre-existing disease, or previous surgery (Zhang & King, 2022). Furthermore, previous studies have shown that approximately 15% of autografts result in stenosis or obstructed vessels within one year of implantation. That is when synthetic vascular grafts emerge as a better solution for the aforementioned problems, in particular Teflon (polytetrafluoroethylene) and Dacron (polyethylene terephthalate) vascular grafts. However, when the diameter of the grafts is less than 6 mm, the synthetic arterial grafts fail due to the formation of thrombosis, low patency, mechanical mismatch, and intimal hyperlapsia (Desai et al., 2011; Li & Henry, 2011; Behrens & Ruder, 2021; Washington & Bashur, 2017). For a vascular graft to remain patent for a long time, its structural and mechanical behavior must match that of an artery. An ideal vascular graft should possess the following attributes:

1. It should have mechanical strength similar to a normal vessel to withstand the hemodynamic stresses.
2. It should be non-toxic and non-immunogenic.
3. It should be biocompatible and easily available in different sizes for emergency care.
4. It should be easily suturable.
5. It should be resistant to thrombosis and infection in vivo.
6. Last but not least, it should have a reasonable manufacturing cost.

(Desai et al., 2011; Zhang & King, 2022; Gokarneshan & Dhatchayani, 2017)

Vascular grafts may be created from a variety of materials and in a wide range of sizes (6–20 mm) (Gokarneshan & Dhatchayani, 2017):

- Synthetic: Nylon, Teflon®, Dacron®, Orlon®
- Synthetic biodegradable polymers include polyglycolic acid (PGA), poly(lactide-co-glycolic) acid (PLGA), polylactic acid (PLA), polycaprolactone, and biodegradable materials like polyurethanes and poly (glycerol-sebacate) (Liu et al., 2018).
- Natural polymers: collagen, gelatin, elastin, fibrin, silk fibroin, and chitosan

To date, synthetic vascular grafts are mainly constructed using manufacturing techniques like weaving, knitting, and electrospinning. A comparison between woven grafts and knitted grafts is shown in Table 12.1.

TABLE 12.1

Comparison between woven and knitted grafts

Manufacturing technique employed	Design/ Structure	Characteristics of the graft manufactured	Limitations
Weaving	Plain, twill, and satin	• Soft textured surface, easy administration and manipulation, inertness, porosity, bursting-strength, easily suturable, and biological therapeutic response (Mehta et al., 2019)	• They are susceptible to grow radially and fray. • During suturing, they get disentangled at the cut ends.
Knitting	Warp and weft	• Knitted materials are smoother, more pliable, acquiescent, highly porous, and are much more convenient as compared to woven materials (Mehta et al., 2019; Calvin et al., 2020). • Warp knitted structures are more dimensionally stable than weft knitted structures since they have less stretch (Mehta et al., 2019). • Their structural resemblance to arteries protects them from undergoing fatigue amplification.	• Knitted structures are more porous than woven fabrics which benefits tissue ingrowth but results in undesirable water permeation (to reduce permeability, knitted materials must be impregnated with collagen or gelatin) (Calvin et al., 2020). • Dacron is the only material which is available in the form of commercial knitted graft (Singh et al., 2015).

12.3.2 Braided Textiles

Braiding is the procedure of interlacing at least three yarns in an angled overlying structure. Braided textiles are robust and flexible, which is why they are readily used in surgical sutures, due to the low crossing profile (0.044–0.058 in) of braided structure that aids in delivery (Huang et al., 2018). Advancements in 3D braiding techniques have led to the formation of complex structures such as "I"-beam solid tubes and hollow tubes. Because of the braided hollow tube's low bending rigidity and its potential to expand unidirectionally, it is used in vascular stents (Chen, 2015). Braided textiles are also used in manufacturing anterior cruciate ligament (ACL) prostheses. The characteristics of a textile material highly depend on its structural design; therefore, to improve the efficiency of a textile material, it can be produced by the incorporation of weaving, knitting, and braiding. For instance, in the construction of PET fabric, the yarns are first knitted, and then the knits are braided together (Calvin et al., 2020).

12.3.3 Now, Let's Discuss the Materials Used in the Creation of Scaffolds

12.3.3.1 Natural Polymers

Extracellular matrix-derived proteins are biocompatible and biostable; consequently, they have become a center of attraction for scientists and researchers since they provide structural complexity with functional groups that act as a chemically active site for cell attachment (Mehta et al., 2019). They can mimic the biostructure of the native blood vessels. ECM proteins that are commonly used in the fabrication of tissue-engineered prostheses include collagen, gelatin, elastin, and fibrin (Carrabba & Madeddu, 2018). Some other natural polymers, including silk fibroin, chitosan, and polysaccharides, for example, cellulose, chitosan, chitin, and alginate, are also used as the base material in the fabrication of scaffolds. Although natural polymers are exceptionally biocompatible and cell cohesive, they still lack the mechanical properties that are necessary for engineering vascular tissues; that is when synthetic polymers emerge as an alternative (Kabirian et al., 2018).

12.3.3.1.1 Cellulose

The major sources of cellulose are plants and agricultural residuals. Biomedical application of cellulose is increasing due to its distinct characteristics like its high tensile strength, antistatic qualities, transparency, abrasion resistance, moisture absorption, and permeability (Zhang et al., 2017; Chen et al., 2016; Teixeira et al., 2019). Cellulose on its own cannot be electrospun, but its fibers can be processed using wet spinning (Miranda et al., 2020). Due to its thrombogenicity, cellulose fibers have been employed as surgical sutures, wound dressings, and hemostats (Calvin et al., 2020).

12.3.3.1.2 Chitosan

Chitosan is obtained from chitin, which is generally procured from the crustacean's shell, insects' cuticles, and the cell walls of fungi which is extensively used as a drug delivery polymer because of its blending ability with a wide range of polymers, aqueous solubility, easy surface changing capacity which easily to turn it into gels, films, or fibers (Malafaya et al., 2007; Rinaudo, 2006; Anitha et al., 2014). Nevertheless, all chitosan polymers are biocompatible, biodegradable, antimicrobial, and have outstanding antitumor and wound healing abilities (Kmiec et al., 2017). Badhe et al. (2017) and Zhang et al. (2006) developed bioresorbable vascular graft scaffolds from chitosan and gelatin using two distinct methods (Toong et al., 2020).

12.3.3.1.3 Collagen

As mentioned earlier, ECM contains a significant amount of collagen; it serves the purpose of limiting strain and providing the required support to blood vessels. Collagen is the most prevalent mammalian protein which has the ability to penetrate lipid-free surfaces and acts as a great surface-active material. Collagen, as compared with other natural polymers, is considerably more preferred in biomedical applications because of its high biodegradability, robustness, superior biocompatibility, and weak reactogenicity (Felgueiras et al., 2014, 2016; Lee et al., 2001; Tangsadthakun et al., 2017). Scaffolds made up of electrospun collagen have high porosity and surface area, which makes them suitable for engineering vascular tissue (Malafaya et al., 2007). Collagen-based fibers have wide biomedical applications; for instance, Jin et al. developed Nerve Guidance Conduits (NGC) with oriented hydrogel arrangements on a PLCL electrospun nanofiber sheet and inferred that the NGC consisting of aligned collagen hydrogel is favorable for peripheral nerve regeneration (Yan et al., 2021).

Martens et al. produced three ultra-small superparamagnetic iron oxide nanoparticles (USPIO) that were instantly settled in collagen scaffolds by chemical cross-linking and employed indirectly as imaging graft scaffolds, which is useful for studying the in vivo degradation cycle (Liu et al., 2022).

12.3.3.1.4 Gelatin

This natural polymer has a high concentration of glycine, proline, and 4-hydroxyproline residues which are extracted from collagen through structural and chemical breakdown. Gelatin has a variety of functional groups in its structure that may act as cell-binding sites or enhance the adhesion of cells which makes it a suitable preference for tissue engineering. It also applies to the manufacture of biocompatible biomolecule delivery systems, coating stents, and the delivery of anti-proliferative drugs and wound dressings (Li & Henry, 2011). They also are used in the delivery of therapeutic active molecules in the targeted sites including adipose tissue, bone, cartilage, etc. through encapsulation (Tamura et al., 2015; Mogoşanu & Grumezescu, 2014; Malafaya et al., 2007). Because of their potential to enhance cell adhesion and cell growth, hybrid hydrogels made from GelMA (gelatin methacrylate) are widely employed in the engineering of cardiovascular tissues (Amal et al., 2022). Electrospinning can be used to fabricate gelatin methacrylate nanofibers by photoinitiator where fibers are interlinked into a network hydrogel in presence of UV rays. Hydrogel nanofibers may be utilized to create extracellular matrix (ECM)-like structures that promote endothelial cell and dermal fibroblast adhesion, proliferation, and migration within scaffolds, hence accelerating vascularization.

Natural polymers lack mechanical strength, flexibility, and toughness while being biocompatible and biodegradable. Comparably, synthetic polymers are much more mechanically robust and thermally stable. They can be easily processed into a variety of shapes and sizes during production. Synthetic polymers tend to be more cost-effective (Liu et al., 2022).

12.3.3.2 Synthetic Polymers

Expanded polytetrafluoroethylene (ePTFE) and polyethylene terephthalate (PET in woven form) are the synthetic materials most often utilized in vascular grafts, commercially known as Dacron which can be easily used with comparably high success for bypass of large arteries (>6 mm) (Zhang & King, 2022; Desai et al., 2011). However, because of thrombosis and intimal hyperplasia, the ePTFE and PET grafts are vulnerable to occlusion and therefore suffer from low patency rates (Behrens & Ruder, 2021; Washington & Bashur, 2017; Elliott et al., 2019), when the vessel diameter is less than 6 mm, as in the case of coronary and infrapopliteal bypass. There is a long-felt need for a non-thrombogenic, viscoelastic, blood-compatible, and biocompatible small-diameter vascular graft; consequently, this is one of the primary motivations for the study of cardiovascular bioengineering (Joseph et al., 2022). Recent research includes anti-thrombogenic modifications with nanoparticles and biomolecules such as growth factors, heparin (as an anticoagulant), cholesterol-lowering agents (statins), anti-inflammatory agents, prophylactic antibiotics, and antimicrobial agents. Moreover, synthetic vascular grafts are now more efficient with the development of surface coatings and tissue-engineered vascular grafts (TEVGs) impregnated with bioactive agents (Amal et al., 2022; Miranda et al., 2020; Li & Henry, 2011). Furthermore, because synthetic grafts do not grow naturally in pediatric patients, multi-surgical intervention may be required for the rest of their lives (Zhang & King, 2022).

12.3.3.2.1 Expanded Polytetrafluoroethylene (Eptfe)

ePTFE is a comparably inert material that was patented as Teflon by DuPont in 1937 (Greco, 1994). ePTFE is a microporous version of PTFE, an inert fluorocarbon polymer, manufactured by its extrusion and sintering. Since it is non-biodegradable and anti-thrombogenic, it is used for lower-limb bypass grafts (7–9 mm) which are stiffer than natural arteries (Desai et al., 2011). Serious drawbacks of such transplant materials are mechanical compatibility and absence of endothelial cells (ECs) and poor patency (Mai & Joseph, 2012). Scientists and researchers proposed a number of promising approaches to increase graft permeability and promote tissue ingrowth and transmural capillary ingrowth for the purpose of enhancing the quality of ePTFE grafts. Meslmani et al. created vascular grafts using poly(lactic-co-glycolic) acid (PLGA) immobilized on polytetrafluoroethylene (ePTFE) films (Meslmani et al., 2017). One of the major drawbacks of conventional ePTFE is suture hole bleeding and sweating, which has been addressed by Sulzer Vascutek's biomedical sealant, which is hydrolyzable gelatin (a water-soluble protein) sealant, also known as SEALPTFE™. As the name suggests, it is applied on the outer surface of ePTFE to minimize sweating and to counter the hole bleeding; moreover, one can achieve excellent handling properties with antibiotic bonding (Radhakrishnan, 2019).

12.3.3.2.2 Petroethylene Terephthalate

PET is a thermoplastic polymer of the polyester family, commonly known as Dacron, manufactured by Maquet Cardiovascular (Mai & Joseph, 2012), with chemical inertness contributing to its biocompatibility. PET has found many applications, one of which is specifically woven or knitted vascular grafts for cardiovascular purposes (He et al., 2022). In the woven grafts, the polyester thread follows the plain weaving pattern, which consequently results in restricted porosity and deformation (under stress) of the final product. However, the knitted Dacron® grafts are constructed by looping the multiple filaments of the PET thread to impart higher porosity and compatibility. In an attempt to enhance the tissue ingrowth, the threads are looped on the surface of the graft. The PET grafts have exquisite mechanical stability for more than 10 years, except for their knitted form, which gets inflated due to their baggy knit pattern (Li et al., 2015). As compared to knitted form, woven PET has smaller pores, consequently reducing blood leakage (Mai & Joseph, 2012). In order to reduce blood and prevent graft infection, PET grafts are often coated with proteins such as albumin, silk fibroin, or collagen (Mai & Joseph, 2012; Li et al., 2015). Further, to prevent mechanical dysfunction and to stimulate tissue incorporation, the surfaces of PET grafts are often crimped, increasing the flexibility, kink resistance, and compliance of the graft. In one of the studies by Yang et al. (2018), it was reported that seamless tubular prostheses created from a blend of polyester and silk yarns had improved mechanical properties and enhanced cytocompatibility as compared to expanded polytetrafluoroethylene (e-PTFE) implants (Li et al., 2015). Similar to ePTFE, PET is also a synthetic material that may cause an immunogenic reaction which promotes the chance of thrombosis and neo-intimal proliferation (Miranda et al., 2020).

The long-term biological response of the non-biodegradable graft materials has emerged as a significant problem, which leads to drastic consequences caused by the foreign body response, such as intimal thickening and chronic thrombotic occlusions. Herein, the biodegradable grafts exhibit properties like biocompatibility and biodegradability that inhibit foreign body response; however, natural polymers lack mechanical stability. Natural polymers have emerged as a promising solution for the non-bioactive nature of synthetic vascular grafts.

12.3.3.2.3 Synthetic Biodegradable

They are capable of a controlled degradation that enables the growth of endothelial cells on the graft's surface by the native cells. With the constant secretion of the components of the ECM, eventually, the endogenous vessels will replace the degraded graft. Biodegradable polymers include polylactic acid (PLA), polyglycolic acid (PGA), poly(lactide-co-glycolic) acid, poly-caprolactone (PCL), polyurethanes, and poly(glycerol-sebacate). One can get a variety of degradation rates of the poly (lactic-co-glycolic acid) (PLGA) polymer by altering the proportions of its constituent polymers, PGA and PLA (Li et al., 2015). Bioresorbable polymers such as polyurethanes (PU) and poly (glycerol-sebacate) have exceptional biocompatibility, blood compatibility, and insignificant thrombogenicity, supporting the development of endothelial cells and the production of elastin (Liu et al., 2018). Synthetic polymers are mechanically fit for the fabrication of vascular grafts but lack the ability of cell proliferation or cytocompatibility; therefore, they should be amalgamated with natural polymers (Toong et al., 2020; Liang et al., 2020; Nguyen & Camci-Unal, 2019), thusly generating a fiber with easy handling and synergistic performance as a vascular prosthesis (Bhuiyan, 2019; Miranda et al., 2020; Yan et al., 2021). Even though these changes result in better materials for engineering vascular grafts or drug delivery systems, fabricating amalgamated fibers requires a variety of manufacturing techniques that can be time-consuming and exhausting. Hence, the development of such a scaffold that can bio-mimic the natural vessels in terms of both mechanical and biological properties is the most pursued goal in the field of vascular graft engineering.

For example, the amalgamation of synthetic polymers and collagen enhances the mechanical strength of the scaffold so formed. Moreover, inserting biomolecules like growth factors into collagen-based scaffolds and gels amplifies their ability to regenerate and heal (Miranda et al., 2020). Another researcher, Sheikh et al., combined silk fibroin and PCL to form a colloidal solution and produced electrospun nanofibers. The resultant nanofibers were hygroscopic in nature and had better mechanical characteristics in comparison to pure silk fibroin nanofibers (Yan et al., 2021; Cunha et al., 2011). Combining marine collagen and PLGA fibers, Jeong et al. fabricated a new collagen-based tubular scaffold that had enhanced mechanical properties in a dry as well as a hydrated environment. It was later revealed that under normal blood circulation, both cell proliferation and alignment along the PLGA fibers were enhanced, and the cells had the ability to maintain their distinctive cell phenotype

(Jeong et al., 2007). Fu et al. observe fibers were produced from a combination of gelatin with PCL and collagen with PLCL for constructing vascular grafts. The resultant fibers exhibited enhanced hydrophilicity and cell adhesion because of the constituent natural proteins. Later on, some in vivo experiments were performed on mice. The researchers concluded from these studies that, when compared to gelatin or PCL scaffolds, tissue regeneration on collagen or PLCL scaffolds was much more homogeneous. Moreover, the modulus of elasticity of the implanted collagen/PLCL scaffold surpassed that of the gelatin/PCL scaffold (Fu et al., 2014). Similarly, Duan et al. engineered vascular tissue by using PCL/collagen core-shell fibers. PCL was included as the core and collagen as the shell; the core has the required mechanical properties, while the shell enhanced the vascular cell attachment (Duan et al., 2016). Joseph et al. constructed a nanotextile-based vascular graft (NanoGraft), exhibiting high flexibility and mechanical robustness, by interlacing nanofibrous threads of poly-L-lactic acid. In the study, the NanoGrafts (4 mm in diameter) and ePTFE graft were first pre-clotted and then implanted in a porcine carotid artery substitute model at the same time. The study demonstrated a patency of 100% and 66% for NanoGraft and ePTFE, respectively, at two weeks, thus, proving the in vivo convenience and safety of NanoGraft and its potential superiority over ePTFE (Joseph et al., 2022).

12.3.3.3 Tissue Engineering in Vascular Grafts

Tissue engineering includes engineering living systems, i.e., constructing an implant that can degrade at a controlled rate in order for cells to heal the damaged tissue and create normal tissue. It includes the election and culture of appropriate cells on 3D scaffolds to promote cell growth and tissue regeneration (similar to native ones) with time (Behrens & Ruder, 2021; Sahar et al., 2017). There are three approaches to modeling tissue-engineered vascular grafts: in vitro (outside of a living body in a controlled environment), in vivo (performed or taking place in a living organism), and in situ (situated on the site) (Sahar et al., 2017; Knight et al., 2014).

In the "in vitro" approach, the engineered tissue is developed in an experimental and controlled manner and then transplanted as a replacement for the native or injured tissue (Radhakrishnan, 2019). In the second and third approaches, the implanted cells work as the "building blocks of neo-tissue" (Knight et al., 2014). In the "in vivo" approach, after the in vitro development of the cells on the scaffold, the scaffold is then implanted in the living body, and the regeneration of the functional tissue takes place within the body. In the "in situ" approach, the substances capable of promoting the gradual secretion of the bioactive molecules and required nutrients are transmitted to the body to allure the body's stem cells or tissue progenitors, and consequently, the regeneration of the functional tissue takes place inside the body (Miranda et al., 2020; Sahar et al., 2017; Brahatheeswaran Dhandayuthapani et al., 2011; Pashneh-Tala et al., 2016). Biocompatibility, biodegradability, mechanical integrity, mechanical strength, porous interconnectivity, and surface properties for cell-cell interaction and cell adhesion are the desired requisites of an ideal material for tissue engineering of a vascular graft (Gentile et al., 2014). The manufacturing technique of a vascular graft may consist of electrospinning, scaffold manufacturing techniques like solvent casting and leaching, gas foaming technology, emulsion freeze drying, and thermally induced phase separation (Pashneh-Tala et al., 2016).

The field of tissue engineering came into existence in 1993 (L'Heureux et al., 1993). This approach has been continuously experimented with for the past two decades due to the urgent and unmet demand for a feasible small-caliber vascular graft (Toong et al., 2020; Zhang & King, 2022). Nikalson et al. used tissue engineering to create a vascular graft by embedding PGA (biodegradable in nature) tubular scaffolds with smooth muscle cells (SMC) (obtained from different individuals of the same species) and culturing them under cyclic radial tension. The graft was decellularized and kept at a temperature of 4°C after the gradual degradation of PGA, and then it was implanted in the body. It exhibited better patency for a brief period of time (1 month–1 year) after implantation in baboon and canine replacement models (Zhang & King, 2022). In another study, to prevent thrombosis in the graft, Matsuzaki et al. blended heparin and PLCL in a methylethylketone/acetone/ethanol solvent. Despite the secretion of 97% of the heparin in not more than the first 24 hours of the implantation, the inclusion of heparin remarkably reduced platelet attachment and thrombosis, hence reducing the thrombotic obstruction rate for the graft from 60% to 0% during one week of implantation (Matsuzaki et al., 2021). In their investigation, Campbell et al. used rabbit and mouse models to study the insertion of a silicon tube into the peritoneal cavity. A uniform layer of SMA-positive cells resembling the tunica medium was seen after two weeks. With the formation of the mesothelium layer, collagen encased the tubes as an adventitia layer (Karkan et al., 2019). To prevent thrombosis, Fengyi et al. produced a heparinized 3D nanofibrous vascular scaffold using chitosan and polycaprolactone. They used "vascular endothelial growth factor (VEGF)" and heparin immobilization to mimic the bioenvironment of the native blood vessels. The study proved that the non-thrombogenicity of these scaffolds increased remarkably with the immobilization of heparin (Karkan et al., 2019). In the search for a better composite vascular graft, silver has been coated on the grafts, preventing postoperative infections (Abdul et al., 2022). In a similar study, sulphate-based coatings have been applied to the grafts, resulting in reduced thrombogenicity and neointimal hyperplasia (Abdul et al., 2022). Diamond-like carbon (DLC) coatings are biocompatible in nature, noncytotoxic, robust, and wear-resistant; thus, they have been used to coat ePTFE-based artificial vascular grafts, ensuring enhanced patency (Orrit-Prat et al., 2021; Fujii et al., 2019). The development of tissue-engineered prostheses is shown in Figure 12.4.

12.3.3.4   Vascular Graft Infection

In general, thrombosis and neointimal membrane formation cause vascular graft infections (Li & Henry, 2011). Vascular graft infections (VGI) occur at a rate of 1–6% and can result in morbidity, mortality, and limb loss in prosthetic vascular surgery (He et al., 2022; Lazic et al., 2022). Accordingly, the task of developing a method for the prevention and effective management of VGIs is of paramount importance. Numerous studies have shown that antibiotic and antiseptic-impregnated grafts can be remarkably effective in the prevention of VGIs, particularly antimicrobial nanofibers and nanoparticles. Nanoparticles and nanofibers have an exceptionally greater surface area, allowing better encapsulation of antibiotics and antiseptics, enabling researchers to create better vascular grafts as compared to conventional antimicrobial grafts (metal-coated, i.e., silver-coated grafts, and rifampin soaked graft) (Ricco & Assadian, 2011; Abdul et al., 2022; Lew &

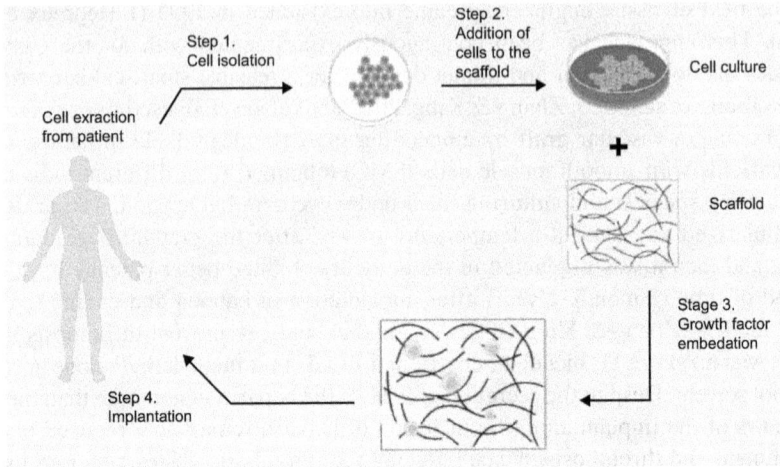

FIGURE 12.4 Development of tissue-engineered prostheses

Moore, 2011; Goëau-Brissonnière et al., 1994); Rifampin, daptomycin, gentamicin, and vancomycin are some of the antibiotics that have been investigated for their applications in synthetic grafts, particularly Teflon and Dacron (Lew & Moore, 2011). Almeida et al. impregnated collagen implants with gentamicin in a related investigation, implanted them in patients with lower limb ischemia, and observed a reduced surgical site infection rate (Almeida et al., 2014). Antiseptics, as compared to antibiotics, generally have a broad range of antimicrobial activity (McDonnell & Russell, 1999). Coating premade vascular grafts with nanofibrous constructs is one of the most effective ways of amplifying the antimicrobial properties of a vascular graft. In an experiment by Liu et al., the nanofibers of PLGA and vancomycin were electrospun onto a vascular graft, and the secretion of vancomycin was observed (Lew & Moore, 2011). Another novel approach to engineering a vascular graft is to embed the antimicrobial materials into the VG; furthermore, it is now possible to blend the drugs or bioactive agents into the electrospinning solution itself (He et al., 2022). A vascular graft for hemodialysis access has been fabricated with PCL as the medial layer and nano spun fibers of type I collagen at the luminal and adventitial sides, ensuring a steady and prolonged release of the drugs used (Radakovic et al., 2017). In another study, distinct gentamicin-coating formulas were applied to ePTFE vascular grafts via dip coating, and their degree of antimicrobial efficacy, blood compatibility, and biocompatibility was evaluated in vitro (Lazic et al., 2022). The results showed a remarkable reduction in surgical site infections in cardiac, general, and orthopedic surgery (Witkowski et al., 2016).

12.3.3.5 Heart Valve

One of the top causes of mortality worldwide, CVD resulted in 17.9 million fatalities in 2019. All illnesses affecting the heart and blood vessels are referred to as cardiovascular diseases (CVDs). They include myocardial infarction (MI), inborn heart disease, pulmonary embolism, coronary heart disease, peripheral arterial disease, and deep vein thrombosis (Sreeniwas & Sinha, 2020).

The human heart contains four valves which allows a unidirectional flow of blood from or towards the heart. There are several reasons for a diseased heart valve, including congenital causes, rheumatic fever, and calcification. Impaired heart valves may result in severe health problems, heart failure, and even death. Replacement with a unique functioning heart valve is the standard therapy for serious heart valve disease. On the basis of the leaflet material, there exist two types of artificial heart valves or heart valve prostheses (Figure 12.5), namely, bioprosthetic heart valves (BHV) and mechanical heart valves (MHV) (Dangas et al., 2016). Generally, to replace the diseased heart valve, these two are employed by means of a surgical or transcatheter approach (Dangas et al., 2016; Li & Henry, 2011).

12.3.3.6 Mechanical Heart Valve

MHVs are more like machines than living tissues; they function as native heart valves but do not have the same microstructure (Shao et al., 2021). Different synthetic materials like polymer, metals such as stainless steel and titanium, ceramics, and carbon, are used in the preparation of mechanical heart valves (Bishop et al., 2017), with mechanically mobile parts, and they have basically three design categories: caged ball valves, tilting disc valves, and bileaflet valves (Khandpur, 2020). MHVs were initially manufactured in the form of an occluder, and then they progressively evolved into modern-day bileaflet valves.

12.3.3.6.1 Caged Ball Valves

In 1960, a surgeon placed the first artificial heart valve to replace a dysfunctional natural mitral valve; moreover, it was a Starr-Edwards caged ball valve (Khandpur,

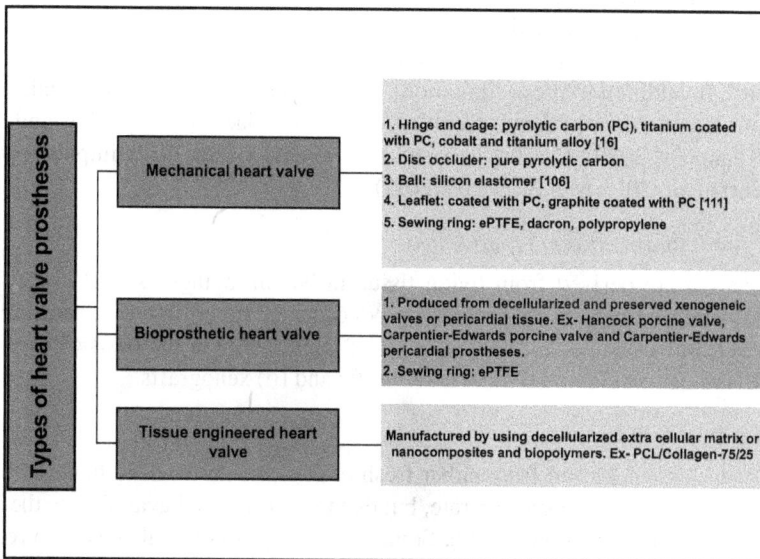

FIGURE 12.5 Prosthetic heart material classification

2020). This valve consists of a ball enclosed within a cage-like structure that is made up of three metal arches. Caged valves are no longer in production (Khandpur, 2020).

12.3.3.6.2   Bileaflet Valves

Bileaflet valves were first used in 1969 and made by attaching two semicircular discs to a sewing ring surrounded by a Teflon or Dacron layer (Khandpur, 2020; Shao et al., 2021). As compared to caged ball or tilting disc implants, leaflet valves ensure better blood flow, and the patient requires a lesser number of anticoagulants to prevent thrombosis. The foremost shortcoming of these valves is that they are susceptible to backflow (Khandpur, 2020).

12.3.3.6.3   Tilting Disc Valves

The Bjork-Shiley valve, commonly known as this, was created in 1969 and has subsequently undergone a number of upgrades. The present-day tilting disc valve consists of a single disc occluder mounted on a metal ring supported by metal struts (Khandpur, 2020). Nowadays, mechanical valve discs and occluders are manufactured from pyrolytic carbon or titanium coated with pyrolytic carbon since they are robust, fatigue- and wear-resistant, non-thermogenic, and exceptionally biocompatible. ePTEE fiber is used over the metal ring to keep the valve secured in its position which aids the sewing of the suture threads with the heart (Khandpur, 2020). The Medtronic-Hall model is the type of tilting disc valve generally used (Khandpur, 2020).

However, mechanical heart valves can last up to the whole lifespan of a patient, but they are prone to thrombosis since blood has a "metal adhesion" tendency (Vellayappan et al., 2015; Mai & Joseph, 2012). Therefore, it is necessary for a patient with a mechanical valve to take anticoagulants for the rest of his life to decrease the risk of embolism and thrombosis formation (Namdari et al., 2017). Moreover, patients with uncontrolled blood pressure, kidney disease, and liver disease cannot take anticoagulants because they have a high risk of bleeding and skin hemorrhage (Dangas et al., 2016). And MHVs can only be implanted via surgery (Dangas et al., 2016). In addition to these limitations, there is an issue of audible sound, which is disturbing to some patients, resulting from a cardiac valve opening and shutting (Khandpur, 2020). On that account, they must consider other implant options (Namdari et al., 2017; Mai & Joseph, 2012).

12.3.3.6.4   Bioprosthetic Heart Valve

These valves are derived from living tissue in human beings as well as animals. Bioprosthetic heart valves are generally produced from decellularized and preserved xenogeneic valves or pericardial tissue (He et al., 2022). On the basis of the tissue used, BHVs can be classified as (i) homografts and (ii) xenografts.

12.3.3.6.5   Homograft

These valves are acquired from either fresh or cryopreserved, dead human bodies. These valves have a high success rate, but due to their limited availability, their use is very restricted (Khandpur, 2020). Sometimes autografts are also used to replace a dysfunctional valve; this generally happens with pediatric patients (Singhal et al., 2013).

12.3.3.6.6   Xenograft

They are made up of chemically treated animal valves and tissues, for example, porcine valves and bovine pericardial valves. They are composed of tissue leaflets supported by a stent and accompanied by a sewing ring made up of Dacron fabric (Singhal et al., 2013; Khandpur, 2020). Also, the pericardial sac (which acts as a mechanical protection for the heart) of some animals, such as cows and horses, is used for tissue accumulation. It has been observed, even after 10 years of implantation, that pericardial valves are more efficient than porcine valves in terms of hemodynamics and durability (Singhal et al., 2013).

12.3.3.6.7   Classification of Xenografts

1. VALVE STENT
   The aortic valves of porcine are obtained from the slaughterhouse and are kept in a frigid saline solution for preservation. Because these valves are readily available and inexpensive and do not necessitate the regular prescription of anticoagulants, they are widely used as a replacement for the diseased valve. These valves are composed of two major parts: (i) porcine valve leaflets; (ii) a metallic or plastic stent enclosed in fabric (of varying sizes); and (iii) a sewing ring. The porcine aortic valves, three in number, are interconnected with each other, and then this structure is arranged on the metallic and plastic stents. The sewing ring is secured at the stent bottom and is employed in sewing the artificial valve (Khandpur, 2020). But a major limitation of these valves is the amplification of the occurrence of stenosis caused by the presence of metallic stents and cuffs (Singhal et al., 2013).
2. STENTLESS VALVE
   Stentless valves are employed to "shunt the limitations of stented valves and to enhance the hemodynamics" (Singhal et al., 2013; Khandpur, 2020). These are produced from an unaltered porcine aortic valve or from a bovine pericardial sac. As compared to stented valves, stentless valves facilitate more efficient orifice areas (Dangas et al., 2016).
3. PERCUTANEOUS/TRANSCATHETER VALVE
   Percutaneous balloon valvuloplasty is reasonable for patients with valvular heart disease; in this procedure, valve tissues are expanded by applying pressure, resulting in calcific deposit fragmentation. These valves are fabricated from biological membranes and sutured onto a self-expandable frame so that they have a small surface area, resulting in easier initiation and establishment of the prostheses (Singh et al., 2015). Some commercial versions of percutaneous valves are Medtronic's CoreValve, transcatheter aortic valve, St. Jude Medical's Portico transcatheter aortic valve, and Edwards' Sapien aortic valve. A transcatheter pulmonary valve has been developed by M/s Medtronic to treat diseased pulmonary valves with unwanted leakage and obstruction (Singhal et al., 2013). Goldstone et al. performed research on patients of different ages (40–49 years, 50–69 years, and 70–79 years) and observed that the patients in the age group of 40–49 years who opted for BHVs had a greater likelihood of mortality

(Goldstone et al., 2017). Furthermore, they concluded that the patient's age is a crucial factor to consider when opting for an artificial heart valve (Goldstone et al., 2017). BHVs may be preferred, especially by younger patients, to avoid any lifetime commitments such as a restricted diet, routine body checkups, regular administration of blood thinners, etc., and women who would like to have kids (Li, 2019).

In general, the following bioprosthetic heart valves are used for clinical application: the Hancock porcine valve, the Carpentier-Edwards porcine valve, and Carpentier-Edwards pericardial prostheses (John et al. Bioprosthetic heart valves are comparably nonthromogenic, and since there is no need for anticoagulants, the risk of bleeding and skin hemorrhage is minimized). Nevertheless, due to tissue degeneration and calcification, BHVs (which can last up to 20 years) are much less durable than MHVs (Rahimtoola, 2003; Chrobak et al., 2006; He et al., 2022).

In addition to these drawbacks, BHVs and MHVs are not capable of self-remodeling; as a consequence, they cannot be used to treat congenital deformities (Namdari et al., 2017). To find an optimal solution, researchers are continuously trying to develop a hemocompatible heart valve that is capable of anti-calcification, self-remodeling, and tissue ingrowth. To engineer an optimal heart valve, the scaffold should (i) be able to imitate mechanical and elastic attributes of the natural heart valves (Masoumi et al., 2013); (ii) imitate the extracellular matrix of the native tissues (Alavi et al., 2013); and (iii) be capable of controlled degradation and should promote tissue regeneration (Sant et al., 2011; Sahar et al., 2017). Subsequently, various researchers utilized nanocomposites, since they provide a high surface area and improved durability and biocompatibility, to develop tissue-engineered heart valves (TEHVs) (Namdari et al., 2017; Vellayappan et al., 2015). Rimer et al. fabricated a valve by stitching two decellularized engineered tissue tubes together in a controlled pattern using a degradable suture and implanting it in the major pulmonary artery of a growing lamb. They observed the deposition of collagen IV, elastin, and endothelial cells on the implanted material (Reimer et al., 2016). Padala et al. proposed to use CardioCel for valve implantation therapy in pediatric patients, which demonstrated good preclinical results (Padala, 2016). In a novel study by Fioretta et al., they fabricated a bis-urea-modified polycarbonate TEHV pre-embedded with BMCs (Bone Marrow Cells) and concluded that its "in vivo" performance as a heart valve replacement was worse than the original TEHV without any modifications (Fioretta et al., 2020). Badrossamay et al. (2014) evaluated the mechanical strength of SANF scaffolds and PCL/Collagen-75/25 and found that their Young's modulus and maximal strain are similar as the cardiac muscles and heart valve leaflets (Padala, 2016; Namdari & Eatemadi, 2016).

12.4 CONCLUSION AND FUTURE PROSPECT

This review demonstrates that there is still an unmet need for (i) a small-caliber vascular graft with biostability, hemocompatibility, and a microstructure similar to extracellular matrix, as well as (ii) a heart valve with long-term durability and the ability to self-remodel for pediatric patients. In the case of vascular scaffolds, both manmade and natural fibers have their own corresponding pros and cons; therefore, a hybrid material may generate a more promising and an "off-the-shelf" solution to these shortcomings. It has been discovered experimentally that an ideal material for a tissue-engineered vascular graft must be biostable, biocompatible, hemocompatible, porous, and have a microenvironment similar to the ECM. Similarly, for an ideal tissue-engineered heart valve, the fabricated material should have non-thrombogenic properties, anti-calcificant properties, long potency, durability, and be easily implantable so that the patient can live a normal life after implantation. With advancements in nanotechnology, the fields of fiber spinning techniques, biopolymer engineering, and surface modification processes have also evolved, paving the way for the development of an ideal vascular graft and an efficient heart valve prosthesis.

Researchers have demonstrated that tissue-engineered vascular grafts and heart valves have immense potential in vitro since they were able to embed them with biomolecules and nanoparticles, but in vivo implantation showed relatively distinct results. Several studies have been conducted to improve the overall quality of TEVGs and TEHVs by seeding the graft material with biomolecules such as collagen, BMCs, endothelial cells, etc. These experiments, however, would be impossible without the electrospinning techniques used to create electrospun nanofibers. The resulting nanofibers had a high surface area, porosity, flexibility, and mechanical strength. These experiments opted for nanotechnology such as nanocoating, nanoencapsulation, nanosurface modifications, etc. to enhance the efficiency of the resultant prostheses. Although these TEVGs and TEHVs were not as efficient as the natural heart vessels and natural heart valves, respectively, they highlighted the immense potential of the field of nanotechnology. The advent of this technology has been a boon to the medical field as well as the field of textiles.

REFERENCES

Abdul, W.Z., Rong, L., Xinbo, W. (2022). Structural design and mechanical performance of composite vascular grafts. *Bio-Des. Manuf.*, 5, 757–785.

Agarwal, S., Wendroff, J.H., Greiner, A. (2008). Use of electrospinning technique for biomedical applications. *Polymers*, 49, 5603–5621.

Alavi, S.H., Ruiz, V., Krasieva, T., Botvinick, E.L., Kheradvar, A. (2013). Characterizing the collagen fiber orientation in pericardial leaflets under mechanical loading conditions. *Annuals Biomed Eng.*, 41, 547–561.

Almeida, C.E.P.C., Reis, L., Carvalho, L., Almeida, C.M.C. (2014). Collagen implant with gentamicin sulphate reduces surgical site infection in vascular surgery: A prospective cohort study. *Int. J. Surg.*, 12, 1100–1104.

Amal, G.K., Rajendra, K.S., Kapil, D.P., Jung-Hwan, L., Hae-Won, K. (2022). Multifunctional GelMA platforms with nanomaterials for advanced tissue therapeutics. *Bioact Mater.*, 8, 267–295.

Andrzej, H., Joanna, G., Saeid, G., Magdalena, S., Jarosław, M., Wirginia, L., Magdalena L., Wojciech, M., Marek, J.L. (2017). Structure and properties of slow-resorbing nanofibers obtained by (Co-axial) electrospinning as tissue scaffolds in regenerative medicine. *PeerJ.*, 5, e4125.

Anitha, A., Sowmya, S., Kumar, P.S., Deepthi, S., Chennazhi, K., Ehrlich, H., Tsurkan, M., Jayakumar, R. (2014). Chitin and chitosan in selected biomedical applications. *Prog. Polym. Sci.*, 39, 1644–1667.

Badhe, R.V., Bijukumar, D., Chejara, D.R., Mabrouk, M., Choonara, Y.E., Kumar, P., du Toit, L.C., Kondiah, P.P.D., Pillay, V. (2017). A composite chitosan-gelatin bi-layered, biomimetic macroporous scaffold for blood vessel tissue engineering. *Carbohydr. Polym.*, 157, 1215–1225.

Badrossamay, M.R., Balachandran, K., Capulli, A.K., et al. (2014). Engineering hybrid polymer-protein super-aligned nanofibers via rotary jet spinning. *Biomaterials*, 35, 3188–3197.

Behrens, M.R., Ruder, W.C. (2021). Biopolymers in regenerative medicine: Overview, current advances, and future trends. In B. Rehm, M.F. Moradali (Eds.), *Biopolymers for Biomedical and Biotechnological Applications* (pp. 357–380). New Jersey, NY: Wiley.

Bhuiyan, Z. (2019). Vascular graft. *Biomaterials Science and Engineering*, 1–19.

Bishop, E.S., Mostafa, S., Pakvasa, M., Luu, H.H., Lee, M.J., Wolf, J.M., Ameer, G.A., He, T.-C., Reid, R.R. (2017). 3-D bioprinting technologies in tissue engineering and regenerative medicine: Current and future trends. *Genes Dis.*, 4, 185–195.

Brahatheeswaran Dhandayuthapani, Y.Y., Maekawa, T., Kumar, S.D. (2011). Polymeric scaffolds in tissue engineering application: A review. *Int. J. Polym. Sci.*, 1–19.

Calvin, C., Brian, G., Natalie, K. L., Zhicheng, Y., Benjamin, S., Martin, W. K., Sangwon, C., Hai-Quan, M. (2020). Medical fibers and biotextiles. In William R. Wagner, Shelly E. SAkiyama-Elbert, Guigen Zhang, Michael J. Yaszemski (Eds.), *Biomaterials Science*, 575–600.

Carrabba, M., Madeddu, P. (2018). Current strategies for the manufacture of small size tissue engineering vascular grafts. *Frontiers in Bioengineering and Biotechnology*, 6, 41.

Chen, J., Xu, J., Wang, K., Cao, X., Sun, R. (2016). Cellulose acetate fibers prepared from different raw materials with rapid synthesis method. *Carbohydr. Polym*, 137, 685–692.

Chen, X. (2015). *Advances in 3D Textiles*. Woodhead Publishing Limited, in association with textile institute.

Chia, H.N., Wu, B.M. (2015). Recent advances in 3D printing of biomaterials. *J. Biol. Eng.*, 9, 4.

Chrobak, K.M., Potter, D.R., Tien, J. (2006). Formation of perfused, functional microvascular tubes in vitro. *Microvasc. Res.*, 71, 185–196.

Cunha, C., Panseri, S., Antonini, S. (2011). Emerging nanotechnology approaches in tissue engineering for peripheral nerve regeneration. *Nanomed. Nanotechnol. Biol. Med.*, 7, 50–59.

Dangas, G.D., Weitz, J.I., Giustino, G., Makkar, R., Mehran, R. (2016). Prosthetic heart valve thrombosis. *J Am Coll Cardiol.*, 68(24), 2670–2689.

Desai, M., Seifalian, A.M., Hamilton, G. (2011). Role of prosthetic conduits in coronary artery bypass grafting. *Eur J Cardiothorac Surg.*, 40(2), 394–398.

Doshi, J., Reneker, D.H. (1995). Electrospinning process and applications of electrospun fibers. *J. Electrost.*, 35(2–3), 151–160.

Duan, N., Geng, X., Ye, L., Zhang, A., Feng, Z., Guo, L., Gu, Y. (2016). A vascular tissue engineering scaffold with core-shell structured nano-fibers formed by coaxial electrospinning and its biocompatibility evaluation. *Biomed Mater*, 11(3), 035007.

Elliott, M.B., Ginn, B., Fukunishi, T., Bedja, D., Suresh, A., Chen, T. (2019). Regenerative and durable small-diameter graft as an arterial conduit. *Proc. Natl. Acad. Sci. U S A.*, 116, 12710–12719.

Felgueiras, H.P., Amorim, M.T.P. (2017). Functionalization of electrospun polymeric wound dressings with antimicrobial peptides. *Colloids Surf*, 156, 133–148.

Felgueiras, H.P., Murthy, N.S., Sommerfeld, S.D., Brás, M.M., Migonney, V., Kohn, J. (2016). Competitive adsorption of plasma proteins using a quartz crystal microbalance. *ACS Appl. Mater. Interfaces*, 8, 13207–13217.

Felgueiras, H.P., Sommerfeld, S.D., Murthy, N.S., Kohn, J., Migonney, V.R. (2014). Poly (NaSS) functionalization modulates the conformation of fibronectin and collagen type I to enhance osteoblastic cell attachment onto Ti6Al4V. *Langmuir*, 30, 9477–9483.

Fioretta, E.S., Lintas, V., Mallone, A., Motta, S.E., Von Boehmer, L., Dijkman, P.E., Cesarovic, N., Caliskan, E., Rodriguez Cetina Biefer, H., Lipiski, M., et al. (2020). Differential leaflet remodeling of bone marrow cell pre-seeded versus nonseeded bioresorbable transcatheter pulmonary valve replacements. *JACC: Basic Transl. Sci.*, 5, 15.

Fu, W., Liu, Z., Feng, B., Hu, R., He, X., Wang, H., Yin, M., Huang, H., Zhang, H., Wang, W. (2014). Electrospun gelatin/PCL and collagen/PLCL scaffolds for vascular tissue engineering. *Int J Nanomedicine*, 9, 2335–2344.

Fujii, Y., Goyama, T., Muraoka, G. (2019). Effects of diamondlike-carbon coating for ePTFE artificial vascular graft as arteriovenous graft. *Eur J Vasc Endovasc Surg.*, 58(6), e419–e420.

Gentile, P., Chiono, V., Carmagnola, I., Hatton, P.V. (2014). An overview of poly (lactic-co-glycolic) acid (PLGA)-based biomaterials for bone tissue engineering. *Int. J. Mol. Sci.*, 15, 3640–3659.

Goëau-Brissonnière, O., Mercier, F., Nicolas, M.H., Bacourt, F., Coggia, M., Lebrault, C., Pechère, J.C. (1994). Treatment of vascular graft infection by in situ replacement with a rifampin-bonded gelatin-sealed Dacron graft. *J. Vasc. Surg.*, 19, 739–744.

Gokarneshan, N., Dhatchayani, U. (2017). Mini review: Advances in medical knits. *J Textile Eng Fashion Technol.*, 3(2), 621–625.

Goldstone, A.B., Chiu, P., Baiocchi, M., Lingala, B., Patrick, W.L., Fischbein, M.P. (2017). Mechanical or biologic prostheses for aortic-valve and mitral-valve replacement. *N. Engl. J. Med.*, 377, 1847–1857.

Greco, R.S. (1994). *Implantation Biology: The Host Response and Biomedical Devices.* CRC Press, Boca Raton, Florida.

Gupta, B.S. (2013). *Shaped Biotextiles for Medical Implants.* In Martin W. King, Bhupender S. Gupta, Robert Guidoin (Eds.), *Biotextiles as Medical Implants*, 113–136, Woodhead Publishing Series in Textiles, Cambridge, UK.

He, E., Serpelloni, S., Alvear, P., Rahimi, M., Taraballi, F. (2022). Vascular graft infections: An overview of novel treatments using nanoparticles and nanofibers. *Fibers*, 10(2), 12.

Huang, C.-H., Lee, S.-Y., Horng, S., Guy, L.-G., Yu, T.-B. (2018). In vitro and in vivo degradation of microfiber bioresorbable coronary scaffold. *J. Biomed. Mater. Res.*, 106, 1842–1850.

Jeong, S.I., Kim, S.Y., Cho, S.K., Chong, M.S., Kim, K.S., Kim, H., Lee, S.B., Lee, Y.M. (2007). Tissue-engineered vascular grafts composed of marine collagen and PLGA fibers using pulsatile perfusion bioreactors. *Biomaterials*, 28, 1115–1122.

Joseph, J., Domenico Bruno, V., Sulaiman, N., Ward, A., Johnson, T.W., Baby, H.M., Kerala Varma, P., Jose, R., Nair, S.V., Menon, D., George, S.J., Ascione, R. (2022). A novel small diameter nanotextile arterial graft is associated with surgical feasibility and safety and increased transmural endothelial ingrowth in pig. *J. Nanobiotechnology*, 20(1), 71.

Joseph, J., Krishnan, A.G., Cherian, A.M., Rajagopalan, B., Jose, R., Varma, P., Maniyal, V., Balakrishnan, S., Nair, S.V, Menon, D. (2018). Transforming nanofibers to woven nanotextiles for vascular application. *ACS Appl Mater Interfaces*, 10(23), 19449–19458.

Jyothirmai, S., Panda, S. (2021). Nanotechnology and its applications in textiles—a review. *IJARIIE*, 7(2).

Kabirian, F., Ditkowski, B., Zamanian, A., Heying, R., Mozafari, M. (2018). An innovative approach towards 3d-printed scaffolds for the next generation of tissue-engineered vascular grafts. *Materials Today: Proceedings*, 5, 15586–15594.

Karkan, S.F., Davaran, S., Rahbarghazi, R., Salehi, R., Akbarzadeh, A. (2019). Electrospun nanofibers for the fabrication of engineered vascular grafts. *J Biol Eng.*, 13, 83.

Khandpur, R.S. (2020). *Compendium of Biomedical Instrumentation*. New York, NY: Wiley.

King, M.W., Gupta, B.S., Guidoin, R. (2013). *Shaped Biotextiles for Medical Implants*.

Kmiec, M., Pighinelli, L., Tedesco, M., Silva, M., Reis, V. (2017). Chitosan-properties and applications in dentistry. *Adv. Tissue Eng. Regen. Med.*, 2, 00035.

Knight, D.K., Gillies, E.R., Mequanint, K. (2014). Vascular grafting strategies in coronary intervention. *Frontiers in Materials*, 1.

Lazic, I., Obermeier, A., Dietmair, B., Kempf, W.E., Busch, A., Tübel, J., Schneider, J., von Eisenhart-Rothe, R., Biberthaler, P., Burgkart, R., Pförringer, D. (2022). Treatment of vascular graft infections: Gentamicin-coated ePTFE grafts reveals strong antibacterial properties in vitro. *J Mater Sci Mater Med.*, 33(3), 30.

Lee, C.H., Singla, A., Lee, Y. (2001). Biomedical applications of collagen. *Int. J. Pharm.*, 221, 1–22.

Lew, W., Moore, W. (2011). Antibiotic-impregnated grafts for aortic reconstruction. *Semin. Vasc. Surg.*, 24, 211–219.

L'Heureux, N., Germain, L., Labbé, R., Auger, F.A. (1993). In vitro construction of a human blood vessel from cultured vascular cells: A morphologic study. *J. Vasc. Surg.*, 17, 499–509.

Li, G., Li, Y., Chen, G., He, J., Han, Y., Wang, X., Kaplan, D.L. (2015). Silk-based biomaterials in biomedical textiles and fiber-based implants. *Adv Healthc Mater*, 4(8), 1134–1151.

Li, K.Y.C. (2019). Bioprosthetic Heart Valves: Upgrading a 50-Year Old Technology. *Front Cardiovasc Med.* 6, 47.

Li, S., Henry, J.J. (2011). Nonthrombogenic approaches to cardiovascular bioengineering. *Annu. Rev. Biomed. Eng.*, 13, 451–475.

Liang, J., Grijpma, D.W., Poot, A.A. (2020). Tough and biocompatible hybrid networks prepared from methacrylated poly (trimethylene carbonate) (PTMC) and methacrylated gelatin. *Eur. Polym. J.*, 123, 109420.

Liu, R.H., Ong, C.S., Fukunishi, T., Ong, K., Hibino, N. (2018). Review of vascular graft studies in large animal models. *Tissue Eng Part B Rev.*, 24, 133–143.

Liu, X., Wang, N., Liu, X., Deng, R., Kang, R., Xie, L. (2022). Vascular repair by grafting based on magnetic nanoparticles. *Pharmaceutics*, 14(7), 1433.

Mai, T.L., Joseph, C.W. (2012). Biomaterial applications in cardiovascular tissue repair and regeneration. *Expert Rev. Cardiovasc. Ther.*, 10(8), 1039–1049.

Malafaya, P.B., Silva, G.A., Reis, R.L. (2007). Natural—origin polymers as carriers and scaffolds for biomolecules and cell delivery in tissue engineering applications. *Adv. Drug Deliv. Rev.*, 59, 207–233.

Masoumi, N., Johnson, K.L., Howell, M.C., Engelmayr, G.C. (2013). Valvular interstitial cell seeded poly(glycerol sebacate) scaffolds: Toward a biomimetic in vitro model for heart valve tissue engineering. *Acta. Biomaterialia*, 9, 5974–5988.

Matsuzaki, Y., John, K., Shoji, T., Shinoka, T. (2019). The evolution of tissue engineered vascular graft technologies: From preclinical trials to advancing patient care. *Appl. Sci.*, 9, 1274.

Matsuzaki, Y., Miyamoto, S., Miyachi, H., Iwaki, R., Shoji, T., Blum, K. (2021). Improvement of a novel small-diameter tissue-engineered arterial graft with heparin conjugation. *Ann Thorac Surg.*, 111, 1234–1241.

McDonnell, G., Russell, A.D. (1999). Antiseptics and disinfectants: Activity, action, and resistance. *Clin. Microbiol. Rev.*, 12, 147–179.

Mehta, P., Zaman, A., Smith, A., Rasekh, M., Haj-Ahmad, R., Muhammad, S.A., van der Merwe, S., Chang, M.-W., Ahmad, Z. (2019). Broad scale and structure fabrication of

healthcare materials for drug and emerging therapies via electrohydrodynamic techniques. *Adv. Ther.*, 2(4), 1800024.

Meslmani, B.M., Mahmoud, G.F., Bakowsky, U. (2017). Development of expanded polytetrafluoroethylene cardiovascular graft platform based on immobilization of poly lactic-
co-glycolic acid nanoparticles using a wet chemical modification technique. *Int. J.
Pharm.*, 529.

Miranda, C.S., Ribeiro, A.R.M., Homem, N.C., Felgueiras, H.P. (2020). Spun biotextiles in
tissue engineering and biomolecules delivery systems. *Antibiotics (Basel)*, 9(4), 174.

Mogoşanu, G.D., Grumezescu, A.M. (2014). Natural and synthetic polymers for wounds and
burns dressing. *Int. J. Pharm.*, 463(2), 127–136.

Morris, H., Murray, R. (2020). Medical textile, *Textile Progress,* 52, 1–127.

Namdari, M., Eatemadi, A. (2016). Nanofibrous bioengineered heart valve—application in
paediatric medicine. *Biomed. Pharmacother.*, 84, 1179–1188.

Namdari, M., Negahdari, B., Eatemadi, A. (2017). Paediatric nanofibrous bioprosthetic heart
valve. *IET Nanobiotechnol.*, 11(5), 493–500.

Nguyen, M.A., Camci-Unal, G. (2019). Unconventional tissue engineering materials in dis-
guise. *Trends Biotechnol*, 38(2), 178–190.

Orrit-Prat, J., Bonet, R., Rupérez, E. (2021). Bactericidal silverdoped DLC coatings obtained
by pulsed filtered cathodic arc codeposition. *Surf. Coat. Tech.*, 15(411), 126977.

Padala, M. (2016). Biomaterials for heart valve replacement: Conjectures and refutations. *J.
Thorac. Cardiovasc. Surg.*, 152, 1175–1176.

Pashneh-Tala, S., MacNeil, S., Claeyssens, F. (2016). The tissue-engineered vascular graft-
past, present, and future. *Tissue Eng. Part B Rev.*, 22, 68–100.

Qian, Y., et al. (2018). Biomimetic domain-active electrospun scaffolds facilitating bone
regeneration synergistically with antibacterial efficacy for bone defects. *ACS Appl.
Mater. Interfaces*, 10(4), 3248–3259.

Radakovic, D., Reboredo, J., Helm, M., Weigel, T., Schürlein, S., Kupczyk, E., Leyh, R.G.,
Walles, H., Hansmann, J. (2017). A multilayered electrospun graft as vascular access
for hemodialysis. *PLoS One*, 12, e0185916.

Radhakrishnan, S. (2019). Application of biotechnology in the processing of textile fabrics. In
S. Senthilkannan Muthu (Ed.) (pp. 277–325). London: Springer Nature.

Rahimtoola, S. (2003). Choice of prosthetic heart valve for adult patients. *J. Am. Coll.
Cardiol.*, 41, 893–904.

Reimer, J., Syedain, Z., Haynie, B. (2016). Implantation of a tissueengineered tubular heart
valve in growing lambs. *Ann. Biomed. Eng.*, 18, 1–13.

Ricco, J.-B., Assadian, O. (2011). Antimicrobial silver grafts for prevention and treatment of
vascular graft infection. *Semin. Vasc. Surg.*, 24, 234–241.

Rinaudo, M. (2006). Chitin and chitosan: Properties and applications. *Prog. Polym. Sci.*, 31,
603–632.

Rychter, M., Baranowska, K.A., Lulek, J. (2017). Progress and perspectives in bioactive agent
delivery via electrospun vascular grafts. *RSC Adv.*, 7, 32164–32184.

Sahar, S., Kharaziha, M., Masoumi, N., Fallahi, A., Tamayol, A. (2017). Medical textiles as
substrates for tissue engineering. In K.L. Mittal, T. Bahners (Eds.), *Textile Finishing:
Recent Developments and Future Trends*. New Jersey, NY: Wiley.

Sant, S., Hwang, C.M., Lee, S.H., Khademhosseini, A. (2011). Hybrid PGS-PCL microfibrous scaffolds with improved mechanical and biological properties. *J. Tissue Eng.
Regenerative Med.*, 5, 283–291.

Shah, Md., Maruf, H., Md. Shahjalal, Jaglul, H.M., Riasat Alam, A. M. (2019). Medical textiles: Application of implantable medical textiles. *Global Journal of Medical Research*,
19(4), 17–24.

Shao, Z., Tao, T., Xu, H., Chen, C., Lee, I.-S., Chung, S., Dong, Z., Li, W., Ma, L., Bai, H., Chen, Q. (2021). Recent progress in biomaterials for heart valve replacement: Structure, function, and biomimetic design. *View*, 2(6), 1–17.

Singh, C., Wong, C. S., Wang, X. (2015). Medical textiles as vascular implants and their success to mimic natural arteries. *J. Funct. Biomater*, 6, 500–525.

Singhal, P., Luk, A., Butany, J. (2013). Bioprosthetic heart valves: Impact of implantation on biomaterials. *ISRN Biomaterials*, 2, 1–14.

Sreeniwas, K., Sinha, N. (2020). Cardiovascular disease in India: A 360 degree overview. *Med. J. Armed Forces India*, 76(1), 1–3.

Tamura, M., Yanagawa, F., Sugiura, S., Takagi, T., Sumaru, K., Kanamori, T. (2015). Click-crosslinkable and photodegradable gelatin hydrogels for cytocompatible optical cell manipulation in natural environment. *Sci. Rep.*, 5, 15060.

Tangsadthakun, C., Kanokpanont, S., Sanchavanakit, N., Banaprasert, T., Damrongsakkul, S. (2017). Properties of collagen/chitosan scaffolds for skin tissue engineering. *Journal of Metals, Materials and Minerals*, 16(1), 37–44.

Teixeira, M.A., Amorim, M.T.P., Felgueiras, H.P. (2020). Cellulose acetate in wound dressings formulations: Potentialities and electrospinning capability. In J. Henriques, N. Neves, P. de Carvalho (Eds.), *XV Mediterranean Conference on Medical and Biological Engineering and Computing—MEDICON 2019* (pp. 1227–1230). IFMBE Proceedings, vol. 76. Cham: Springer.

Toong, D.W.Y., Toh, H.W., Ng, J.C.K., Wong, P.E.H., Leo, H.L., Venkatraman, S., Tan, L.P., Ang, H.Y., Huang, Y. (2020). Bioresorbable polymeric scaffold in cardiovascular applications. *Int J Mol Sci.*, 21(10), 3444.

Tucker, N., Stanger, J.J., Staiger, M.P., Pazzaq, H., Hofman, K. (2012). The history of the science and technology of electrospinning from 1600 to 1995. *J. Eng. Fibers Fabr.*, 7, 63–73.

Vellayappan, M.V., Balaji, A., Subramanian, A.P., John, A.A., Jaganathan, S.K., Murugesan, S., Mohandas, H., Supriyanto, E., Yusof, M. (2015). Tangible nanocomposites with diverse properties for heart valve application. *Sci Technol Adv Mater.*, 16(3), 033504.

Wagner, W.R., Sakiyama-Elbert, S.E., Zhang, G., Yaszemski, M. J. (2020). *Biomaterials Science: An Introduction to Materials in Medicine*. Elsevier, Amsterdam, The Netherands.

Wang, M., Zhao, Q. (2019). *Electrospinning and Electrospray for Biomedical Applications* (pp. 330–344). Elsevier, Amsterdam, The Netherlands.

Washington, K.S., Bashur, C.A. (2017). Delivery of antioxidant and anti-inflammatory agents for tissue engineered vascular grafts. *Frontiers in Pharmacology*, 8, 659.

Witkowski, J., Wnukiewicz, W., Reichert, P. (2016). Polymers as carriers of gentamicin in traumatology and orthopedic surgery—current state of knowledge. *Polim w medycynie*, 46(1), 101–104.

Yan, Y., Yao, R., Zhao, J., Chen, K., Duan, L., Wang, T., Zhang, S., Guan, J., Zheng, Z., Wang, X., Liu, Z., Li, Y., Li, G. (2021). Implantable nerve guidance conduits: Material combinations, multi-functional strategies and advanced engineering innovations. *Bioact Mater*, 11, 57–76.

Yang, G., et al. (2018). From nano to micro to macro: Electrospun hierarchically structured polymeric fibers for biomedical applications. *Polym. Sci.*, 81, 80–113.

Zhang, F., King, M.W. (2022). Immunomodulation strategies for the successful regeneration of a tissue-engineered vascular graft. *Adv. Healthc. Mater.*, 11(12), e2200045.

Zhang, L., Ao, Q., Wang, A., Lu, G., Kong, L., Gong, Y., Zhao, N., Zhang, X. (2006). A sandwich tubular scaffold derived from chitosan for blood vessel tissue engineering. *J. Biomed. Mater. Res. Part A*, 77, 277–284.

Zhang, X., Peng, X., Zhang, S.W. (2017). Biodegradable medical polymers: Fundamental sciences. In X. Zhang (Ed.) *Science and Principles of Biodegradable and Bioresorbable Medical Polymers: Materials and Properties* (pp. 1–33). Cambridge, NY: Woodhead Publishing.

13 Nanofibrous Textile Scaffolds
A New Innovation in Nanotechnology for Tissue Engineering

Srijita Sen and Om Prakash Ranjan

13.1 INTRODUCTION

Surgical replacements of tissues or organs in irreversible organ failure, different diseases or injuries like burns, pressure sores, liver cirrhosis, venous stasis ulcer, and many more with donated tissues or organs has been found to be clinically successful in the middle era of the 19th and 20th century. The stepwise progress in advanced transplantation was very challenging mainly because of implantation rejection by the host immune system against the foreign transplant. In the long-term outlook, there is still a lack of organs or tissues available which can meet the demands of the increased population, although many initiatives have been taken for encouraging organ donations and their better utilization. As an alternative solution, engineered tissue came to the forefront for functional replacement where new tissues will be self-regenerated from the seeded living cells on a configured scaffold. Especially, tissue engineering has been found to be effective to repair congenital malformation of any organ or tissues like rib cage or ear cartilage, craniofacial defects or valve defects, etc. in children without multiple surgeries. However, the earliest scaffolds faced a dilemma of improper suppliance of nourishments to tissues. To overcome this improper mass transfer issue, scaffolds should have a porous interconnecting network for desired biological response. In the modern scientific discipline, nanofibrous-based porous scaffolds are emerging as tissue engineering templates having a high surface area-to-volume ratio favoring interaction with cells and cell respiration by creating a suitable microenvironment. In addition, the nanofibrous structure can control the release of bioactive agents for hours, days to months to regulate the target cell phenotypes (Barhoum et al., 2018). At the scale of nano to the micro range, nanofiber organization into hierarchical helix yarn and fabricating a scaffold of aligned, twisted yarn can be a prototype of load-bearing stretchable micro tissues. On application of large mechanical strains, such nanofibrous scaffolds have been shown to shield seeded cells, protecting them from DNA damage, nuclear envelope rupture, and apoptosis as a consequence. Such kind of nano affine deformation behavior added a high value to the usage of nanofiber as a tissue engineering scaffold building block, although build-up of bulk complex tissues is challenging using only nanofiber constructs (Li et al., 2019). Studies also reported that reinforcement of nanoyarns in composite scaffolds can be a better choice to augment tissue rehabilitation (Vijayamohan et al., 2018).

In the same direction of organ reconstruction and renovation of their functioning, textile technology has brought revolutions in the patterning and orientation of fiber-made yarns into scaffolds. These aid in the improvement of the cell adhesion more than nanofibers being more similar in dimensionality to the extracellular matrix of native tissues, enhanced biostability of adhered cells, and self-stability in biological fluids. Despite these facts, textile technology was bounded to the use of fibers of microscale lacking superiority in surface properties as well as mechanical, optical, biological, and electrical performances (Wu et al., 2022). Fibers of more than 10-micrometer size are larger than the native extracellular matrix which hinders effective cellular attachments. These factors suggest the needed tissue engineering scaffold must integrate traditional textile manufacturing techniques with nanofibrous arrays. In fact, the combined use of nano and micro-sized fibers in scaffolds has been shown to expand the advantages of nanofiber substrates (Karbasi et al., 2016; Cai et al., 2020).

13.2 DIFFERENT TYPES OF TEXTILE PATTERNS AND THEIR APPLICATION IN TISSUE ENGINEERING

Fibers are arranged in different ways because the number of fibers in multifilament yarn, twisted or straight yarn, level of twisting, running direction of fibers over other fibers, fiber density, and many more factors can dramatically affect the physical and mechanical properties of textile scaffolds. Even if the same type of yarn is used, depending on the design the scaffold performance gets changed. Therefore, the systemic study should be done to establish a relationship in alliance with the novel nanofiber textile pattern and their tissue regenerative performances. Even tensile testing, stiffness, bursting stress, and tear stress of individual types of yarn configurations can be accomplished (McCullen et al., 2010). To date, researchers have explored mostly conventional patterns. However, with technological advancements, many modifications have been made. Few conclusions have been drawn from different pieces of research on the suitability of a specific textile design for a particular tissue engineering application. Some of these have been discussed in the following.

13.2.1 WOVEN PATTERN TEXTILE SCAFFOLD

Nanofibers/microfibers, nanoyarn/microyarn, or their combination are interlaced to each other at a right angle. Weaving density and the warp-weft component can be altered according to the requirement of the site of application. Apart from the ordinary weaving, more asymmetric weaving patterns are twill and satin. In twill, weft passes diagonally in an alternate sequence as 2 up-2 down or 2 up-1 down pattern, over and under multiple warps. Whereas in the latter one warp passes over 4 or more wefts and thus the long interlocking gaps create a more smooth, soft, and elastic textile. This asymmetry is important to consider as warp and weft will possess different degrees of affinity toward cell adhesion. The mechanical stress resistance of these textile patterns is more similar to the human soft tissues (Jiang et al., 2021a). With the improvement of textile processing machinery, three-dimensional designs like orthogonal, multilayer, and interlock patterns have been explored which can mimic the complex hierarchical tissue structure, withstand higher loads, and be flexible to body movement. In particular, cubic three-dimensional fabric from angle interlock patterned textile for intervertebral disk engineering (exert biomimetic stress-strain behavior, good delamination resistance, nonrestricted dynamic motion) (Shikinami et al., 2021), honeycomb pattern with tubular weave for cardiac tissue engineering (encourage myocardial cell alignment) (Engelmayr et al., 2008), orthogonal weave for bone and cartilage tissue engineering (enhance the production of mineralized extracellular tissue matrix and mesenchymal stem cells differentiation into osteoblast-lineage) (Person et al., 2018) have proven the promising effect of 3-D textile technology. Moreover, an interlocking weaving loom can be infiltered with a hydrogel matrix to favor the homogeneous distribution of progenitor cells (Akbari et al., 2016).

13.2.2 Knitted Pattern Textile Scaffold

Interconnecting loops are prepared by knitting warp or weft fibers or yarn(s) in the vertical or horizontal direction, respectively. Warp and weft knitted textile scaffolds show distinct features in flexibility and porousness, although all types of knitted textile scaffolds are great contenders for other textile patterns to engineer load-bearing tissues (Akbari et al., 2016). Rotational rectangle knits, compacted V knits, and re-entrant hexagon knits are great candidates for this purpose (Jiang et al., 2021a). These also possess auxetic properties; upon stretching they become thicker and have high resistance to fracture and indentation (Ma et al., 2016). This is suitable for repairing tendons and arteries. Advanced patterns of knitting like "seamless knitting" can fulfill the requirement for connective tissue engineering (Jiang et al., 2021a). Therefore, ideal knitted patterns must be systematically evaluated for the highest compatibility with biological tissues.

13.2.3 Braided Pattern Textile Scaffold

Three or more fiber threads are overlapped by inter-twining each other which gives the scaffold a unique feature of withstanding different loads in both axial and radial directions. This feature made it superior to knitted and woven textile being able to stand firm against torsion, bending, or traction as well as abrasion. A braided scaffold can be bent to 180° at any direction without any structural deformation or breakage. The structural stability is not compromised by the scaffold flexibility, and therefore it is an avant-grade component for articular and connective tissue engineering (Akbari et al., 2016) but is not useful for complex tissue reconstruction (Jiang et al., 2021a, 2021b). Nanoyarns can be braided in different angles to change its mechanical parameters. The number of interyarn pores is tailored by varying the number of yarns, braiding layers, as well as braiding angle. A hollow braided pattern has an advantage over solid braids due to adequate spaces for cellular growth. Such patterns have been evaluated for vascular tissues, nerves, and urethral tissue regeneration (Jiang et al., 2021b; Mi et al., 2015; Aibibu et al., 2016). These kinds of patterns suffer from limited radial compressive properties which restrict their applicability for healing and regeneration of long-distance tissues (Jiang et al., 2021a, 2021b).

13.3 APPLICATION OF NANOFIBROUS TEXTILE SCAFFOLDS IN HARD TISSUE ENGINEERING

The bone tissue engineering scaffold should demonstrate the equity between osteo-inductive potential as well as stable supportive strength. However, it is notoriously challenging in real circumstances to manufacture such a scaffold describing complete biomechanical similarity to the bone. Recently, textile technology has emerged to fabricate weaved multi-layered scaffolds from nanofibers which can simulate complex fibrillar matrix of native bone. Appropriate selection of textile scaffold components, for example polylactic acid (PLA) and tussah silk fibroin (TSF), can promote significantly higher gene expression of ALP (catalyzes calcium apatite formation) along with Col I which in turn improves MSC differentiation into osteoblasts in an early phase of bone formation. The design of the scaffold fabric also plays a key role in accelerating new bone formation. The vertical interweaving of parallel warp and weft nanofiber yarn when joined together into a multi-layered structure possesses close similarity to that of lamellar bone as parallel nanofiber yarns mimic the collagen fibrils. In osteogenesis late phase, PLA/TSF woven scaffold has been shown to support OCN gene expression, leading to three times greater cell growth on the 3-D space of the scaffold than the nonwoven scaffold structure. In terms of mechanical performance, woven textile scaffold of the same nanofiber yarns exhibits higher Young's modulus and lower compression deformation than nonwoven textile scaffolds (Shao et al., 2016). However, three-dimensional net-like nonwoven textile based on solid free forming technique can meet up with the prerequisite of bone tissue engineering scaffold. Further light has been shed on this type of micro fibrous textile by functionalizing nanofibers throughout the textile layers. This hybrid technology combines the supremacy of the 3D interconnecting network of the textile as well as nanofiber mesh. Based on this novel concept, thin gelatine nanofibers have been incorporated into the knitted scaffold of chitosan. Chitosan micro threads of this composite textile have exquisite strength. On the other side, porousness is controlled by nanofiber depositions which upgrade the cellular regeneration property of the scaffold furnished with adequate surface area for cell membrane receptor binding (Hild et al., 2013). For stronger imitation of the natural bone fibril matrix, nanofiber textiles preparation can be subjected to a biomineralization process. Evidently, when vertically interwoven fabric of polylactic acid and tussah silk fibroin nanofibers is subjected to induced growth of Hydroxyapatite over its surface, a highly ordered construct is formed with a better modulus of compression. The protein adsorption also gets amplified with an improved hydrophilic balance of the fabric (Gao et al., 2018).

13.4 APPLICATION OF NANOFIBROUS TEXTILE SCAFFOLDS IN INTERFACIAL SOFT TO HARD TISSUE ENGINEERING

Accidental injury, chronic inflammation, and age-related degeneration in the tendon-to-bone interface suffer from inferior healing despite tendon transplantation due to lower vascularity and cellularity in the affected zone. Restoration of such soft to hard tissue integrity needs the reproduction of transitional architecture of mineralized to non-mineralized tissue to mimic the interfacial zones between tendons and bone (Figure 13.1). Such a transitional construction of nano-hydroxylapatite (HA) gradient scaffold has been developed with substantial efforts combining nanofabrication and textile manufacturing process. A varying amount of HA has been added into the electrospinning solution of poly(L-lactide-co-ε-caprolactone) and silk fibroin to get the nanofibrous structure of different HA-grade. This will wrap polylactic acid microfiber core to get a single strand of the textile building block to allow optimal cell adherence. Spatial HA gradient has been shown to release calcium and simultaneous mineralized matrix development favoring mouse embryo osteoblast precursor cells (MC3T3-E1) proliferation as well as osteogenic differentiation and phenotype regulation of rat bone marrow stem cells. On the other hand, the HA-less yarn segments have been shown to induce tenogenic differentiation of rBMSCs. Thus, scaffold component variation has been found to be great for restoring the tendon to bone integrity without hampering the flexibility. This fibrous scaffold also has the potential to be used for tissue engineering of ischiofemoral, iliofemoral, and pubofemoral ligaments. However, this novel scaffold has proven to be physiologically relevant, for tissue engineering in-depth in-vivo degradation character of the scaffold must be evaluated with varying implant site and physiological conditions as the degradability of HA is highly variable in different conditions (Xie et al., 2021).

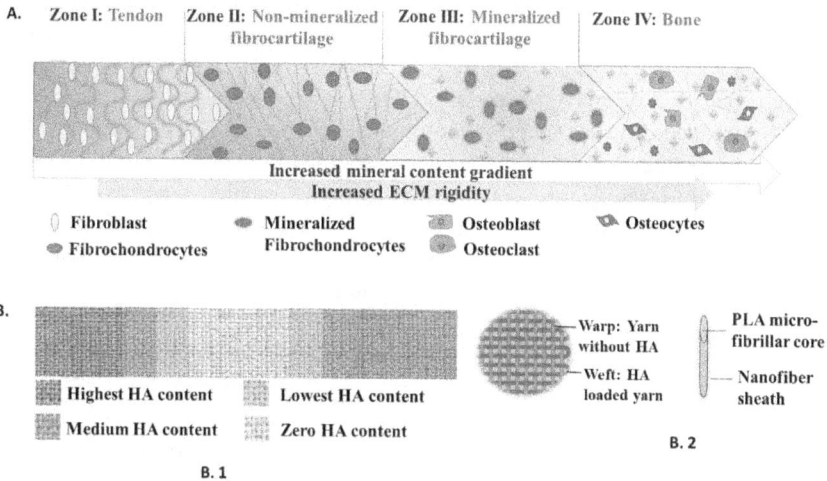

FIGURE 13.1   A: Complex ECM microenvironment between tendon to bone interface, B.1: Woven textile scaffold architecture, B.2: Microstructure of textile yarn

13.5 APPLICATION OF NANOFIBROUS TEXTILE SCAFFOLDS IN SOFT TISSUE ENGINEERING

13.5.1 NANOFIBROUS TEXTILE SCAFFOLD IN TENOGENIC DIFFERENTIATION AND LIGAMENT TISSUE ENGINEERING

Gestures, motions, and movements are an integral part of body actions that are severely affected by ligaments and tendon injury. Successful surgical reconstruction of these damaged tissues can promote rapid healing and delay the chances of permanent tissue dysfunctionality, but it is challenging. However, after multiple failures with the conventional fibrous mat, the textile scaffold has come into the TE platform to deal with the poor inherent healing of tendons. One major limitation to the unsuccessful tissue regeneration is the unpropitious biological reaction due to stress-shielding arising from mismatched stiffness between scaffold and ligament/tendon tissue. Braided nanofibrous scaffolds with different degrees of stiffness and flexibility can be engineered to support the target tissue's mechanical property by varying the nanofiber strands and braiding angle (Barber et al., 2013). A novel PLLA scaffold has been designed by twisting braided structure which permits the strain at minimum stresses and thus lowers the risk of scaffold fatigue-associated failures. Additional twisting imparts elasticity similar to that of anterior cruciate ligament tissue (Freeman et al., 2009). Although cell infiltration through the highly ordered braided architecture is limited, it may favor heterogeneous matrix deposition over the scaffold. However, the stacking pattern of the nanofibrous sheet has been reported to support the homogeneous distribution of more cells over the scaffold surface in the direction of aligned fibers. The deposition of collagen and sulfated glycosaminoglycan gradually increases with the increased cell count to facilitate supplementation for tenogenic differentiation. These differences in biomechanical properties in terms of tenogenic marker expression, extracellular matrix protein deposition, and stress-strain modulus can be overcome by combining microfibrils with nanofibers in scaffold fabrication (Rothrauff et al., 2017). Such a structure is made from a repeated tri-layer structure of polydioxanone (PDO) nanofiber-adhesive polycaprolactone nanofiber-weaved polydioxanone monofilament (Figure 13.2) and is mechanically robust to mimic the strength of the tendon, especially in the human rotator cuff tendons. This multi-layered fabric combination of highly oriented nanofibrous structure and grooved, less oriented woven structure has demonstrated different substratum for cell adhesion with an improved response for the latter one, although the former ensures 20 times more tensile strength, matching the tendon property. The rationale of each layer in the tissue repairmen has been described in Figure 13.2. The versatility of the multiple-layer thickness and porosity encourages smart textile development to repair a hernia (Hakimi et al., 2015).

One of the major complications after tendon surgery is peri-tendinous adhesion delaying the rehabilitation by inflammations. Nanofiber-based textile has shown accelerated repairing of injured flexor digitorum profundus and restoration of its normal pull-out force in a rabbit tendon repair model. The engineering membrane was based on hyaluronic acid-polycaprolactone composite nanofibers treated with silver nanoparticles. When it has been used to wrap the tendons, no adhesion to the surrounding

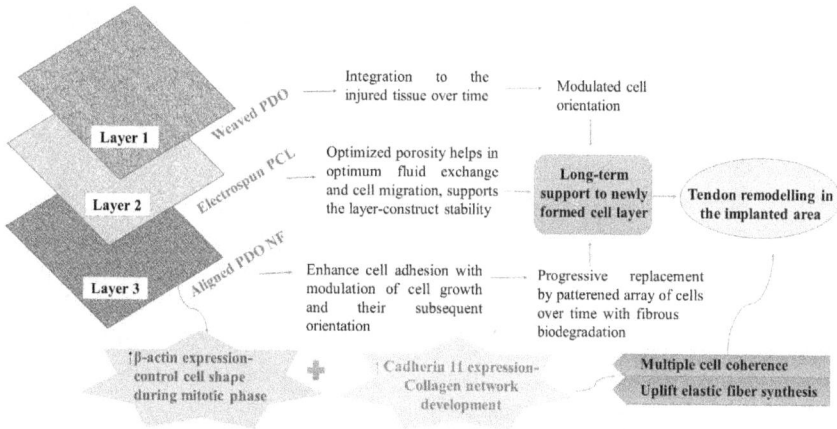

FIGURE 13.2 Tri-layered textile scaffold and its functioning for tendon regeneration

tissues was observed. The core-sheath design of the nanofibers allows the fast release of anti-inflammatory silver nanoparticles from the outer sheath, whereas the slow release of hyaluronic acid from the core allows smooth gliding of the tendons. Hyaluronic acid is a natural constituent of the inner synovial layer of a tendon. Therefore, this scaffold acts as a biomimetic tendon sheath without hindering the nutritional exchange. Thus, the nanofibrous textiles can elicit a great tissue repair response to a higher extent when material selection is proper (Chen et al., 2015).

13.5.2 Nanofibrous Textile Scaffold in Vascular Remodeling

Smooth muscle cells align circumferentially in blood vessels which confers higher strength circumferentially rather than longitudinally. To mimic this complex mechanical attribute nanotextile technologies has come into the scenario. At first, nano yarns are made by twisting hundreds to thousands of nanofibers. For the inter-weaving of the yarns, longitudinal and circumferential or transverse yarns can be constructed by bundling a different number of yarns to achieve strength withstand-ing the anisotropic stress-strain properties of the blood vessels (Babu et al., 2021). Along with that, the porosity of the woven textile can also be tuned by varying the number of longitudinal yarns to regulate cell migration. A woven conduit made from hierarchical bundling of 12 longitudinal and four circumferential nano yarns of PLLA, PCL, and collagen has been found to favor the serum proteins uptake through capillary action and their subsequent entrapment within the nanochannels in the direction of yarn alignment. This plays a significant role in promoting endothelization. However, the protein-biotextile interaction is governed by the hydrophilicity of the textile surface. Notably, the hydrophilic character of PLLA gets improved in a nanofibrous woven scaffold in comparison to a nonwoven scaffold. These observa-tions have been found to be promising to engineer vascular tissue using nanofiber textile scaffolds as a template (Joseph et al., 2018). A triple-layered nanofibrous graft

has been developed combining electrospun and braiding textile technology, which
can imitate all three layers (Figure 13.3) of vascular ECM microstructure as well as
the blood vessel macrostructure (Zhang et al., 2017).

13.5.3 Nanofibrous Textile Scaffold in Cardiac Tissue Repairing and Heart Valve Engineering

With time, there are a lot of changes in lifestyle and food habits that ultimately
welcome cardiac diseases and this is now the most common cause of early death.
At the end stage of cardiac disease, heart transplantation becomes the only option.
However, it is important to note that, according to certain data, 87% of heart transplant recipients may have a life expectancy of approximately one year after the procedure. At this time, the tissue engineering technique is considered a boon although
there is a snag to replicating the anisotropy of cardiac tissue with individual traditional electrospun or microfiber textile scaffolds. For example, an aligned nanofiber
scaffold can replicate that anisotropy, but it is difficult to shape complex valve anat-
omy and trileaflets geometry with simple nanofiber organizations. CorCap (Acorn
Cardiovascular, Inc., St. Paul, Minn.), a cardiac restraint device with a knitted multifilament polyester yarn design, had been shown to possess anisotropic compliance
when placed circumferentially around the heart from the apex to the atrioventricular
groove. It has been shown to possess withstanding power against ventricular wall
stress. The impressive results of clinical studies in advanced heart failure, focusing
on cardiac remodeling, have proven the suitability of knitted textiles (Walsh, 2005;
Mann et al., 2012; Oliveira, 2014).

As an upshot, there is transforming research to intertwine textile engineering with
nanofiber technology for cardiac tissue engineering. When the uniaxially aligned
nanofiber yarn (UANY) is processed into a predesigned woven fabric and subsequently embedded into a hydrogel layer, a tissue engineering template is created.
This template is ready to be laden with cells with the aid of biological glue. On such
bioactive hydrogel/PAN UANY and micro yarn composite templates, seeded cells
of human aortic valve interstitial and human aortic root smooth muscle have been

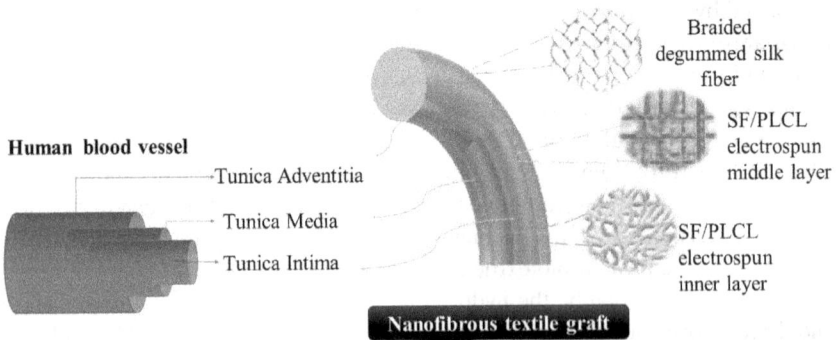

FIGURE 13.3   Human blood vessel mimetic nanofibrous textile scaffold

shown to proliferate to the aligned direction of fibrous constructs. On biochemical stimulation, these can generate heart valve-associated markers revealing that the functionality of these cells is preserved (Wu et al., 2016).

An anisotropic flat, knitted template has been reported to be made from poly(lactic-co-glycolic) acid and polycarbonate-urethane (Bionate) electrospun over cotton or polyester base. Upon adhesion of cardiomyocytes (isolates of neonatal rats) to these templates, the spontaneous beating of individual cells in a synchronous fashion was observed. Quantification of the heartbeats with "Motion Analysis Software" has revealed that the cells on Bionate/PE textile can exert more sustained contractility with fewer fluctuations and therefore can be considered as a physiologically relevant cardiac tissue engineering material as a proof of concept (Şenel Ayaz et al., 2014). However, the longevity of the engineered heart valve is dependent on several factors like textile type (woven/nonwoven), fiber arrangements and orientation (pain weave/satin/twill/diamond mesh, etc.), the building block of the textile (nanofiber monofilament/multifilament nano yarn), and textile processing as well (Liberski et al., 2017).

In a recent study, nanofiber electrospun is transformed into three-dimensional yarn textile coated with α-mangostin. In-vitro culture of cardiac cells has shown the expression of different cardiac markers. Improved angiogenesis by this biocompatible woven textile can be a potential candidate for cardiac tissue engineering (Arthi & Rama, 2022).

13.5.4 NANOFIBROUS TEXTILE SCAFFOLD IN SKIN TISSUE ENGINEERING

Unique strain-stiffening properties of human skin tissue are associated with the helical patterns of different fibrillar proteins. Therefore, tissue engineering scaffolds should also reproduce the same pattern for the highest compatibility. Textile-based electrospun sandwich has been explored to match the sufficient mechanical strength as a prerequisite for healing full-thickness skin wounds. In this study, a crochet fabric mat is placed in between two layers of electrospun fibers. The middle crochet textile was designed to simulate the interconnected collagen fiber structure of the skin, whereas the outer fibrous layers are highly customizable to fit the physical and mechanical characteristics of different skin types. Therefore, it is more expedient as a skin tissue engineering scaffold. To match the tissue physic mechanical patterns of different regions of the body, other nanofibrous materials and different textile patterns can be explored. For example, more curved textile patterns will be used for skin tissue engineering of the toe region (Jiang et al., 2021a). Recently, textile-based sensor devices could stimulate the healing of wound areas with continual assessment of the wound condition based on pH, temperature, and other biomarkers of the injured area. It can be a minimally invasive real-time approach to provide quantitative information about the condition of chronic wounds (ElSaboni et al., 2022). It can give the flexibility for remote controlling of the further healing process by controlling the rate of delivery of therapeutic agents. Nanofibrous textiles will be a great player to make such advanced wound healing devices of lightweight material, and the tunable flexibility will allow placing the material in the proper position of the wound regardless of the location.

13.5.5 Nanofibrous Textile Scaffold in Nerve Tissue Engineering

In recent decades, multifarious approaches have been tried to reconstruct injured nerve tissues including modification of the intraluminal architecture, incorporation of intraluminal extracellular matrix fillers, neurotrophic factors, etc. Despite that, no engineered nerve conduit is able to support the complete functional recovery of peripheral nerves having an injury length of more than 3 cm gap (Luca et al., 2015). Nerve conduits made from tubular hollow structures possess a higher tendency to break in a longer length. In this situation, braided textile is found to be important to make larger conduits, as these constructions can withstand any kind of stress even up to a longer length of 15 to 20 cm. without visible damage (Pillai et al., 2020). The high kink resistance and flexibility of nanofibrous braid textile is a satisfactory candidate for further modifications like the integration of electrical cues. The nano yarn bundles have more similar artifacts to the natural nerve trunk, and individual nanofiber can closely mimic the longitudinal alignment of axons in fascicles (Wu et al., 2019). Some bioactive polymers have been exploited to manufacture electrospun nano yarn. Among these MeGel and laminin-based nanofibrous constructs have demonstrated sufficient compressive mechanical support and good in-vivo migration of Schwann cells along the longitudinal axis of nanofiber yarns (Wu et al., 2019; Wu et al., 2017). Thus, synergistic effects of biological cues and topological cues (nano yarn morphology) provide hope for promising nerve tissue engineering materials.

13.6 ELECTROACTIVE NANOFIBROUS SCAFFOLDS AS A PROMISING TEXTILE MATERIAL IN TISSUE ENGINEERING

With the emergence of the conducting polymer as a new member, integration of the biological cues to the electrical cues has made headway toward the development of smart tissue engineering textiles. Polyaniline (PANI), polythiophene, Poly (3,4-ethylene dioxythiophene) [PEDOT], polypyrrole (PPY), and some other intrinsically conducting polymers have been shown to stimulate attachment and proliferation of myoblasts, Schwann cells, fibroblasts, primary cardiomyocytes, cardiac cells, and mesenchymal stem cells in form of hydrogels or as microfiber/nanofiber composite (Balint et al., 2014). These interesting outcomes may be due to the induced electrical coupling between cells by the electroactive substrates, stimulation of protein adsorption to that substrate, and altered surface hydrophilicity/hydrophobicity of the substrate (Lee, 2013). Most interestingly, few conducting polymers that encourage self-healing can be explored for restoration of native functionality and biomechanical properties of the damaged tissue in the applied area by enhanced electrical resistance with increased heat. This is guided by their polymeric chain entanglement and other dynamic molecular features facilitating the generation of the charge transport pathway. However, single use of conducting polymer is not able to provide the desired strength of the engineered three-dimensional scaffold and therefore is copolymerized with other polymers for the betterment of mechanical characteristics as well as processibility. Electroactive nanofiber textile scaffolds can be either designed from intrinsically conducting polymers and their composites or the textile matrix can be modified by embedding conducting fillers like silver nanowires, carbon nanotubes, and PEDOT microspheres to control the tissue regeneration signaling from externally applied stimulation (Sen et al., 2022).

It was witnessed that the conductive polymer-based nanofiber scaffolds encourage the adhesion of human mesenchymal stem cells. PEDOT: PSS (polystyrene sulfonate) scaffold stimulates differentiation of osteogenic precursor cells (Shahini et al., 2014). Nanofiber mesh constructed from different conducting polymer(s) combinations like PLA-PANI, PLGA-PANI, PPY-PCL, etc. has shown elevated cardiomyocyte viability and enhanced maturation. An additional feature of such scaffolds is the ability to perk up the rate of calcium wave propagation which is needed for the normal functioning of the heart (Sen et al., 2022). In skeletal muscle tissue engineering, conductive fibrous scaffolds were found to improve the expression of myogenin, troponin T, and genes for myosin heavy chain, which is helpful for myotube formation (Jun et al., 2009; Ford & Chandra, 2012). Several research activities have shown that conductive biomaterials can effectively upregulate the gene expression of epidermal growth factors, and vascular endothelial growth factors. This stimulates collagen deposition and granulation in the injured tissue (Sen et al., 2022). Some conducting polymers also exhibit antimicrobial properties which are advantageous in skin tissue engineering (Korupalli et al., 2021). In nerve tissue engineering, electrical stimulation can significantly increase the maturation of Schwann cells-like cells and induce secretion of several important nerve growth factors on the electroactive scaffolds. A co-woven nerve conduit scaffold from PPY coated poly-(L-lactic acid) yarn can assist in enhanced neurite outgrowth and axonal differentiation (Gopalakrishnan-Prema et al., 2020). All these existing studies reflect that there is a need to utilize conducting nanofibers as a textile scaffold substrate for future applications.

13.7 CHALLENGES AND FUTURE CONSIDERATIONS

A nanofibrous textile scaffold as regenerative medicine has drawn attention for its multifarious unique properties overcoming problems associated with the conventional nanofibrous scaffold, like precise control over the scaffold porosity, balancing between scaffold firmness, toughness, flexibility, and durability. Although the field of textiles is growing gradually as a new advent for the development of superior tissue engineering material, challenges are being faced especially with the existing machines available for nano yarn processing that are not capable to produce complex structures other than small prototypes. To meet clinical needs, it is an emergency to design a machine with high processing efficiency. Simultaneously, there is also a need for improvement in spinning technology to ameliorate the production of long, continuous nano yarn that can meet the biological characteristics. Currently, there are very few automatic machines available to design a textile pattern with a predefined program namely Raschel, Tricot, flatbed, and circular. These can construct complex two-dimensional and three-dimensional scaffold structures on a large scale (Akbari et al., 2016). So, attention should be given to automation to aid the larger productivity of all types of textile patterns. Still, there are very restricted types of textile designs available. As no single scaffold is ideal for all types of tissues as organs, much more experimentation is needed at the nanoscale level of design. The help of computer-aided design (CAD) (Mbise et al., 2015) and deep learning-based design software (Jiang et al., 2021a, 2021b) can be taken for better designing of optimized textile patterns. For high-accuracy prediction of nano yarn or their textile scaffold mechanical behavior, intelligent neural network (INN) application will add a significant value (Naghashzargar et al., 2013).

For the designing of future scaffolds, stimuli-responsive nanofibrous biotextile must be taken into consideration as there are many effective outputs that are available to show the significant enhancement in cell adherence, proliferation, and differentiation in response to the thermal or mechanical stimuli application. Region-specific biophysical cues are an interesting possibility that can be taken into consideration to combine with this nanotechnology to regulate the phenotype of the seeded cells. Apart from the design concern, more focus should be given to the in-vivo long-term compatibility of the textile scaffold. Novel biodegradable polymers can be explored in the future to construct absorbable regenerative medicines, as the most commonly used electrospinning process has given relaxation to a variety of natural and synthetic polymers to make nanofiber-containing webs and nano yarns (Liu et al., 2022). Some studies have inferred that the degradation rate of tissue engineering scaffolds strongly influences cellular metabolism and consequently the genesis of stem cells, and angiogenesis (Park et al., 2010; Sung et al., 2004). At the same time, it should be examined that the degradation rate of the textile scaffold is not putting the newly regenerated tissue into stress shielding (Freeman et al., 2007).

Clinical relevancy of the nanofibrous textile upon human application has shown to be less promising despite optimistic in-vitro and ex-vivo results. This might be due to the use of small animal models rather than larger animals having more similar hierarchical tissue features. Therefore, to increase the possibility of clinical translation larger animal models must be used for a better understanding of the underlying mechanisms of tissue regeneration, inflammation, and calcifications during the mending tenure (Shiroud et al., 2021). Last but not least, systemic study on the behaviors of progenitor cells and structure-induced regeneration should be performed simultaneously to attain maximally functional tissue development. In fact, microfluidics that can manipulate the geometry, dielectric properties, and polarizability of suspended cells and fluids in a non-destructive way, can be collaborated with nanofiber-textile nanotechnology (Afsaneh & Mohammadi, 2022).

13.8 CONCLUSION

Most of the research involves the application of nanofibrous textile scaffolds for different soft tissues. However, there are several successful results available for nanofiber matrix and nanofiber-reinforced scaffolds in hard tissue repair and remodeling. Therefore, it is a great opportunity to explore the textile springboard of nanofibers in the improvement of hard tissue engineering. In this context, nanofiber fabrics may be designed to deliver growth factors externally to speed up the critically defective tissue repairmen (Huang et al., 2020). There is a hope to expand this nanotechnology from the aforementioned tissues to a broader class including the cornea, pancreas, lungs, and larynx. It is obvious that a set of new obstacles will come when the applications of this innovation try to move forward from in-vitro research to the public arena. More attention should be given to scale-up manufacturing and proper regulation by authentic committees or government authorities so that the significant efforts of these new research can be translated into actual therapies. The market penetration of these new innovations will remarkably depend on the cheaper and less complicated alternative solutions for storage conditions, and the shelf-life of the products over the available tissue-engineered products. Continued collaborative efforts through interdisciplinary research and industry partnerships can bring nanofibrous textile scaffolds to the general public in the near future.

REFERENCES

Afsaneh, H., Mohammadi, R. (2022). Microfluidic platforms for the manipulation of cells and particles. *Talanta Open*, 5, 100092.

Aibibu, D., Hild, M., Cherif, C. (2016). An overview of braiding structure in medical textile. In Yordan Kyosev (Ed.) *Advances in Braiding Technology* (pp. 171–190). Woodhead Publishing, Cambridge, UK.

Akbari, M., Tamayol, A., Bagherifard, S., Serex, L., Mostafalu, P., Faramarzi, N., Mohammadi, M.H., Khademhosseini, A. (2016). Textile technologies and tissue engineering: A path toward organ weaving. *Adv Healthc Mater*, 6, 5(7), 751–766.

Arthi, S.R., Rama, S.V. (2022). Antioxidant α-mangostin coated woven polycaprolactone nanofibrous yarn scaffold for cardiac tissue repair. *ACS Applied Nano Materials*, 5075–5086.

Babu, R., Reshmi, R.C., Joseph, J., et al. (2021). Design, development, and evaluation of an interwoven electrospun nanotextile vascular patch. *Macromolecular Materials and Engineering*, 2100359.

Balint, R., Cassidy, N.J., Cartmell, S.H. (2014). Conductive polymers: Towards a smart biomaterial for tissue engineering. *Acta Biomaterialia*, 10(6), 2341–2353.

Barber, J.G., Handorf, A.M., Allee, T.J., and Li, W.-J. (2013). Braided nanofibrous Scaffold for Tendon and ligament tissue engineering. *Tissue Engineering Part A*, 19(11–12), 1265–1274.

Barhoum, A., Rasouli, R., Yousefzadeh, M., Rahier, H., Bechelany, M. (2018). Nanofiber technology: History and developments. In Ahmed Barhoum, Mickhael Bechelany, Abdel salam Hamby Makhlouf *Handbook of Nanofibers* (pp. 2–18). Springer, New York.

Cai, J., Xie, X., Li, D., et al. (2020). A novel knitted scaffold made of microfiber/nanofiber core-sheath yarns for tendon tissue engineering. *Biomaterials Science*, 16, 4413–4425.

Chen, C.-H., Chen, S.-H., Shalumon, K.T., Chen, J.-P. (2015). Dual functional core-sheath electrospun hyaluronic acid/polycaprolactone nanofibrous membranes embedded with silver nanoparticles for prevention of peritendinous adhesion. *Acta Biomaterialia*, 26, 225–235.

ElSaboni, Y., Hunt, J.A., Stanley, J., et al. (2022). Development of a textile-based protein sensor for monitoring the healing progress of a wound. *Scientific Reports*, 12(1), 7972.

Engelmayr, G.C., Jr., Cheng, M., Bettinger, C.J., Borenstein, J.T., Langer, R., Freed, L.E. (2008). Accordion-like honeycombs for tissue engineering of cardiac anisotropy. *Nat Mater*, 7(12), 1003–1010.

Ford, S.J., Chandra, M. (2012). The effects of slow skeletal troponin I expression in the murine myocardium are influenced by development-related shifts in myosin heavy chain isoform. *J. Physiol.*, 590(23), 6047–6063.

Freeman, J.W., Woods, M.D., Cromer, D.A., Wright, L.D., Laurencin, C.T. (2009). Tissue engineering of the anterior cruciate ligament: The viscoelastic behavior and cell viability of a novel braid—twist scaffold. *Journal of Biomaterials Science, Polymer Edition*, 20(12), 1709–1728.

Freeman, J.W., Woods, M.D., Laurencin, C.T. (2007). Tissue engineering of the anterior cruciate ligament using a braid—twist scaffold design. *Journal of Biomechanics*, 40(9), 2029–2036.

Gao, Y., Shao, W., Qian, W., et al. (2018). Biomineralized poly (1 -lactic- co -glycolic acid)-tussah silk fibroin nanofiber fabric with hierarchical architecture as a scaffold for bone tissue engineering. *Materials Science and Engineering: C*, 84, 195–207.

Gopalakrishnan-Prema, V., Mohanan, A., Shivaram, S.B., Madhusudanan, P., Raju, G., Menon, D., Shankarappa, S.A. (2020). Electrical stimulation of co-woven nerve conduit for peripheral neurite differentiation. *Biomed Mater.*, 15(6), 065015.

Hakimi, O., Mouthuy, P. A., Zargar, N., Lostis, E., Morrey, M., Carr, A. (2015). A layered electrospun and woven surgical scaffold to enhance endogenous tendon repair. *Acta Biomaterialia*, 26, 124–135.

Hild, M., Toskas, G., Aibibu, D., et al. (2013). Chitosan/gelatin micro/nanofiber 3D composite scaffolds for regenerative medicine. *Composite Interfaces*, 21(4), 301–308.

Huang, C., Yang, G., Zhou, S., Luo, E., Pan, J., Bao, C., Liu, X. (2020). Controlled delivery of growth factor by hierarchical nanostructured core-shell nanofibers for the efficient repair of critical-sized rat calvarial defect. *ACS Biomaterials Science & Engineering*, 6(10), 5758–5770.

Jiang, C., Wang, K., Liu, Y., Zhang, C., Wang, B. (2021a). Application of textile technology in tissue engineering: A review. *Acta Biomaterialia*, 128, 60–76.

Jiang, C., Wang, K., Liu, Y., Zhang, C., Wang, B. (2021b). Textile-based sandwich scaffold using wet electrospun yarns for skin tissue engineering. *Journal of the Mechanical Behavior of Biomedical Materials*, 119, 104499.

Joseph, J., Krishnan, A.G., Cherian, A.M., et al. (2018). Transforming nanofibers into woven nanotextiles for vascular application. *ACS Applied Materials & Interfaces*, 10(23), 19449–19458.

Jun, I., Jeong, S., Shin, H. (2009). The stimulation of myoblast differentiation by electrically conductive sub-micron fibers. *Biomaterials*, 30(11), 2038–47.

Karbasi, S., Fekrat, F., Semnani, D., Razavi, S., Zargar, E.N. (2016). Evaluation of structural and mechanical properties of electrospun nano-micro hybrid of poly hydroxybutyrate-chitosan/silk scaffold for cartilage tissue engineering. *Adv. Biomed. Res.*, 28(5), 180.

Korupalli, C., Li, H., Nguyen, N., et al. (2021). Conductive materials for healing wounds: Their incorporation in electroactive wound dressings, characterization, and perspectives. *Advanced Healthcare Materials*, 10(6), e2001384.

Lee, J.Y. (2013). Electrically conducting polymer-based nanofibrous scaffolds for tissue engineering applications. *Polymer Reviews*, 53(3), 443–459.

Li, Y., Guo, F., Hao, Y., et al. (2019). Helical nanofiber yarn enabling highly stretchable engineered microtissue. *Proceedings of the National Academy of Sciences*, 116(19), 9245–9250.

Liberski, A., Ayad, N., Wojciechowska, D., et al. (2017). Weaving for heart valve tissue engineering. *Biotechnology Advances*, 35(6), 633–656.

Liu, J., Li, Tao, Zhang, H., et al. (2022). Electrospun strong, bioactive, and bioabsorbable silk fibroin/poly(L-lactic-acid) nanoyarns for constructing advanced nanotextile tissue scaffolds. *Materials Today Bio*, 14, 1002432.

Luca, A.C.D., Wassim, R., Francesco, G., et al. (2015). Tissue-engineered constructs for peripheral nerve repair: Current research concepts and future perspectives. *Plastic and Aesthetic Research*, 2213–2219.

Ma, P., Yuping, C., Boakye, A., Jiang, G. (2016). Review on the knitted structures with auxetic effect. *The Journal of the Textile Institute*, 108(6), 947–961.

Mann, D.L., Kubo, S.H., Sabbah, H.N., et al. (2012). Beneficial effects of the CorCap cardiac support device: Five-year results from the Acorn trial. *J. Thorac. Cardiovasc. Surg.*, 143(5), 1036–1042.

Mbise, E., Dias, T., Hurley, W. (2015). Design and manufacture of heated textiles. In T. Dias (Ed.), *Electronic Textiles* (pp. 117–132). Woodhead publishing series in textile. Amsterdam, The Netherlands: Elsevier.

McCullen, S.D., Haslauer, C.M., Loboa, E.G. (2010). Fiber-reinforced scaffolds for tissue engineering and regenerative medicine: Use of traditional textile substrates to nanofibrous arrays. *Journal of Materials Chemistry*, 20(40), 8776.

Mi, H.-Y., Jing, X., Yu, E., McNulty, J., Peng, X.-F., Turng, L.-S. (2015). Fabrication of triple-layered vascular scaffolds by combining electrospinning, braiding, and thermally induced phase separation. *Materials Letters*, 161, 305–308.

Naghashzargar, E., Semnani, D., Karbasi, S., Nekoee, H. (2013). Application of intelligent neural network method for prediction of mechanical behavior of wire-rope scaffold in tissue engineering. *The Journal of the Textile Institute*, 105(3), 264–274.

Oliveira, G.H., Al-Kindi, S.G., Bezerra, H.G., Costa, M.A. (2014). Left ventricular restoration devices. *Journal of Cardiovascular Translational Research*, 7(3), 282–291.

Park, S.-H, Gil, E.S., Kim, H.J., Lee, K., David, K.L. (2010). Relationships between degradability of silk scaffolds and osteogenesis. *Biomaterials*, 31(24), 6162–6172.

Person, M., Lehenkari, P.P., Berglin, L., et al. (2018). Osteogenic differentiation of human mesenchymal stem cells in a 3D woven scaffold. *Scientific Reports*, 8, 10457.

Pillai, M.M., Kumar, G.S., Houshyar, S., Padhye, R., Bhattacharyya, A. (2020). Effect of nanocomposite coating and biomolecule functionalization on silk fibroin based conducting 3D braided scaffolds for peripheral nerve tissue engineering. *Nanomedicine*, 24, 102131.

Rothrauff, B.B., Lauro, B.B., Yang, G., Debski, R.E., Musahl, V., Tuan, R.S. (2017). Braided and stacked electrospun nanofibrous scaffolds for tendon and ligament tissue engineering. *Tissue Eng Part A.*, 9–10, 378–389.

Sen, S., Bal, T., Rajora, A.D., Sharma, S., Sharma, S.R., Sharma, N. (2022). Conducting polymers as efficient materials for tissue engineering. In R.K. Gupta (Ed.), *Conducting Polymers*. Boca Raton, NY: CRC Press.

Şenel Ayaz, H.G., Perets, A., Ayaz, H., Gilroy, K.D., Govindaraj, M., Brookstein, D., Lelkes, P.I. (2014). Textile-templated electrospun anisotropic scaffolds for regenerative cardiac tissue engineering. *Biomaterials*, 35(30), 8540–8552.

Shahini, A., Yazdimamaghani, M., Walker, K.J., Eastman, M.A., Hatami-Marbini, H., Smith, B.J., Ricci, J.L., Madihally, S.V., Vashaee, D., Tayebi, L. (2014). 3D conductive nanocomposite scaffold for bone tissue engineering. *Int J Nanomedicine*, 9, 167–181.

Shao, W., He, J., Han, Q., et al. (2016). A biomimetic multilayer nanofiber fabric fabricated by electrospinning and textile technology from polylactic acid and Tussah silk fibroin as a scaffold for bone tissue engineering. *Materials Science and Engineering: C*, 67, 599–610.

Shikinami, Y., Kawabe, Y., Yasukawa, K., Tsuta, K., Kotani, Y., Abumi, K. (2021). A biomimetic artificial intervertebral disc system composed of a cubic three-dimensional fabric. *The Spine Journal*, 10(2), 141–152.

Shiroud, H.B., Ruan, R., De-Juan-Pardo, E.M., Zheng, M., Doyle, B. (2021). Biofabrication and signaling strategies for tendon/ligament interfacial tissue engineering. *ACS Biomater Sci Eng.*, 7(2), 383–399.

Sung, H.J., Meredith, C., Johnson, C., Galis, Z.S. (2004). The effect of scaffold degradation rate on three-dimensional cell growth and angiogenesis. *Biomaterials*, 25, 5735–5742.

Vijayamohan, M., Anitha, A., Menon, D., Iyer, S., Nair, S.V., Nair, M.B. (2018). Nanofibrous yarn-reinforced HA-gelatin composite scaffolds promote bone formation in critical-sized alveolar defects in rabbit model. *Biomedical Materials (Bristol, England)*, 13(6), 065011.

Walsh, R.G. (2005). Design and features of the Acorn CorCap cardiac support device: The concept of passive mechanical diastolic support. *Heart Failure Reviews*, 10(2), 101–107.

Wu, S., Dong, T., Li, Y., et al. (2022). State-of-the-art review of advanced electrospun nano-fiber yarn-based textiles for biomedical applications. *Applied Materials Today*, 27, 101473.

Wu, S., Duan, B., Liu, P., Zhang, C., Qin, X., Butcher, J.T. (2016). Fabrication of aligned nanofiber polymer yarn networks for anisotropic soft tissue scaffolds. *ACS Applied Materials & Interfaces*, 8(26), 16950–16960.

Wu, S., Ni, S., Jiang, X., Kuss, M.A., Wang, H.-J., Duan, B. (2019). Guiding mesenchymal stem cells into myelinating schwann cell-like phenotypes by using electrospun core-sheath nanoyarns. *ACS Biomaterials Science & Engineering*, 5, 5284–5294.

Wu, T., Li, D., Wang, Y. (2017). Laminin-coated nerve guidance conduits based on poly(l-lactide-co-glycolide) fibers and yarns for promoting Schwann cells' proliferation and migration. *Journal of Materials Chemistry B*, 5(17), 3186–3194.

Xie, X., Cai, J., Yao, Y., et al. (2021). A woven scaffold with continuous mineral gradients for tendon-to-bone tissue engineering. *Composites Part B: Engineering*, 212, 108679.

Zhang, Y., Li, X.S., Guex, A.G., et al. (2017). A compliant and biomimetic three-layered vas-cular graft for small blood vessels. *Biofabrication*, 9(2), 025010.

14 Use of Nanoparticles in Fabrication of Antimicrobial Biofilms Derived From Natural Resources for Wound Dressing

Rakesh Kumar

14.1 INTRODUCTION

Soy protein matrix is a biodegradable polymer that falls in the category of protein based natural biopolymers. The major advantages include easy availability, by-product of soy oil industry and its biodegradable nature. Soy protein is composed of two globular protein subunit fractions called 7S (β-conglycinin) and 11S (glycine) (Rani et al., 2021). Based on the protein contents, soy protein exists in three forms, i.e., soy flour (SF), soy protein concentrate (SPC) and soy protein isolate (SPI). For research purposes, scientists use SPI as a base material and in some cases SPC. SPI can be fabricated into films and fibres and both forms can be explored extensively. Soy protein has globular structure, and it is different from other proteinous material. Due to its globular nature, soy protein is resistant to hydrolysis and hence suitable for biomedical applications. Reddy and Yang in 2009 developed soy protein fibres of 50–150 mm in absence of any additives or cross-linking material. Soy protein based fibres supported the growth of mouse fibroblasts for the duration of seven days (Reddy & Yang, 2009).

Bacterial cellulose (BC) is a natural biodegradable polymer synthesized as a secondary metabolite through the fermentation process in presence of bacteria such as *Acetobacter xylinum, Pseudomonas sp., Gluconacetobacter sp.* and others (Pandit & Kumar, 2021). BC possesses high crystallinity and high water absorbing capacity. It is nontoxic and biodegradable in nature. High water capacity is attributed to its unique three dimensional network structure and presence of several hydroxyl groups on BC (Zmejkoski et al., 2018), which make it an ideal candidate for its use in wound healing or antibacterial dressings (Kumar et al., 2019b).

DOI: 10.1201/9781003331612-17

Nanotechnology has been greatly explored in the area of medical science. Several nanoparticles such as silver, montmorillonite (MMT), titanium oxide, multiwalled carbon nanotubes (MWNTs), zinc selenide and zinc sulphide can be incorporated into soy protein matrix to create bionanocomposites (Kumar et al., 2019a, 2019c). Silver is the most widely used metal for the fabrication of bionanocomposite materials. In ancient times also, the use of silver as an antimicrobial material has been demonstrated (Shameli et al., 2011). Silver is effective against all kinds of microbes including bacteria, fungi, algae and viruses (Fei et al., 2013). Nowadays, silver nanoparticles can be incorporated in either soy protein or BC matrix so that the resulting materials can be used as wound dressings or for drug delivery (Wei et al., 2011). Antimicrobial silver nanoparticles had been incorporated in SPI to form (AgNPs)/SPI films through in-situ synthesis (Zhao et al., 2013).

The commercially available layered silicate clay that has been explored widely in research is MMT. By solution intercalation, MMT has been incorporated in SPI to fabricate SPI/MMT nanocomposites (Echeverria et al., 2014). Multiwalled carbon nanotubes (MWNTs) can also be incorporated into glycerol plasticized SPI film to form MWNT/soy protein nanocomposite plastics (Xiang et al., 2017). Wang et al. fabricated SPI/titanium dioxide films which had the capability to kill *E. coli* and *S. aureus* (Wang et al., 2014). In addition, many inorganic and metal nanoparticles had been explored to increase the shelf-life of food (Hoseinnejad et al., 2017).

SPI and BC based biomaterial can be fabricated in the form of hydrogels. These materials have been explored for the delivery of drugs, contact lenses, and wound dressings. Structural and mechanical characteristics of the SPI and BC based hydrogels are important for exploring their application as biomaterial. In absence of any additives soy protein hydrogels were fabricated by Chien et al., with possible application for tissue engineering and drug delivery as well as for wound healing (Chien et al., 2014). SPI based hydrogels increased at higher content of SPI. It was also observed that SPI based hydrogels with high content of SPI released a low amount of fluorescein over a period of one week (Chien et al., 2014).

14.2   NANOPARTICLES INCORPORATED SOY PROTEIN ISOLATE

SPI films are prepared using the solution-casting method. Generally, 5 to 7% SPI (w/v wrt) are slowly dissolved in water maintained at 60–65°C and pH of around 9 to 9.5. Then the plasticizer (glycerol, 30% w/w, relative to SPI) is added to fabricate SPI films. Glyoxal (1% w/w, wrt SPI) and gentamycin (1% or 3% w/w, wrt to SPI) were added as cross-linking agent and drug, respectively to the SPI suspension, and the suspension was subjected to constant stirring so as to prepare drug incorporated SPI film for controlled release of drugs that can kill bacteria in a continuous manner. The pH was maintained as 7.2 for 30 min (Peles et al., 2013). Prusty et al. synthesized the soy protein polyacrylamide incorporated nano silver nanocomposite hydrogel by in situ polymerization process. This hydrogel can be used for the release of drugs such as ciprofloxacin (Prusty et al., 2019).

SPI suspension with 10% SPI powder in water was prepared by maintaining the same condition as discussed earlier. To prepare hydroxyethyl cellulose (HEC) slurry, one can take 2 wt% of HEC and dissolve it in distilled water under stirring conditions. After that, both HEC slurry and SPI suspension were mixed in a weight ratio of 3:7 followed by stirring for another 6 h so as to obtain homogenous slurry. In the homogenous slurry of HEC and SPI, 100 mg/mL MMT dispersion was added under constant stirring for 12 h. Epichlorohydrin (ECH) solution, as cross-linker, was added dropwise for 30 min to the MMT incorporated cross-linked HEC and SPI dispersion so that it can be casted to obtain a porous scaffold followed by freeze dry-ing of the resulting material. The resulting material was then immersed in 5% acetic acid solution for 30 min and then neutralized with alkali followed by second time freeze drying of the sample. All the processes, except freeze drying, were carried at room temperature to obtain cross-linked MMT-modified HEC/SPI nanocomposite scaffolds. The obtained samples were designated as EHSS-1%M, EHSS-2%M, and EHSS-3%M (Wu et al., 2021). Here there is variation of MMT as 1% w/v, 2% w/v, and 3% w/v in the sample. EHSS-0%M that represented the absence of MMT was prepared the same way as discussed and was used as a control. A schematic diagram of the preparation of the two types of porous scaffolds is presented in Figure 14.1.

14.3 NANOPARTICLES INCORPORATED BACTERIAL CELLULOSE

Lignin nanoparticles have been incorporated in BC to reduce the rate of biodegrada-tion of the composite material (Tian et al., 2021). The inoculum for fermentation was prepared by growing *Acetobacter xylinum* or *G. xylinus* in 25 mL of standard fruc-tose medium at 30°C for three days. 2 g L^{-1} lignin obtained from different sources were added and dispersed in the standard fructose medium, respectively. BC-lignin nanocomposite production was achieved by further inoculating small volume of inoculum to large volume of inoculum and the media were subjected to static fer-mentation for 15 days at 30°C.

Since BC hydrogels do not show any antibacterial properties, their application in wound dressings is limited and hence silver nanoparticles have been introduced as

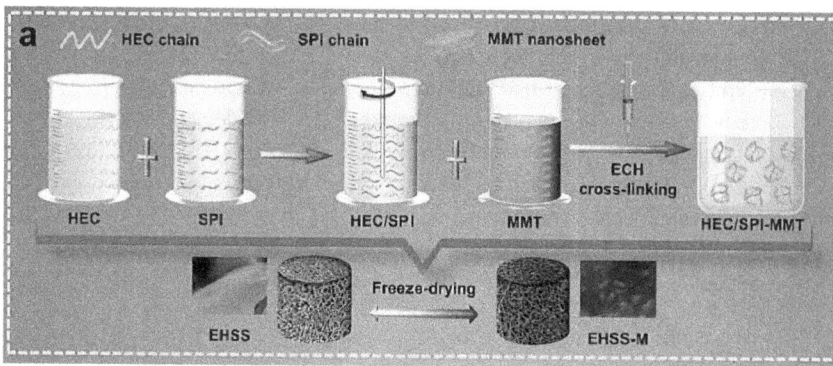

FIGURE 14.1 Preparation of MMT-incorporated SPI and HEC cross-linked nanocompos-ite scaffolds. (Reproduced from the permission from Wu et al. (2021). Nanoclay mineral-reinforced macroporous nanocomposite scaffolds for in situ bone regeneration: in vitro and in vivo studies. *Materials & Design* 2021, 205, 109734, Copyright (2021) Elsevier).

antibacterial agents into solution of polyvinyl alcohol (PVA)/bacterial cellulose (BC) (Song et al., 2021). The incorporation of silver nanoparticles was carried out in two steps. *Acetobacter xylinum* was cultured in an HS medium with pH being maintained at 6.4, and the fermentation was carried out at 28°C for seven to 10 days. To remove the residual medium and other impurities, the upper BC film was collected after 10 days and placed in a 0.1 M NaOH solution at 80°C for 40 min and then it was subjected to freeze drying. The BC dry film was converted into BC powder via mechanical grinding to prepare transparent BC solution in presence of NaOH/water mixture. The hydrogels were prepared by taking 0, 1, 2 and 4 mM of $AgNO_3$ into 10% PVA and BC solutions (1:1, v/v). The solutions were 60°C for 1 h to get the resulting hydrogels that were abbreviated as PVA/BC, PVA/BC-Ag1, PVA/BC-Ag2 and PVA/BC-Ag3 (Song et al., 2021).

Silymarin-zein (SMN-Zein) nanoparticles were prepared in which BC is prepared according to the earlier mentioned process. BC films prepared from BC powder were preswollen in at 40°C for 24 h. After that the swollen BC films were dipped in 200 mL of SMN-Zein nanoparticle suspensions which was colloidal in nature under shaking condition at 30°C for 4 h (Tsai et al., 2018). 1% aqueous suspension of ZnO nanoparticles was prepared under continuous stirring for 30 min. Then BC-ZnO nanocomposites were prepared by immersing prepared BC films into suspension of ZnO nanoparticles. The shaking condition of 150 rpm was maintained at 50°C for 24 h. The resulting BC-ZnO nanocomposites were lypholized (Khalid et al., 2017).

Biocomposites based on BC and chitosan membranes incorporated with poly(*N*-isopropylacrylamide)/polyvinyl alcohol nanoparticles that exhibited antimicrobial behaviour were prepared and reported. These drug-loaded polymeric biomaterials can be explored as wound dressing having antibacterial property (Stanescu et al., 2021).

Preparation of HEC/BC based cryogel that had been incorporated with both silver and titanium oxide nanoparticles designated as Ag@TiO_2NPs has been reported (El-Naggar et al., 2020). The cryogel was prepared using three steps:

(i) Sol formation—10g of HEC was dissolved in 90 mL H_2O under mechanical stirring for 2 h at room temperature. Side by side 1% BC suspension was also prepared by dissolving 1 g BC in 100 mL distilled water under mechanical stirring. Both HEC and BC solutions were then mixed at different ratios at room temperature for 1 h at 800 rpm. Finally, sol was prepared by using different volumes of the dispersed silver and titanium oxide nanoparticles.

(ii) Gel formation—To produce gel, glyoxal as chemical cross-linker was added dropwise. Continuous mechanical stirring was maintained for 30 min so that the gels could be set. Care was taken to remove the air bubbles if any from the viscous solution that is gel.

(iii) Cryogel—The gel obtained in the second step was freeze dried to get cryogel.

The CQD-TiO_2 NPs solution was sprayed on wet BC at room temperature so as to incorporate CQD-TiO_2 NPs into BC (Malmir et al., 2020). The moisture from the composite was totally removed by using the heat press machine and after drying for two days at 40°C. Also to incorporate graphene oxide (GO), BC was prepared by fermentation technique after seven days of fermentation as described earlier. The traditional Hummers method was used to prepare GO (Hou et al., 2020). The BC (GO) composite film of 4.0 cm diameter and 1.00 mm thickness was formed by blending

BC and GO. The film was neutralized with alkali after giving alkali treatment for 2 h at 80°C to remove growth medium and cells adhered to BC (GO) composite film. The BC (GO) composite film was freeze dried to get 0.17 mm BC(GO) film. In 2 mg mL^{-1} of dopamine (DA), the prepared BC (GO) composite film was immersed followed by soaking in 1 mM AgNO$_3$ solution to get Ag-pDA (rGO) composite film having thickness of about 0.20 mm (Zhang et al., 2021).

14.4   PROPERTIES

14.4.1   MECHANICAL

Peles et al. prepared three types of yellowish, transparent, homogeneous, soy protein films with thickness of 0.5 mm designated as SPI (neat protein films), SPI–gly (cross-linked SPI films) and SPI–gly–th (cross-linked and thermally treated SPI films at 80°C for 24 h min) (Peles et al., 2013). The tensile properties of the three types of prepared films are given in Figure 14.2. SPI–gly–th showed highest tensile strength

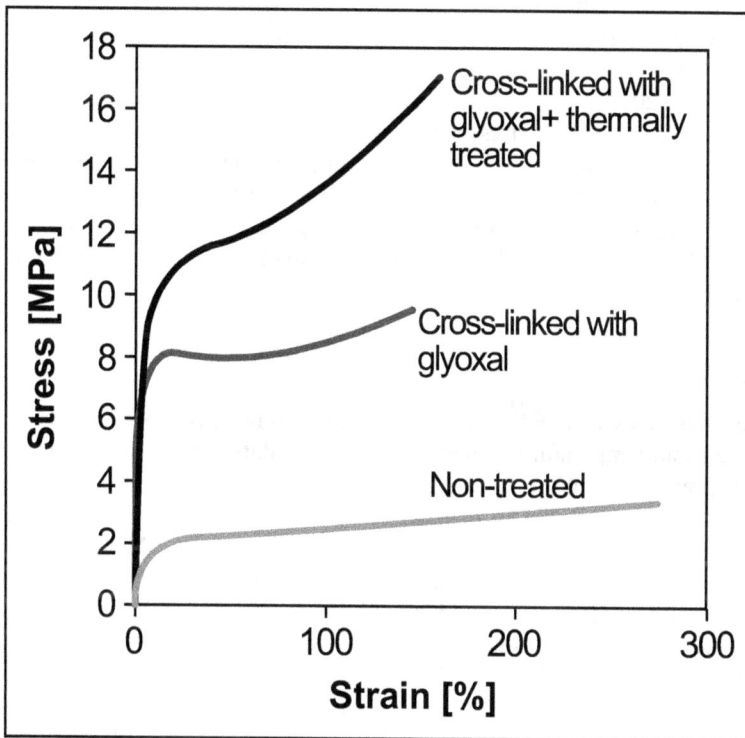

FIGURE 14.2   Tensile properties of SPI films (5% w/v) plasticized with glycerol (50% w/w) cast from pH 7.2, 55°C solutions are indicated in the inset of the Figure 14.2. (Reproduced from the permission from Peles et al. (2013). Soy protein films for wound-healing applications: antibiotic release, bacterial inhibition and cellular response. *Journal of Tissue Engineering and Regenerative Medicine* 2013, 7, 401–412, Copyright (2013) Wiley).

of 16.0 ± 1.5 MPa and elongation at break of 145 ± 25%. This is attributed to the fact that glyoxal acts as a cross-linker. The presence of free amine groups in SPI is responsible for cross-linking with glyoxal that contained aldehydes and higher temperature facilitates cross-linking in SPI by the presence of cysteine groups leading to S–S associations (Peles et al., 2013).

Wu et al. reported that as the MMT concentration increased in the EHSS-2%M and EHSS-3%M groups, the nanocomposite scaffolds presented higher mechanical strength (Wu et al., 2021). The data of compressive modulus of sample prepared are given as 0.29 ± 0.07 MPa for pure EHSS; 0.55 ± 0.03 MPa for EHSS containing 1% MMT; 2.01 ± 0.87 MPa for EHSS containing 2% MMT; 2.1 ± 0.93 MPa for EHSS containing 3% MMT. The results show that with the increasing concentration of MMT there is increase in compressive modulus of the nanocomposite scaffolds, and in absence of MMT the nanocomposite showed very less compressive modulus.

The incorporation of Ag in PVA/BC resulted in the formation of PVA/BC-Ag hydrogels. It was reported that PVA/BC-Ag showed higher stress-at-break and elongation-at-break compared to PVA/BC without the addition of Ag. Also, it has been noted that with the addition of AgNPs, the mechanical properties of PVA/BC-AgNPs initially increased and then showed decreasing trend (Song et al., 2021). The decrease in mechanical properties may be due to agglomeration of AgNPs at higher content. The addition of CQD-TiO$_2$ in BC increased the tensile strength and the Young's modulus, and this is attributed to coherence between NPs and BC (Malmir et al., 2020).

Zhang et al. reported the stress-strain curves of BC based composite films in presence of graphene oxide i.e., BC(GO), dopamine i.e., pDA/BC(GO) and silver ions i.e., Ag-pDA/BC (rGO). The maximum tensile strength of 1.2 MPa was observed for the BC film and its composite in the wet state. Tensile properties increased for freeze-dried, dopamine-added and silver ions-loaded BC based composites (Zhang et al., 2021).

14.4.2 WATER UPTAKE

The scaffolds fabricated by Wu et al. were immersed in a PBS solution over a period of 24 h at room temperature (Wu et al., 2021). The data show that swelling ratio of scaffolds prepared by Wu et al. increased with time. The large pore sizes and pore distribution was responsible for penetration of a large amount of the solvent leading to higher swelling rate. It has been reported that in presence of MMT the scaffolds reached equilibrium after 4 h of immersion in PBS solution. The values as reported were 1670 ± 101%; 1593 ± 199%; 1376 ± 139% for 1%, 2% and 3% MMT in EHSS, respectively. After 24 h of immersion in PBS the water absorption increased slowly and it reached the value of 1913 ± 252%. This is attributed to the fact that MMT acts as barrier for water molecules and that is the reason one could see reduced water absorption at higher contents of MMT in EHSS. Due to low water absorption MMT-containing scaffolds maintain structural integrity so it can be used as structural support for bone regeneration.

BC, PVA/BC and PVA/BC-Ag hydrogels as prepared by Song et al. were immersed in an SBF solution for 24 h to study their water absorption capacity

(Song et al., 2021). After the addition of PVA in BC, PVA/BC and PVA/BC-Ag hydrogels showed good water absorption performance. It has been reported that PVA/BC, PVA/BC-Ag hydrogels absorbed better than the PVA/BC hydrogel, and the swelling rate of PVA/BC-Ag3 was reported as 1604.9 ± 58.2%. The incorporation of AgNPs in PVA/BC increased the pore size so water holding capacity increased and was maximum for PVA/BC-Ag3. It has also been reported that the water retention capacity of the hydrogels showed a decreasing trend over time. Water retention capacity of PVA/BC showed ~24.19%, and incorporation of Ag nanoparticles decreased the water retention values which are given as 20.84%, 17.49%, 12.38% for PVA/BC-Ag-1, PVA/BC-Ag-2 and PVA/BC-Ag-3 hydrogels, respectively after air exposure for 6 h. This may be due to the highly porous structure of PVA/BC-Ag hydrogel.

After 1800 min, air-dried and freeze-dried SMN1.0-Zein1.0/BC composite films reach equilibrium upon being subjected to water uptake studies (Tsai et al., 2018). Due to incorporation of zein, SMN1.0-Zein1.0/BC lower swelling degrees when compared to neat BC film which is attributed to the hydrophobic nature of zein protein.

14.5   APPLICATIONS

14.5.1   Wound Dressing

Generally, acute wounds take eight to 12 weeks for complete healing. On the other hand, chronic wounds persist beyond 12 weeks, with the possibility to reoccur. The repair process of wound healing occurs in several steps starting from hemostasis, inflammation, proliferation and lastly maturation or remodelling. In the first step of the healing process, fibrin clot is formed by aggregation of platelets at the wound site. The formation of fibrin clot depends on the wound depth, size, type, location and also infection state. SPI (soy protein isolate) and BC (bacterial cellulose)-based natural biopolymers, because of their biodegradability and biocompatibility are attractive as wound dressing materials. SPI has been also shown to facilitate the blood clot and stimulate collagen deposition for enhancing wound healing.

BC-ZnO nanocomposites were explored as wound healing material by subjecting the measurements of the wound after 0, 5, 10 and 15 days after the application of the BC-ZnO nanocomposites on the affected area (Figure 14.3). The data show the shrinkage in wound size. In BC-ZnO nanocomposites treated group, day 0 wound size was 289 ± 0 mm^2 and it reduced to 98.3 ± 7.6 mm^2 on day 15. Thus 7% and 66% healing was observed for this group. In 1% silver sulfadiazine treated group, day 0 wound size was 289 ± 0 mm^2 and it reduced to 66.6 ± 5.7 mm^2 on day 15. This was taken positive control in this 1%, and 77% healing was observed. In the negative control treated group, day 0 wound size was 289 ± 0 mm^2 and it reduced to 234.6 ± 5.7 mm^2 on day 15. In this 0% and 18% healing was observed. So it has been stated that BC-ZnO nanocomposites healing process may have occurred by effecting fibroblast proliferation and keratinocytes. The data suggest that positive control showed better wound healing nature than BC-ZnO nanocomposites.

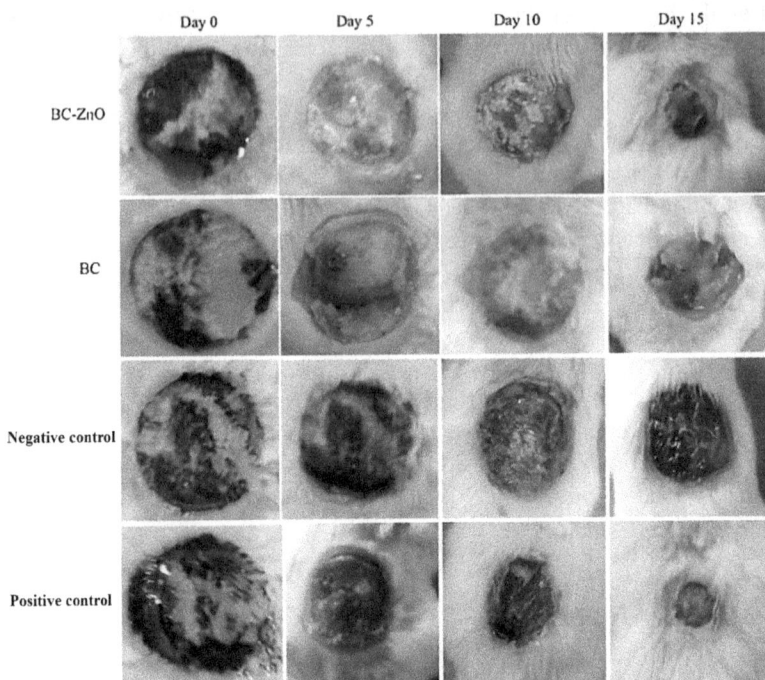

FIGURE 14.3 Wound photographs of BC-ZnO nanocomposites treated group in comparison with negative control, BC and positive control group on different treatment days. (Reproduced from the permission from Khalid et al., 2017. Bacterial cellulose-zinc oxide nanocomposites as a novel dressing system for burn wounds. *Carbohydrate Polymers* 2017, 164, 214–221, Copyright (2017) Elsevier).

14.5.2 ANTIBACTERIAL

The three bacterial strains *S. albus*, *S. aureus* and *P. aeruginosa* were tested against the drug loaded SPI films prepared by Peles et al. All the three bacteria were effective against the drug gentamicin. Among all three bacterial strains the most sensitive was *S. albus* while *P. aeruginosa* showed highest resistance against the drug. For at least 14 days, two bacteria except *P. aeruginosa* were effectively inhibited. On the other hand, *P. aeruginosa* was effectively inhibited till the third day. 3% gentamicin incorporated SPI film showed larger zones of inhibition when compared with 1% gentamicin incorporated SPI film.

Escherichia coli, Shigella flexneri, Bacillus cereus and Listeria inuaba were used as the test bacteria to observe the antibacterial behaviour of polyacrylamide-soy protein (PAM-SP) and silver nanoparticles embedded PAM-SP (PAM-SP@Ag) nanocomposite hydrogels (Prusty et al., 2019). *Bacillus cereus* bacteria had more resisting power, and *Shigella flexneri* showed lowest antibacterial property. In PAM-SP@Ag nanocomposite hydrogels silver nanoparticles restricted the growth of bacteria in nanocomposite hydrogels which is attributed to hydrogen bonding interaction among the amide group of acrylamide chains and silver nanoparticles.

E. coli and *S. aureus* are the most common skin infection species. The PVA/BC hydrogel is deprived of antibacterial activity. However with the addition of Ag in PVA/BC, the PVA/BC-Ag hydrogels showed antibacterial ability. The bactericidal rates of PVA/BC-Ag1 were 65.63 ± 2.63% for *E. coli* and 51.17 ± 1.49% for *S. aureus*, and for PVA/BC-Ag3 it increased to 99.72 ± 0.14% and 99.38 ± 0.48%, respectively (Song et al., 2021).

Bacterial populations of the SMN1.0-Zein1.0/BC nanocomposite films-treated bacterial cultures were significantly less compared to the alkaline-treated BC films-treated groups. Air-dried SMN1.0-Zein1.0/BC nanocomposite showed inhibitory ratios against *E. coli*, *S. aureus* and *P. aeruginosa* as 21.6 ± 2.8%, 62.1 ± 1.9%, 28.2 ± 4.9%, respectively. On the other hand, freeze-dried SMN1.0-Zein1.0/BC nanocomposite film showed less inhibitory ratio as 17.4 ± 3.6%, 53.5 ± 2.3% and 23.5 ± 5.4% against *E. coli*, *S. aureus* and *P. aeruginosa* (Tsai et al., 2018).

In burn wounds the two common pathogens *P. aeruginosa* and *S. aureus* are found. It is important to see the effect of the nanocomposites against the said bacteria. The antibacterial activity of BC and BC-ZnO nanocomposites was assessed against wound infection. *E. coli*, *C. freundii*, *P. aeruginosa* and *S. aureus* were used to assess the effectiveness of these composites against the three bacteria. BC-ZnO nanocomposites showed 90%, 90.9%, 87.4% activity against *E. coli*, *C. freundii*, *P. aeruginosa* falling under Gram negative bacterial strains as well as 94.3% for *S. aureus* falling under Gram positive category (Khalid et al., 2017).

Ag@TiO$_2$NPs based cryogels were tested against the infectious microbial strains. The increase in Ag and TiO$_2$ nanoparticle concentration enhanced parallelly the antimicrobial activity against *E. coli*, *P. aeruginosa*, *S. aurous*, *B. subtilis* and unicellular fungi *C. albicans* (El-Naggar., 2020). The presence of a smaller amount of nanoparticle showed no antimicrobial activity. From this study, the author reported that TiO$_2$NPs and AgNPs showed synergistic nature and hence it was more effective than the use of only one nanoparticle either TiO$_2$NPs or AgNPs.

As already reported, neat BC film and BC films blended with graphene oxide had almost zero inhibition on almost all the bacteria reported in this research paper (Zhang et al., 2021). After immersing both types of film in dopamine, the composite biofilms showed a slight antibacterial activity. The bactericidal zone reached to 6.3 mm when both the films were impregnated with AgNO$_3$. Actually AgNO$_3$ releases AgNPs that increase antibacterial activity of the composite biofilms (Zhang et al., 2021) (Figure 14.4). It has been reported that BC-Ag, the composite film with BC, GO and Ag nanoparticles, has excellent antibacterial properties and due to which wound healing is accelerated (Zhang et al., 2021).

14.5.3 Drug Release

SPI has been explored extensively in delivery systems for bioactive ingredients. A delivery system is designed in such a way so as to retain sensitive compounds with degradable characteristics to control the release of drugs (Tian et al., 2018). Soy protein-based hydrogels are explored for capturing, protecting and providing various bioactive ingredients in the pharmaceutical industries. Soy protein-based biopolymer

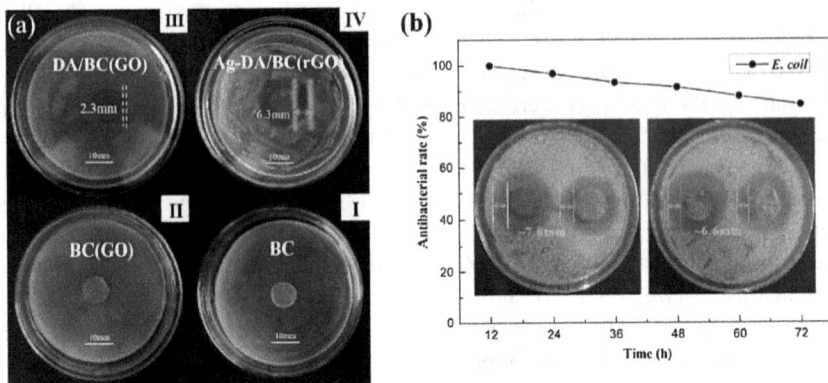

FIGURE 14.4 Antibacterial activity of various composite films in presence and absence of silver nanoparticles. (Reproduced from the permission from Zhang et. al., 2021. Zhang, L., Yu, Y., Zheng, S., et al. Preparation and properties of conductive bacterial cellulose-based graphene oxide-silver nanoparticles antibacterial dressing. *Carbohydrate Polymers* 2021, 257, Article 117671, Copyright (2021) Elsevier).

nanocarriers can effectively protect drugs from harsh process and environmental conditions. In this way, drugs can be safely delivered to target organs and cells.

Peles et al. used two SPI films that they had prepared for the release studies, SPI–gly and SPI–gly–th (Peles et al., 2013). 1% w/w or 3% gentamicin was incorporated in SPI–gly and SPI–gly–th films. The drug release kinetics was studied for about 60 days. The cumulative release profiles of the four types of samples are presented in Figure 14.5. The release profiles were divided into three main stages:

(a) In first 6 h, burst release.
(b) During the first week, there is decrease release rate of drug which is exponential in nature.
(c) During the second week, there is constant release rate of drug.

Gentamicin release profile for SPI–gly and SPI–gly–th was studied. The thermal treatment showed a significant effect on the release profile of the drugs. SPI–gly–th films showed 40% higher burst effect and release of total quantity drug during the first week.

Release of ciprofloxacin (CFX) drugs from PAM-SP hydrogel and PAM-SP@Ag nanocomposite has been reported under various pH conditions (Prusty et al., 2019). It was observed that in basic pH (higher in pH 7.5), the drug release rate was faster whereas it was slower in acidic pH (pH 1.2–6.5) in both of hydrogels and nanocomposite hydrogels. With the increase in time from 0 to 6 h the amounts of drug released from PAM-SP@Ag nanocomposite hydrogels showed an increase in value from 75.4% to 95.27%.

14.6 CONCLUSION

Polymer reinforcement technology of SPI or BC with AgNPs, ZnO, TiO_2 and CDs offers an opportunity to alter the physical and mechanical properties of biopolymers

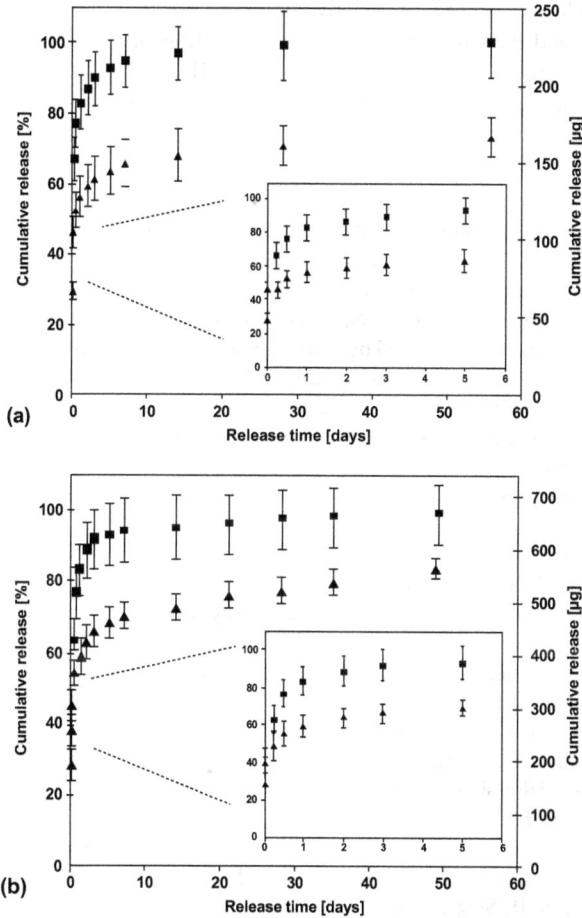

FIGURE 14.5 Gentamicin release profile from SPI films plasticized with glycerol (50% w/w) and SPI–gly: ■, non-treated; ▲, thermally treated (80°C, 24 h); (a) films loaded with 1% w/w gentamicin; (b) films loaded with 3% w/w gentamicin. (Reproduced from the permission from Peles et al. (2013). Soy protein films for wound-healing applications: antibiotic release, bacterial inhibition and cellular response. *Journal of Tissue Engineering and Regenerative Medicine* 2013, 7, 401–412, Copyright (2013) Wiley).

than can be explored as tissue engineering scaffold, antibacterial films, wound healing materials and many other biomedical devices. SPI films had been loaded with gentamicin for bacterial inhibition in presence of silver nanoparticles. SPI as scaffolds or their bioactive degradation products on wound healing in vivo has been demonstrated. Most of the products currently available to surgeons cannot show all the essential characteristics for biodegradable biomaterials. The BC or SPI based hydrogels had porous structures, high swelling capacities, and good water retention abilities that absorb the exudate and hence keep the wound surface moist so that it can be widely used as wound dressing materials. Researchers had explored the nanoparticles incorporated SPI/BC biomaterials in treating infections and it has been observed that there was no sign of infection in bionanocomposite treated groups. Thus it can be finally concluded that AgNPs, ZnO, TiO_2 and CDs incorporated SPI/BC biomaterials can be successful in combating infection.

REFERENCES

Chien, K.B., Chung, E.J., Shah, R.N. (2014). Investigation of soy protein hydrogels for biomedical applications: Materials characterization, drug release, and biocompatibility. *Journal of Biomaterials Applications*, 28(7), 1085–1096.

Echeverria, I., Eisenberg, P., Mauri, A.N. (2014). Nanocomposites films based on soy proteins and montmorillonite processed by casting. *Journal of Membrane Science*, 449, 15–26.

El-Naggar, M.E., Hasanin, M., Youssef, A.M. (2020). Hydroxyethyl cellulose/bacterial cellulose cryogel dopped silver@ titanium oxide nanoparticles: Antimicrobial activity and controlled release of tebuconazole fungicide. *International Journal of Biological Macromolecules*, 165, 1010–1021.

Fei, X., Jia, M., Du, X., et al. (2013). Green synthesis of silk fibroin-silver nanoparticle composites with effective antibacterial and biofilm disrupting properties. *Biomacromolecules*, 14(12), 4483–4488.

Hoseinnejad, M., Jafari, S.M., Katouzian, I. (2017). Inorganic and metal nanoparticles and their antimicrobial activity in food packaging applications. *Critical Reviews in Microbiology*, 44(2), 1–21.

Hou, Y.G., Lv, S.H., Liu, L.P., et al. (2020). High-quality preparation of graphene oxide via the hummers' method: Understanding the roles of the intercalator, oxidant, and graphite particle size. *Ceramics International*, 46, 2392–2402.

Khalid, A., Khan, R., Ul-Islamc, M., et al. (2017). Bacterial cellulose-zinc oxide nanocomposites as a novel dressing system for burn wounds. *Carbohydrate Polymers*, 164, 214–221.

Kumar, R., Anjum, K.A., Rani, S., et al. (2019a). Material properties of ZnS nanoparticles incorporated soy protein isolate biopolymeric film. *Plastic Rubber and Composites: Macromolecular Engineering*, 48(10), 448–455.

Kumar, R., Kumari, P., Singh, P., et al. (2019b). Fabrication of poly lactic acid incorporated bacterial cellulose adhered flax fabric biocomposites. *Biocatalysis and Agricultural Biotechnology*, 21, Article No. 101277.

Kumar, R., Praveen, R., Rani, S., et al. (2019c). ZnSe nanoparticles reinforced biopolymeric soy protein isolate film. *Journal of Renewable Materials*, 7(8), 749–761.

Malmir, S., Karbalaei, A., Pourmadadib, M., et al. (2020). Antibacterial properties of a bacterial cellulose CQD-TiO_2 nanocomposite. *Carbohydrate Polymers*, 234, Article no. 115835.

Pandit, A., Kumar, R. (2021). A review on production, characterization and application of bacterial cellulose and its biocomposites. *Journal of Polymers and the Environment*, 29, 2738–2755.

Peles, Z., Binderman, I., Berdicevsky, I., et al. (2013). Soy protein films for wound-healing applications: Antibiotic release, bacterial inhibition and cellular response. *Journal of Tissue Engineering and Regenerative Medicine*, 7, 401–412.

Prusty, K., Biswal, A., Biswal, S.B. (2019). Synthesis of soy protein/polyacrylamide nanocomposite hydrogels for delivery of ciprofloxacin drug. *Materials Chemistry and Physics*, 234, 378–389.

Rani, P., Yu, X., Liu, H., et al. (2021). Material, antibacterial and anticancer properties of natural polyphenols incorporated soy protein isolate: A review. *European Polymer Journals*, 152, Article No 110494.

Reddy, N., Yang, Y. (2009). Soy protein fibers with high strength and water stability for potential medical applications. *Biotechnology Progress*, 25, 1796–1802.

Shameli, K., Bin Ahmad, M., Zargar, M., et al. (2011). Synthesis and characterization of silver/montmorillonite/chitosan bionanocomposites by chemical reduction method and their antibacterial activity. *International Journal of Nanomedicine*, 6, 271–284.

Song, S., Liu, Z., Abubaker, M.A., et al. (2021). Antibacterial polyvinyl alcohol/bacterial cellulose/nano-silver hydrogels that effectively promote wound healing. *Materials Science & Engineering C*, 126, Article no. 112171.

Stanescu, P.-O., Radu, I.-C., et al. (2021). Novel chitosan and bacterial cellulose biocomposites tailored with polymeric nanoparticles for modern wound dressing development. *Drug Delivery*, 28, 1932–1950.

Tian, D., Guo, Y., Huang, M., et al. (2021). Bacterial cellulose/lignin nanoparticles composite films with retarded biodegradability. *Carbohydrate Polymers*, 274, Article no. 118656.

Tian, H.F., Guo, G.P., Fu, X.W., et al. (2018). Fabrication, properties and applications of soy-protein-based materials: A review. *International Journal of Biological Macromolecules*, 120, 475–490.

Tsai, Y.H., Yang, Y.N., Ho, Y.C., et al. (2018). Drug release and antioxidant/antibacterial activities of silymarin-zein nanoparticle/bacterial cellulose nanofiber composite films. *Carbohydrate Polymers*, 180, 286–296.

Wang, Z., Zhang, N., Wang, H.Y. (2014). The effects of ultrasonic/microwave assisted treatment on the properties of soy protein isolate/titanium dioxide films. *LWT-Food Science and Technology*, 57(2), 548–555.

Wei, B., Yang, G., Hong, F. (2011). Preparation and evaluation of a kind of bacterial cellulose dry films with antibacterial properties. *Carbohydrate Polymers*, 84(1): 533–538.

Wu, M., Chen, F., Wu, P., et al. (2021). Nanoclay mineral-reinforced macroporous nanocomposite scaffolds for in situ bone regeneration: In vitro and in vivo studies. *Materials & Design*, 205, Article no. 109734.

Xiang, A., Guo, G., Tian, H. (2017). Fabrication and properties of acid treated carbon nanotubes reinforced soy protein nanocomposites. *Journal of Polymers and the Environment*, 25(3), 519–525.

Zhang, L., Yu, Y., Zheng, S., et al. (2021). Preparation and properties of conductive bacterial cellulose-based graphene oxide-silver nanoparticles antibacterial dressing. *Carbohydrate Polymers*, 257, Article no.117671.

Zhao, S., Yao, J. R., Fei, X. (2013). An antimicrobial film by embedding in situ synthesized silver nanoparticles in soy protein isolate. *Materials Letters*, 95, 142–144.

Zmejkoski, D., Spasojević, D., Orlovska, I., et al. (2018). Bacterial cellulose-lignin composite hydrogel as a promising agent in chronic wound healing. *International Journal of Biological Macromolecules*, 118, 494–503.

Index

For Product Safety Concerns and Information please contact our EU
representative GPSR@taylorandfrancis.com
Taylor & Francis Verlag GmbH, Kaufingerstraße 24, 80331 München, Germany

www.ingramcontent.com/pod-product-compliance
Lightning Source LLC
Chambersburg PA
CBHW060812220326
41598CB00022B/2596